A Handbook on Counseling African American Women

Recent Titles in
Race and Ethnicity in Psychology

A Handbook on Counseling African American Women

Psychological Symptoms, Treatments, and Case Studies

KIMBER SHELTON,
MICHELLE KING LYN,
AND MAHLET ENDALE,
EDITORS

Foreword by Rosie Phillips Davis

Race and Ethnicity in Psychology
Jean Lau Chin, Yolanda E. Garcia, and Arthur W. Blume,
Series Editors

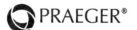 PRAEGER®

An Imprint of ABC-CLIO, LLC
Santa Barbara, California • Denver, Colorado

Library of Congress Cataloging-in-Publication Data

Names: Shelton, Kimber, editor. | King Lyn, Michelle M., editor. | Endale, Mahlet, editor.
Title: A handbook on counseling African American women : psychological symptoms, treatments, and case studies / Kimber Shelton, Michelle King Lyn, and Mahlet Endale, editors ; foreword by Rosie Phillips Davis.
Description: First edition. | Santa Barbara, California : Praeger, 2022. | Series: Race and ethnicity in psychology | Includes bibliographical references and index.
Identifiers: LCCN 2021025303 (print) | LCCN 2021025304 (ebook) | ISBN 9781440875953 (cloth) | ISBN 9781440875960 (ebook)
Subjects: LCSH: Mentoring—United States. | African American women—Counseling of. | Cross-cultural counseling—United States. | Social work with women—United States.
Classification: LCC BF637.M45 H363 2022 (print) | LCC BF637.M45 (ebook) | DDC 305.48/896073—dc23
LC record available at https://lccn.loc.gov/2021025303
LC ebook record available at https://lccn.loc.gov/2021025304

ISBN: 978-1-4408-7595-3 (print)
       978-1-4408-7596-0 (ebook)

26 25 24 23 22   1 2 3 4 5

This book is also available as an eBook.

Praeger
An Imprint of ABC-CLIO, LLC

ABC-CLIO, LLC
147 Castilian Drive
Santa Barbara, California 93117
www.abc-clio.com

This book is printed on acid-free paper (∞)
Manufactured in the United States of America

This book discusses treatments (including types of medication and mental health therapies), diagnostic tests for various symptoms and mental health disorders, and organizations. The authors have made every effort to present accurate and up-to-date information. However, the information in this book is not intended to recommend or endorse particular treatments or organizations, or substitute for the care or medical advice of a qualified health professional, or used to alter any medical therapy without a medical doctor's advice. Specific situations may require specific therapeutic approaches not included in this book. For those reasons, we recommend that readers follow the advice of qualified health care professionals directly involved in their care. Readers who suspect they may have specific medical problems should consult a physician about any suggestions made in this book.

Contents

Foreword

Rosie Phillips Davis

The image of the White policeman's knee on George Floyd's neck for 9 minutes and 29 seconds as he cried out, "I can't breathe," in May 2020 will live in my memory forever. I was so shaken that I could not talk. In my predominantly White neighborhood, I walk about five days a week, speak to all the neighbors, and encourage their walking. I am a member of our neighborhood garden club. And yet when Floyd was killed, no one said anything to me. No one called. When I finally mentioned it, people seemed surprised by my feelings. I hardly heard from any of my White friends and colleagues, even though I was serving as immediate past president of the American Psychological Association. Interestingly, as I served on a dissertation committee for an African American doctoral student, part of her study included conversations about the strong Black woman. The literature that she used questioned what such labeling did to Black/African American women. Strangely, the discussion made me rediscover the strong Black woman in me. I decided to stop waiting on someone to save me. I began to find my voice.

I wonder what I would have done had I had women like Drs. Shelton, Lyn, and Endale around or any of the women writers in this book? I suspect the time it took to regain my voice may have been shorter. Oh, I have seen therapists over the years, but the problems I took to them were so definable. They were usually about my family and my relationships. But what about the societal stressors that Black women face just because they live in the United States of America? Throughout this book the authors call that fact to the reader's attention. They talk about the intersectionality of being Black and female. They talk about being poor; being LGBTQ/PAN/ nonconforming/nonbinary; having a disability; experiences in higher education. They add all of the identities that make the Black/African American woman the individual that she is in the context in which she lives. Drs. Shelton, Lyn, Endale and their colleagues tell all of us that it is perfect for that woman to be whom she is. Their book lets us know that Black women are welcome in their offices and can be welcome in your office too.

It was Kimberle Crenshaw (1989) who coined the term *intersectionality*, and we began to understand gendered racism. But that was just the beginning. Shelton et al. now tell the reader about the kinds of mental health problems that are layered on the multiple identities of Black women. African American women have depression, anxiety, bipolar, substance abuse issues, eating disorders, suffer from partner violence, have loneliness, and every other issue that the entire population deals with. These writers tell us that there are those out there who can serve these Black women and even more can serve if they just have enough training. In this book the authors demonstrate numerous mental health challenges and add case descriptions of African American women in order to help the practitioner understand how to apply interventions with Black women who are dealing with PTSD or alcoholism or whatever comes through the door. Consistent throughout their descriptions is the call to create safe environments that empower and give permission to African American women to be themselves and heal. In individual, couple and family, or group counseling, or in residential treatment, this book will help the practitioner learn how to intervene with African American women.

REFERENCE

Crenshaw, K. (1989). Demarginalizing the intersection of race and sex: A Black feminist critique of antidiscrimination doctrine, feminist theory and antiracist politics. *University of Chicago Legal Forum*: Vol. 1989, Article 8. http://chicagounbound.uchicago.edu/uclf/vol1989/iss1/8

Preface

Kimber Shelton
Michelle King Lyn
Mahlet Endale

The intent of this book is to further mental health practitioners' awareness, understanding, and ability in providing competent mental health care to Black and African American women. Post slavery, Jim Crow, Black suffrage and civil rights, gendered racism, and other forms of oppression continue to impact the mental wellness of African American women, their relationships, and their families. Our hope is that readers will take away conceptual knowledge, concrete skills and tools in affirmative practice, and increased motivation to advocate and participate in systemic change bettering the mental well-being of Black and African American women.

Black and African American women are deserving of mental health services that empower and honor them, that invite challenge to internalized and externalized forms of oppression, and that foster personal and familial growth. However, practitioners are often ill prepared in creating therapeutic environments of safety, challenge, and respect for Black and African American women. For one, mental health professionals continue to be undertrained in working with Black and African Americans. Although there have been improvements in the number of diversity-focused courses offered at the graduate level, mental health practitioners continue to express being underprepared for work with ethnic minority groups.

Two, mental health practitioners are not immune from internalizing negative and dehumanizing societal messages targeting Black and African American women. As all other Americans are, mental health professionals

are exposed to political rhetoric that demoralizes Black women; legal precedent that penalizes Blackness; misogynoir (anti-Black misogyny) messages that label Black women as dangerous, aggressive, angry, and ugly;
and the accepted violence against Black women and their bodies.

Third, White and male supremacy continue in psychological research.
With multiculturalism and social justice being adopted as the fourth and
fifth forces of psychology, the psychological community has far to go in
changing psychological narratives and translating research to practice.
Black women scholarship continues to be devalued and underutilized,
pushing the current movement of #citeblackwomen. Take, for example,
the fact that Black women scholars such as Drs. Beverly Green, Beverly Tatum, and Janet Helms and emerging Black women scholars such
Drs. Jioni Lewis, Bryana French, Della Mosley, and Candice Hargons have
extensively written about anti-blackness and gendered racism, while one
of the top selling anti-racism books is written by a White woman, Robin
DiAngelo.

This book is written for all mental health professionals serving Black
and African American women. Shared ethnicity, race, and gender may
help Black and African American women mental health practitioners
better appreciate and connect with Black and African American women.
However, shared identity status does not automatically translate to competent care. Black and African American mental health professionals
receive much of the same psychological training as their White and male
counterparts; thus, many must also develop awareness and skill in providing culturally competent practice.

Non-Black and African American women and men benefit from this
book by gaining clinical information, an insider's view of the therapy room
with African American women clinicians working intimately with their
clients, and support for racial and gender justice advocacy. In recent years
as Black Lives Matter activism has forced the nation to face how it treats
Black and African American members of this society, many non-Black and
African American people, mental health clinicians included, have come to
understand and own their deficits in understanding and supporting the
Black experience in this country. Many have made a concerted effort to
increase their multicultural awareness and anti-racist approaches to their
clinical work. This text will serve as a great resource in these endeavors.

WHO ARE BLACK AND AFRICAN AMERICAN
WOMEN?

In this book, the terms African American, Black, and Black American
are used synonymously to represent women and gender-expansive folx
within the United States who are the descendants of the fourth African
diasporic stream. This book speaks specifically to the descendants of
individuals brought out of Africa to what is now the United States in the

Atlantic slave trade. Content is also relevant for people of African descent who themselves or whose ancestors more recently immigrated voluntarily to the United States; however, this book does not fully explore the experiences of more recently immigrated communities of African descent. We use identity markers in shared solidity, while encouraging readers to recognize the unique and diverse ethnic, cultural, and geographical differences between Black and African American women.

The book editors and the majority of the contributing chapter authors identify as Black and/or African American women. The editors and contributors are personally and professionally committed to improving the therapy experience of Black and African American women. Having attended psychotherapy themselves and with client caseloads comprised primarily of African American women, the book editors understand both the challenges African American women face in obtaining competent care, and the healing and transformative benefits of quality care. Ideally, this book supports readers' investment in recognizing and challenging their own beliefs and biases, reducing barriers to treatment, and demystifying and decolonizing the therapy process.

ORGANIZATION

This book is organized in four parts. Part One introduces a general contextualization of intersectionality and cultural competence related to serving Black and African American women. Part Two examines clinical considerations commonly experienced by Black and African American women. Chapters detail symptoms and treatments related to depression, anxiety, trauma, severe and chronic mental health issues, alcohol and drug addiction, and eating disorders. Part Three details treatment approaches to working with Black and African American women. Individual, couples and family, group therapy, inpatient and rehabilitation treatment approaches, and cultural adaptations are explored. Finally, Part Four addresses mental health and treatment needs of African American sexual orientation and gender identity minorities, women with disabilities, college students, and women with multiracial identities.

ACKNOWLEDGMENTS

During the time this book was written and reviewed, Kobe Bryant, Chadwick Boseman, and civil rights leader John Lewis died; Atatiana Jefferson, Elijah McClain, Ahmaud Arbery, Breonna Taylor, George Floyd, and Jacob Blake were murdered; and COVID-19 continues to kill a disproportionate number of Black Americans, while subsequently amplifying the burden of childcare and work Black women endure. Despite the historical nomination of an African American and South Asian woman, Senator Kamala Harris, as vice president on a major party ticket, the political climate has been oppressive and dismissive of the experiences of Black and African American women.

This has been a year of perpetual mourning, rage, and frustration for the Black community. It has also been a year of activism and social justice momentum. We appreciate the authors' dedication through this process, as we know that the state of U.S. affairs has compromised our collective mental well-being. This book is focused on counseling African American women and improving the mental wellness of African American women; however, note, many of our mental health needs will absolve when Black Women Matter.

Black Women—We are you. We hear you. We see you. We honor you. We do better for you.

CHAPTER 1

Intersectionality in Therapy for African American and Black Women

Candice Nicole Hargons
Natalie Malone
*Chesmore Montique**

Black women's identities—the social groups they claim membership in and the personal meaning they make from them—inform their lived experience. Beyond the two identities of Blackness and womanhood, other social locations such as age, ethnicity, sexuality, and socioeconomic status influence how Black women are treated, how they understand the world, and how they act (Collins, 2000). Clinically, treatment that isolates their identity to one defining identity, rather than the intersection of many, misses the mark. This has been a long-standing critique of theory and therapies applied to Black women.

During the second wave of feminism, women were striving for equal rights. However, discussions continued to develop around the question of which women were being considered. The origins of intersectionality emerged from Black women realizing mainstream feminism was about middle-class, educated, White women. In 1977, the Combahee River Collective, a group of Black feminists, articulated the need for an interlocking understanding of racism, sexism, and classism for Black women (Combahee River Collective, 1995). They saw the need for a framework that

---

* All coauthors contributed equally to the writing of the manuscript; thus, the authorship order reflects alphabetical organization by last name.

incorporated the various experiences of diverse women, most notably, women of different races (e.g., Black women). Black feminist scholars began to challenge sociological research lacking examination of people's experiences with multiple forms of oppression. As we will comment, this challenge extends to psychotherapy models and treatments related to Black women's mental health.

HISTORY OF INTERSECTIONALITY

Hancock (2015) notes that the origin of intersectional thought dates back to 1823 in Maria Stewart's criticism of the racial, gender, and economic components of the U.S. system. Stewart, a free Black woman living in Boston, was an activist whose impact on social movements was minimal due to gendered backlash in the Black community and economic oppression from White business owners. In her writings, Stewart reprimanded those who complied with the U.S. systems of racial–economic and racial–gendered apartheid. Predating Karl Marx's (1843) ideas on political emancipation, Stewart intended to illuminate the latent oppressive systems using multiple axes of power (Hancock, 2015). Stewart serves as early documented evidence for intersectional thought.

Leading critical race scholars Patricia Hill Collins and Kimberlé Crenshaw saw the need to replace single-axis frameworks with an orientation that acknowledges the nuance of social identity interactions (Collins, 2000; Crenshaw, 1989). Collins recognized the need for a model that integrates social identities. This way of thinking removes the idea that identities must be ranked by importance, recognizing that they all interact, informing what an individual does or does not experience. Likewise, Crenshaw (1989) coined the construct *intersectionality*, which provides a framework addressing how social identities are constitutive and undividable on both individual and systemic levels. In short, the theory of intersectionality provides the space to explore the interaction of social identities and how it shapes experiences of oppression.

Applications of Intersectionality

An intersectional framework recognizes the distinctions within oppressed groups, emphasizing the qualitative differences among social positionings. For example, the experience of a particular gender may be dissimilar for different racial identities (e.g., Black women and White women). With intersectionality, we emphasize that it is not as valuable to talk about identities separately, because it omits the multiplicative experience of identities. Intersectional theory is useful for interrogating the interaction of various social locations such as ability, ethnicity, religion, class, and sexual orientation. Previous single-axis theories do not appreciate the interaction of social identities that integrate into one's experience.

Intersectional theory recognizes the compounding feature of identities, rather than exclusive characteristics that do not interact.

Intersectional theory has become a central tenet to feminist theory and transformed the way we conceptualize gender (Shields, 2008). Moreover, intersectionality is utilized by policy makers, human rights activists, and political figures around the world. Yet, despite recognition of the importance of intersectionality, many fields that value rigorous methodologies have lagged on the practical implementation of this perspective (Shields, 2008)—its application to therapy has been limited.

The Misuse of Intersectionality

The reach of intersectionality's application is undeniable. However, as the theory attracts a broader audience, concerns of how the core tenets are being utilized exist (Shields, 2008). Bilge (2013) discusses how current cultures of neoliberalism neutralize the political potential of the framework. "Commonplace discourses assume that western societies have largely overcome problems of racism, sexism, and heterosexism/homophobia" (Bilge, 2013, 407). This culture leads individuals to employ a "language of diversity" to acknowledge social locations (Bilge, 2011), without the implementation of intersectional interventions. Intersectionality then becomes a buzzword to validate one's level of awareness of diverse experiences. People overlook the systemic work necessary to accomplish social equity. Bilge (2011) refers to this as ornamental intersectionality, utilizing it opportunistically to gain intellectual, moral, and political capital. Consequently, ornamental intersectionality neutralizes radical social justice politics.

Therapy is a site where intersectionality can be reclaimed for healing. For therapy to be intersectional, it must address structural inequalities and the complicated relationship between marginalized and privileged identities. When therapists lack comprehension of the core features of intersectionality, the therapeutic impact can be minimal and superficial. This mishap leaves intersectionality only to be addressed as "multiple identities" (Grzanka & Miles, 2016), diminishing the theory back to the predated single-axis model. This shallow understanding negates the interactive component, where facets of self cannot be considered exclusively. It is crucial we transcend superficial identity politics, moving from viewing diversity as a demographic to an intersectional orientation (Grzanka & Miles, 2016). For Black women, the intersectional construct of gendered racism is an important starting point in therapy.

GENDERED RACISM

Sociologist Philomena Essed (1991) defined gendered racism as forms of oppression due to the inextricable nature of racism and sexism embedded in Black women's experiences. Black women may share racial oppression with other racial or ethnically marginalized groups. However, the process of racism alone does not account for potential gender oppression Black women encounter. Both forms of oppression independent of one another insufficiently capture experiences of power struggle and silencing for Black women. Thus, gendered racism accounts for the "double burden" of racism and sexism (Essed, 1991). Understanding how gendered racism operates and informs Black women's coping styles is critical for therapists working with this population.

Recognizing Gendered Racism

Some forms of gendered racism are more recognizable than others. For example, the #SayHerName campaign highlights the pervasive, yet overlooked, police victimization of Black girls and women and calls for a more gender-inclusive interpretation of race-based violence. These overt experiences of gendered racism brim into therapeutic work in the form of cultural mistrust, stigma, and underutilization of services by Black women (Curtis-Boles, 2019), and require therapists to navigate Black women's experiences with gendered racism.

Still, gendered racism manifests in subtle ways such as gendered racial microaggressions, stereotypes, and racialized sexual objectification (Lewis & Neville, 2015; Szymanski & Lewis, 2016). These experiences are rooted in the historical dehumanization and attenuated devaluing of Black women (Collins, 2000). It is critical that therapists, particularly those conducting cross-racial therapy, understand the conditions for Black women. A therapist's ability to navigate overt and covert gendered racism with Black female clients will ultimately inform the therapeutic relationship and level of satisfaction experienced by the client.

Gendered Racial Microaggressions. Sue (2010) refers to racial microaggressions as subtle slights and insults, verbal and nonverbal, delivered by members of dominant groups. Racial microaggressions become gendered at the intersection of race and gender (Lewis et al., 2013). Gendered racial microaggressions in professional settings include microinsults (e.g., assuming a lack of intelligence; questioning a Black woman's position of authority, being held to higher standards, and exclusion [Lewis & Neville, 2015; Sue, 2010]). Often therapists are unaware of their microaggressive behavior and may be anxious to address their actions with clients. For example, a therapist attempting to encourage a Black woman about her professional role may inadvertently microaggress the client by insinuating it is remarkable for her to have her position. A comment such as "your job is impressive" may be interpreted as a microinsult by the client. Lewis and Neville's (2015) Gendered Racial Microaggressions Scale (GRMS) provides a useful measure for researchers and clinicians interested in assessing Black women's experiences with gendered racial microaggressions.

Based on the development of the GRMS, Black women experience silencing and marginalization, controlling imagery or stereotypes, and a reduction to physical qualities (Lewis & Neville, 2015).

Silencing and Marginalization. Black women are often rendered insignificant and invisible, which complicates their workplace and professional experiences. Therapists should be aware of marginalizing behavior occurring during therapeutic interventions with Black women. For example, silencing may occur in therapy when a therapist minimizes a Black female client's emotional reaction to a sexist experience tied to race by referencing all women's experiences with gender discrimination. Instead, therapists may empower Black female clients to name experiences of silencing or marginalization during therapy, as a means of establishing voice and an egalitarian relationship. In the example above, using process comments or inviting interpersonal feedback from the client could mend the therapeutic relationship and allow the therapist to process potential anxiety or discomfort arising in the present moment.

Stereotypes. Therapists working with Black women may increase cultural competence and treatment outcomes with Black female clients by understanding the sociopolitical context of Black women's stereotypes (Watson-Singleton, 2017). Collins's (2000) *Black Feminist Thought* highlighted sociohistorical images of Black women. These controlling images include Mammy, Jezebel, and Welfare Mother. Other imagery includes the Superwoman schema and Angry Black Woman stereotype (Collins, 2000; Woods-Giscombé, 2010). Black women's endorsement of these stereotypes reveals some benefits. For example, enacting the Superwoman schema (e.g., displaying strength, being independent) helps some Black women survive despite barriers and limited resources (Woods-Giscombé, 2010). However, the benefits associated with endorsing stereotypes are at the expense of Black women's mental health. Black women's stereotypes are associated with increased psychological distress, increased anxiety, and depressive symptoms (Watson-Singleton, 2017). Moreover, Black women's stereotypes may negatively impact help-seeking behaviors. Despite being at risk for physical and mental health concerns, Black women underutilize treatment services (Ward, Clark, & Heidrich, 2009). In addition to stigma and cultural mistrust, characteristics of Black women's stereotypes, such as displaying strength, serve as barriers to treatment therapists should be aware of.

Racialized Sexual Objectification. Sexual objectification refers to a process of dehumanization that reduces people to sexual objects (Szymanski, Carr, & Moffitt, 2011). Black women are often reduced to their physical attributes, receiving undesired and uninvited sexualized comments, catcalls, body viewing and touching, and sexual advances (Lewis et al., 2013).

Black women's sexual objectification is associated with hypervigilance to physical threat, self-objectification, psychological consequences such as lowered self-esteem and internalization of sexualized messages (Watson et al., 2012; West, 1995). Therapists should consider how sexual objectification informs clients' presenting concerns. Additionally, therapists identifying as men should consider their position of power based on gender identity and seek to navigate power differentials potentially manifesting with Black female clients (Szymanski, Carr, & Moffitt, 2010).

Mental Health Consequences of Gendered Racism

Black women's experiences with racial and gender discrimination across their life span have the ability to predict the magnitude of other life stressors Black women experience and their well-being (Perry, Harp, & Oser, 2013). Therefore, therapists must consider the mental health consequences of gendered racism and how it compounds Black women's objectives in therapy. Broadly, gendered racism is associated with higher rates of anxiety and depression, fear, and restlessness (Watson-Singleton, 2017). Gendered racism is also associated with higher levels of psychological distress and PTSD among Black women (Lewis & Neville, 2015).

Coping with Gendered Racism

Black women need a variety of adaptive coping strategies to combat the consequences of gendered racism. Black women may utilize passive or active coping strategies (Szymanski & Lewis, 2016). Passive strategies Black women may use to cope with gendered racism include avoidance and internalization (Szymanski & Lewis, 2016). For example, some Black women may make light of sexualized comments related to their physical attributes to avoid conflict or for fear of being subjected to the "angry Black woman" stereotype. Seeking social support is another option some Black women may use to cope with gendered racism. Potential social support systems for Black women include family members, partners, same-racial/ethnic women, and professional networks and organizations centralizing Black women. In treatment, Black women may benefit from same-racial/ethnic group therapeutic support for coping. Lastly, some Black women may cope with gendered racism through acts of resistance (Lewis et al., 2013). Shorter-Gooden (2004) qualitatively examined resistance coping strategies among Black women. In practice, resistance may include relying on spirituality or ancestral support, avoiding triggering people or spaces, or challenging the problem (Shorter-Gooden, 2004). Black women may also resist through a radical hope practice emphasizing understanding the history of Black women's oppression, envisioning equity, and adopting a social justice orientation (Mosley et al., 2020). Intersectional therapy with Black women can emphasize the adaptive coping responses

Black women have developed, while also introducing new strategies for coping and resisting.

ADDITIONAL ASPECTS OF INTERSECTIONALITY

Intersectionality is typically presented as race, gender, and class. Other identities such as ethnic identity, socioeconomic status, and sexual identity, among others, contribute to the complexity of Black women's experiences and likely result in compounded forms of gendered racism (Bowleg, 2008). Below we briefly address lesser discussed, but equally valued, aspects of identity as they relate to Black women.

Ethnic Identity

Ethnicity refers to social identification among people of a common culture or origin. Women of the African diaspora encompass myriad ethnicities including African American, African, Afro-Latinx, and Black or Afro-Caribbean. Black women indicating an African or Caribbean ethnic identity may prefer to identify by nation (e.g., Kenyan, Bahamian, Haitian) or tribe (e.g., Nigerian women may identify as Igbo, Yoruba, or Hausa-Fulani). Ethnicity is often invisible due the societal reduction of Black women to a set of common cultural characteristics. However, because Blackness is not a monolith, attention should be given to Black women of various ethnic identities. Black women who do not ethnically identify as African American may have differing perceptions of Black womanhood and experiences with gendered racial oppression. Intersectional therapy should use the intake process to elicit ethnic identity and make ongoing connections to ethnocultural identities.

Socioeconomic Status (SES)

SES undoubtedly intersects with race and gender, considering discrimination and marginalization may influence the upward mobility of Black women. The literature on Black higher education reveals greater college enrollment and degree attainment by Black women as compared to Black men (Garibaldi, 2014). Still, gendered racism persists in Black women's careers and may require navigating SES privilege due to education while also experiencing gendered racial oppression. Black women in poverty also experience gendered racism similar to upper-SES Black women, but their resources may require that they navigate this gendered racism differently. For example, the gender wage gap affects Black women of all education and socioeconomic statuses and could contribute to financial and psychological concerns brought to therapy. However, Black women in poverty are at increased risk for homelessness, trauma, interpersonal violence, and depression (Jones, 2008; Stockman, Hayashi, & Campbell, 2015).

Sexual Identity

Sexual identity features the related but distinct components of sexual orientation, gender identity, and romantic orientation that intersect and inform how individuals think of themselves as romantic and sexual beings. In addition to gendered racism, Black sexual minority women navigate stigma and discrimination from society at large, as well as the Black community, for their sexual identity (Calabrese et al., 2015). Black sexual minority women report increased psychological distress, depression, anxiety, and alcohol and substance use dependence (Calabrese et al., 2015; Szymanski & Stewart, 2010). Black sexual minority women may feel pulled to choose between their Blackness and sexual identity, especially when religious identities interact with sexual identities.

Spirituality and Religious Identity

Religion has served as a source of strength and solidarity within the Black community and among Black women (Reed & Neville, 2014). Black women's navigation of religious institutions reveals positive and negative experiences. Religious institutions positively influence Black women's well-being and resiliency (Reed & Neville, 2014). However, Black religious institutions may operate within a male-dominated hierarchy that situates Black women as lesser or submissive (Heard Harvey & Ricard, 2018).

Spirituality is commonly referred to as a connection or relationship with a higher power and mediates the relationship between Black women's religiosity and psychological well-being (Reed & Neville, 2014). Thus, it seems Black women's spirituality and religiosity may influence behavior, beliefs, and health. Spirituality may provide Black women with an avenue to dissociate from conservative religious views that are sexist, heteronormative, or other prejudice, while maintaining a relationship with a higher power.

Age

Ageism refers to stereotypes or discrimination based on age. According to Nelson (2016), from perceived age, "we infer social and cognitive competencies, political and religious beliefs, and physical abilities" (3). The literature provides limited insight into the experiences of older adult Black women. Generational differences should also be noted, considering the potential differing values and behaviors of older adult Black women. Older adult Black women navigate additional stereotypes related to age that may be positive (e.g., wisdom) or negative (e.g., fragility) (Chrisler, Barney, & Palatino, 2016). Black women's navigation of ageism may be connected to appearance, body esteem, and psychological distress (Sabik, 2015).

Ability

Broadly, disabilities may be physical, learning oriented, or psychiatric, and visible or hidden. According to DuMonthier, Childers, and Milli (2017), Black women are the second-largest group of women reporting disabilities. Black women experience many consequences due to disability. Consequences may include additional discrimination due to disability, earning less money than Black women without a disability, and physical and mental consequences such as drug-related symptoms (Perry, Harp, & Oser, 2013; Stuart, 1992).

A lesser acknowledged contribution to Black women's perceptions of ability are the subtle distinctions between weakness and strength prevalent among Black women (Hobson, 2019). Black women with disabilities may be perceived as incapable due to their inabilities to endorse or maintain stereotypical abilities. Disability is often stigmatized and hidden, resulting in further erasure of Black women.

Size

Sizeism, or weightism, refers to discrimination based on a person's size or weight. Sizeism is an understudied area among Black women (Smith, 2019). This form of oppression may be understudied for two reasons. First, the current literature on Black women and body size is on Black women's comparison to other racial/ethnic groups of women. This pattern in the literature may mask curvy Black women's experiences of size discrimination and separate Black women from sociocultural factors related to body image (Watson, Lewis, & Moody, 2019). Alternatively, sizeism may be understudied due to greater social acceptance of higher body weight and body satisfaction among Black women (Watson, Lewis, & Moody, 2019). Still, the disproportionate prevalence of obesity among Black women (Marinos et al., 2017) may result in fat stigma and prejudice.

Taken together, various aspects of Black women's identities, starting with race and gender, but including other potential marginalized identities such as socioeconomic status, sexual identity, spirituality, age, ability, and size, must be considered throughout the therapy process. Therapists should understand the cumulative impact of the stress associated with each point of marginalization as they conceptualize the case and plan treatment. However, the intersection of both privileged and marginalized identities allows therapists to recognize what unearned benefits and resources some Black women may have access to based on the way their privileges operate in their specific contexts. Therapy attending to the strengths emerging from both marginalized and privileged identities, as well as the vulnerabilities, is better set up to affirm, heal, and empower Black women clients.

INTERSECTIONALITY IN THERAPY FOR BLACK WOMEN

Intersectionality within therapy emphasizes how systemic, institutional, and structural oppression impact individual and community mental health (Lewis & Grzanka, 2016). Integrating intersectionality into counseling provides therapists an enriched framework from which multiculturalism is conceptualized. This amalgamation renders a robust understanding of Black women as clients. This influence manifests systemically, in the development of the competencies for various psychological and counseling associations and social justice movements everywhere.

Implications for the Therapeutic Care of Black Women

Research about Black women's experiences informs better therapeutic care. A crucial therapeutic benefit of understanding the impact and experiences of multiple marginalized identities is empathy for Black women. This level of informed care dismantles the deficit hypothesis practiced in conventional therapy that suggests nonwhite family structures and practices are pathological (Holmes et al., 2011). Adopting an approach that emphasizes individual and collective strengths proves most effective in reducing distress symptoms.

Feminist Therapy

Feminist perspectives in therapy incorporate many of the intersectional tenets. Feminist models provide a strength-based approach that empowers the client, promoting agency and restoring power that may have been taken away from them (French et al., 2019). Pioneering scholars such as Patricia Hill Collins (2000), Kimberlé Crenshaw (1989), and the Combahee River Collective (1995) informed the evolution of feminist therapy into multicultural feminist therapy. Adding multiculturalism to feminism integrates core concepts of intersectionality into therapeutic practice. Enns and Byars-Winston (2010) elaborate on how the tenants of multicultural feminist therapy can be found in *Guidelines for Psychological Practice with Girls and Women* (2007). The guidelines call on practitioners to (a) rely on practices that are effective for diverse groups of girls and women, (b) foster relationships that lead to empowerment, (c) use unbiased and appropriate assessments, (d) consider the sociopolitical context in which problems occur for the client, (e) acquaint themselves with community and educational resources, and (f) work to change institutional biases. Feminist methods also shift the locus of the problem from the individual to the environment (Holmes et al., 2011). It takes into account the systems and institutions involved that have disempowered the client. For additional literature specific to Black feminism, Jones and Harris (2019) outline a blueprint for using Black feminism in therapy by providing recommendations for clinicians to develop their skills in practice with Black women.

Radical Healing

To move past individual-level approaches, the framework of radical healing was fashioned (French et al., 2019). Informed by theories of intersectionality, ethnopolitical psychology, psychology of liberation, and Black psychology, the structure of radical healing is a multisystemic approach that acknowledges the role of intersectional oppression on people of color and Indigenous individuals' lives based on race, gender, class, religion, nationality, ability, and more (French et al., 2019). French et al. define radical healing as "being able to sit in a dialectic and exist in both spaces of resisting oppression and moving toward freedom" (2019, 11). It requires both acknowledgment of and active resistance to oppression as well as a vision for future freedom and wellness. The framework is grounded in five components that lead to healing: collectivism, critical consciousness, radical hope, strength and resistance, and cultural authenticity and self-knowledge. Healing denotes a collectivism perspective that involves a deep connection to one's community rather than individualistic coping strategies to get by (French et al., 2019). This also parallels research that has shown the success of group therapy for Black women within the context of attending a historically White institution where they may experience intersecting oppressions daily (Jones & Pritchett-Johnson, 2018). It moves individuals from a frame of coping—surviving to get by—into a model of healing—thriving in society and resisting racism—rather than reacting to racial trauma.

Research on Black women has come a long way due to the integration of intersectionality, systemically and throughout practice and research. The universality of intersectionality is evident in the versatility of its application, yet the emphasis on Black women's experiences remains a fundamental component that is often overshadowed. Unremitting self-reflection for clinicians, and on the field at large, will continue to help enhance the quality of care offered to Black women who often need therapeutic services the most, but seldom receive the care.

INTERSECTIONALITY-INFORMED THERAPY

Outreach

Intersectionality-informed therapy begins with the process by which we invite Black women to receive therapy services. Given what the research above has taught us about systemic and stereotypical barriers Black women may face, therapists should seek to establish relationships with communities, places, and organizations that attract Black women.

For example, engaging in monthly outreach at local churches, beauty salons, Black women's organizations, communities that house primarily Black women, and social media pages relevant to Black women's experiences will establish nontherapeutic relationships with Black women that may later lead to therapy. Recently, the first author was a guest speaker at her local church's women's conference, where over 100 Black adolescent girls and women were in attendance. As a therapist, this is more than a potential referral strategy. This outreach was guided by awareness of the intersecting identities that Black women in the community hold (i.e., Black, woman, Christian, married), and it was an intentional strategy to connect and reduce barriers to help-seeking by establishing rapport outside of the therapy setting.

In addition to the locations where outreach should occur, the topics of outreach should be informed by the above-mentioned research on what affects Black women from an intersectional lens. Topics related to Black beauty standards, spiritual/religious identity, relationships and sex, money and mental health, stress and strength, and navigating or resisting gendered racism at work and school may attract Black women. From an intersectionality-informed lens, a radical healing approach recognizes resistance as a possible therapeutic outlet. Further, being a Black woman mental health provider willing to talk openly about the various issues Black women experience puts a face to therapy that looks familiar and potentially more inviting.

Intake

Following outreach, Black women may initiate therapy with a variety of presenting concerns. Given some Black women's endorsement of the Superwoman schema or Strong Black Woman stereotype, this initial session may require a delicate balance of affirming the strength it took to pursue therapy and introducing the possibility that to be strong at all times may not be healthy either. This will occur during the typical clinical interview portion, but the interview questions should also incorporate an intersectional lens. Specifically, ensuring that the above dimensions of identity (race, gender, class, sexual identity, age, body size, ability, etc.) are included on initial paperwork and in the interview protocol is the first step. Clinicians invite Black women to bring their intersecting identities into the therapy room with comments such as, "I encourage you to bring all of your identities into this space" and "I am interested in learning about how all parts of your identity impact your reality and world." Second, invite clients to describe how those identities work together, rather than as individual aspects of their identity. Potential questions may be: "Sometimes it may feel like it isn't just your race or just your body size that impacts you. How does being a Black woman of larger size affect your life?" or "Tell me what it is like for you to walk into your chemistry lab and be the only Black Muslim woman in the room?"

The interviewer may also explicitly name some of the stereotypes about Black women and invite clients to discuss how they adopt, experience, navigate, or resist those stereotypes. Knowing whether they have subscribed to the stereotypes or whether they actively resist them can inform the case conceptualization and treatment planning. Lastly, ending with what the client likes most about being a Black woman with their unique variety of intersecting identities concludes the initial appointment with self-affirmation and uplift, which are culturally relevant protective factors for Black women (Stevens-Watkins et al., 2012). The therapist may then indicate how they'd like to use these valued aspects of self throughout the therapy process.

Case Conceptualization

As the therapist determines diagnoses and conceptualizes the case, maintaining an intersectional lens requires knowing which marginalized and privileged identities are most salient for the client, which are less obviously salient but still impactful, and which may not be in the client's awareness yet. For example, if a highly educated Black woman who is married to a woman comes in for relationship issues, her privileged socioeconomic status, Blackness, womanness, and sexual identity may all be salient. Or she may not recognize how her Blackness is salient. Reading research, as well as Black women's media outside of academic texts, relevant to the most salient identities will bolster empathy and understanding of how the client's social locations intersect and inform their presenting concerns. Holding the conceptualization as a hypothesis or one potential way of viewing the client's experience, rather than a definitive truth, will allow therapeutic flexibility as the therapist creates a treatment plan. Furthermore, if the therapist is also a Black woman, being mindful of the ways the therapist's and client's life align and depart is helpful to use commonalities appropriately while avoiding overidentification.

Treatment

Treatment should be mutually informed by an intersectional lens and best practices from the limited research about Black women, as well as the client's goals. From an intersectional lens, the therapist should remain attentive to the systemic imposition of gendered racism and other potential oppressions that may exacerbate the client's symptoms or present barriers to treatment. For example, an elderly Black woman client may have grown up in an era where Black women were more often relegated to low-paying service positions with fewer benefits. She may still be working, despite being over retirement age and in physical pain related to her work. If she does not have the financial means to stop working, the therapist will need to collaboratively create other outlets to reduce her stress and help her manage pain. The research on pain management and stress reduction may be useful, but the therapist will also need to consider how the client's identities as a Black woman may influence her willingness and ability to try and adhere to a variety of strategies. She should partner with the client to determine the most feasible and relevant stress reduction strategies.

Using potential cultural values related to family, spirituality, authenticity, strength, and common sense may also be useful in an intersectionality-informed therapy approach for Black women. Group therapy with 7 to 12 Black women at a local church may incorporate spirituality and mental health in a culturally congruent way. Or, if Black Vernacular English (BVE) is your mother tongue, using that dialect as well as Standard American English (SAE), rather than exclusive use of psychological jargon and SAE, may represent authenticity. Furthermore, cultivating skills and identifying resources that can be useful once the therapy relationship has ended will support the Black woman client who values independence. These skills may include deep breathing, guided meditation, Black woman–specific affirmations, listening to or creating music, journaling, or media. For example, *Therapy for Black Girls* by Dr. Joy Harden Bradford is a podcast and social media enterprise that focuses on issues that address the Black woman's experience. Listening to these podcasts or engaging in the social media community may enhance the client's sense of connection and well-being, without feeling overly reliant or burdensome.

Termination

Because the Black community may be small in some areas, therapy with Black women may not adhere to strict boundaries around termination and multiple relationships. These should be addressed throughout the therapeutic relationship, but they may become especially salient when it is time for termination. If the therapist is also a Black woman, the client and therapist may share one or more social connections. Asking the client how they would like to approach these relationships during and after the therapy relationship has ended is important. Further, whereas the current American Psychological Association Ethics Code (2017) indicates that clients and therapists should refrain from establishing a friendship, the cultural norms and social networks of Black women may require a discussion about how and whether this is an appropriate ethic within Black women's lives. As an example, a coauthor of this chapter received therapy services from one of the editors of this book in 2008. Since then, they have shared several professional networks, prompting the need for a discussion around multiple relationships and the applicability of that principle to their lives and their willingness to collaborate on projects, engage each other socially, and establish a friendship. Similar to research on rural communities and multiple relationships (Campbell & Gordon, 2003), they found that it was neither realistic nor preferable that they would avoid each other or refrain from collaboration when they shared similarities in professional identity and social location. Black women therapists and clients may rework the informed consent and ethics to fit their cultural norms.

CONCLUSION

Although intersectionality as a theory for understanding the way marginalized identities interact and compound the experience of oppression is not a new concept, its recent popularity and usefulness are welcome in the application to therapy with Black women. As a concept emerging from Black women's epistemology, or ways of knowing, few frameworks better explain the unique position Black women occupy in the world. Therapists reading this chapter have now received an introduction and overview of intersectionality as a theory, a discussion of how it has been used in research on therapy with Black women, and the application of it to therapy practice. It is important to note that this is not an exhaustive representation of how intersectionality-informed therapy may be done, but one of many possibilities depending on the therapist's profession and training, the client's myriad identities, the therapy site resources, and the surrounding community. A primary strength of Black women is creativity (Evans, 2015), and that should be embedded in any use of intersectionality-informed therapy with them.

REFERENCES

American Psychological Association. (2017). *Ethical principles of psychologists and code of conduct.* Washington, DC: Author.

Bilge, S. (2011). Doing critical intersectionality in an age of popular and corporate diversity culture. *International Colloquium on Intersecting Situations of Domination, from a Transnational and Transdisciplinary Perspective.* Paper presented at the International Colloquium on Intersecting Situations of Domination, from a Transnational and Transdisciplinary Perspective, Université de Paris 8, Paris, June 8, 18p.

Bilge, S. (2013). Intersectionality undone: Saving intersectionality from feminist intersectionality studies. *Du Bois Review: Social Science Research on Race, 10*(2), 405–424. https://doi.org/10.1017/S1742058X13000283

Bowleg, L. (2008). When Black + lesbian + woman ≠ Black lesbian woman: The methodological challenges of qualitative and quantitative intersectionality research. *Sex Roles: A Journal of Research, 59*(5–6), 312–325. https://doi.org/10.1007/s11199-008-9400-z

Boyd-Franklin, N. (1987). Group therapy for Black women: A therapeutic support model. *American Journal of Orthopsychiatry, 57*(3), 394–401.

Calabrese, S. K., Meyer, I. H., Overstreet, N. M., Haile, R., & Hansen, N. B. (2015). Exploring discrimination and mental health disparities faced by Black sexual minority women using a minority stress framework. *Psychology of Women Quarterly, 39*(3), 287–304. https://doi.org/10.1177/0361684314560730

Campbell, C. D., & Gordon, M. C. (2003). Acknowledging the inevitable: Understanding multiple relationships in rural practice. *Professional Psychology: Research and Practice, 34*(4), 430–434. https://doi.org/10.1037/0735-7028.34.4.430

Chrisler, J. C., Barney, A., & Palatino, B. (2016). Ageism can be hazardous to women's health: Ageism, sexism, and stereotypes of older women in the healthcare system. *Journal of Social Issues, 72*(1), 86–104. https://doi.org/10.1111/josi.12157

Collins, P. H. (2000). *Black feminist thought: Knowledge, consciousness, and the politics of empowerment.* New York, NY: Routledge.

Collins, P. H. (2005). *Black sexual politics: African Americans, gender, and the new racism.* New York, NY: Routledge.

Combahee River Collective. (1995). Combahee River Collective statement. In B. Guy-Sheftall (Ed.), *Words of fire: An anthology of African American feminist thought* (pp. 232–240). New York, NY: New Press.

Crenshaw, K. (1989). Demarginalizing the intersection of race and sex: A Black feminist critique of antidiscrimination doctrine, feminist theory, and antiracist politics. *Feminist Legal Theory, 1989*(1), 57–80. https://doi.org/10.4324/9780429500480-5

Curtis-Boles, H. (2019). Living in the margins: Intersecting identities and clinical work with Black women. *Women & Therapy, 42*(3–4), 430–446. https://doi.org/10.1080/02703149.2019.1622904

DuMonthier, A., Childers, C., & Milli, J. (2017). The status of Black women in the United States. *Washington, DC: Institute for Women's Policy Research.* https://iwpr.org/wp-content/uploads/2020/08/SOBW_ExecutiveSummary_Digital-2.pdf

Enns, C. Z., & Byars-Winston, A. M. (2010). Multicultural feminist therapy. In H. Landrine & N. F. Russo (Eds.), *Handbook of diversity in feminist psychology* (pp. 367–388). Springer Publishing Company.

Essed, P. (1991). *Understanding everyday racism: An interdisciplinary theory.* Newbury Park, CA: Sage Publications.

Evans, S. Y. (2015). Healing traditions in Black women's writing: Resources for poetry therapy. *Journal of Poetry Therapy: The Interdisciplinary Journal of Practice, Theory, Research, and Education, 28*(3), 165–178. https://doi.org/10.1080/08893675.2015.1051286

Ford, K. A. (2012). Thugs, nice guys, and players: Black college women's partner preferences and relationship expectations. *Black Women, Gender+ Families, 6*(1), 23–42. https://doi.org/10.5406/blacwomegendfami.6.1.0023

French, B. H., Lewis, J. A., Mosley, D. V., Adames, H. Y., Chavez-Dueñas, N. Y., Chen, G. A., & Neville, H. A. (2019). Toward a psychological framework of radical healing in communities of color. *The Counseling Psychologist, 48*(1), 14–46. https://doi.org/10.1177/0011000019843506

Garibaldi, A. M. (2014). The expanding gender and racial gap in American higher education. *Journal of Negro Education, 83*(3), 371–384. https://doi.org/10.7709/jnegroeducation.83.3.0371

Grzanka, P. R., & Miles, J. R. (2016). The problem with the phrase "intersecting identities": LGBT affirmative therapy, intersectionality, and neoliberalism. *Sexuality Research and Social Policy: A Journal of the NSRC, 13*(4), 371–389. https://doi.org/10.1007/s13178-016-0240-2

Hancock, A. M. (2015). Intersectionality's will toward social transformation. *New Political Science*, *37*(4), 620–627. https://doi.org/10.1080/07393148.2015.1089049

Heard Harvey, C. C. C., & Ricard, R. J. (2018). Contextualizing the concept of intersectionality: Layered identities of African American women and gay men in the Black church. *Journal of Multicultural Counseling and Development*, *46*(3), 206–218. https://doi.org/10.1002/jmcd.12102

Hobson, J. (2019). Of "sound" and "unsound" body and mind: Reconfiguring the heroic portrait of Harriet Tubman. *Frontiers: A Journal of Women Studies*, *40*(2), 193–218. https://doi.org/10.5250/fronjwomestud.40.2.0193

Holmes, K. Y., White, K. B., Mills, C., & Mickel, E. (2011). Defining the experiences of Black women: A choice theory®/reality therapy approach to understanding the strong Black woman. *International Journal of Choice Theory and Reality Therapy*, *31*(1), 73–83.

Jones, L. V. (2008). Preventing depression: Culturally relevant group work with Black women. *Research on Social Work Practice*, *18*(6), 626–634. https://doi.org/10.1177/1049731507308982

Jones, L. V., & Harris, M. A. (2019). Developing a Black feminist analysis for mental health practice: From theory to praxis. *Women & Therapy*, *42*(3–4), 251–264. https://doi.org/10.1080/02703149.2019.1622908

Jones, M. K., & Pritchett-Johnson, B. (2018). "Invincible Black women": Group therapy for Black college women. *Journal for Specialists in Group Work*, *43*(4), 349–375. https://doi.org/10.1080/01933922.2018.1484536

Lewis, J., Mendenhall, R., Harwood, S., & Browne Huntt, M. (2013). Coping with gendered racial microaggressions among Black women college students. *Journal of African American Studies*, *17*(1), 51–73. https://doi.org/10.1007/s12111-012-9219-0

Lewis, J. A., & Neville, H. A. (2015). Construction and initial validation of the Gendered Racial Microaggressions Scale for Black women. *Journal of Counseling Psychology*, *62*(2), 289–302. https://doi.org/10.1037/cou0000062

Lewis, J. A., & Grzanka, P. R. (2016). Applying intersectionality theory to research on perceived racism. In A. N. Alvarez, A. N., C. T. H. Liang, & H. A. Neville (Eds.), *Cultural, racial, and ethnic psychology book series. The cost of racism for people of color: Contextualizing experiences of discrimination* (pp. 31–54). Washington, DC: American Psychological Association.

Marinos, A., Gamboa, A., Celedonio, J. E., Preheim, B. A., Okamoto, L. E., Ramirez, C. E., . . . & Shibao, C. A. (2017). Hypertension in obese Black women is not caused by increased sympathetic vascular tone. *Journal of the American Heart Association*, *6*(11), e006971. https://doi.org/10.1161/JAHA.117.006971

Mosley, D. V., Neville, H. A., Chavez-Dueñas, N. Y., Adames, H. Y., Lewis, J. A., & French, B. H. (2020). Radical hope in revolting times: Proposing a culturally relevant psychological framework. *Social and Personality Psychology Compass*, *14*(1), e12512. https://doi.org/10.1111/spc3.12512

Nelson, T. D. (2016). Ageism. In T. D. Nelson (Ed.), *Handbook of prejudice, stereotyping, and discrimination* (pp. 337–353). New York, NY: Psychology Press.

Perry, B. L., Harp, K. L. H., & Oser, C. B. (2013). Racial and gender discrimination in the stress process: Implications for African American women's health and well-being. *Sociological Perspectives: Official Publication of the Pacific Sociological Association*, *56*(1), 25–48. https://doi.org/10.1525/sop.2012.56.1.25

Reed, T. D., & Neville, H. A. (2014). The influence of religiosity and spirituality on psychological well-being among Black women. *Journal of Black Psychology, 40*(4), 384–401. https://doi.org/10.1177/0095798413490956

Sabik, N. J. (2015). Ageism and body esteem: Associations with psychological well-being among late middle-aged African American and European American women. *Journals of Gerontology: Series B: Psychological Sciences and Social Sciences, 70*(2), 189-199. https://doi.org/10.1093/geronb/gbt080

Shields, S. A. (2008). Gender: An intersectionality perspective. *Sex Roles, 59*(5–6), 301–311. https://doi.org/10.1007/s11199-008-9501-8

Shorter-Gooden, K. (2004). Multiple resistance strategies: How African American women cope with racism and sexism. *Journal of Black Psychology, 30*(3), 406–425. https://doi.org/10.1177/0095798404266050

Smith, C. A. (2019). Intersectionality and sizeism: Implications for mental health practitioners. *Women & Therapy, 42*(1–2), 59–78. https://doi.org/10.1080/02703149.2018.1524076

Stevens-Watkins, D., Perry, B., Harp, K. L., & Oser, C. B. (2012). Racism and illicit drug use among African American women: The protective effects of ethnic identity, affirmation, and behavior. *Journal of Black Psychology, 38*(4), 471–496. https://doi.org/10.1177/0095798412438395

Stockman, J. K., Hayashi, H., & Campbell, J. C. (2015). Intimate partner violence and its health impact on ethnic minority women. *Journal of Women's Health, 24*(1), 62–79. https://doi.org/10.1089/jwh.2014.4879

Stuart, O. W. (1992). Race and disability: Just a double oppression? *Disability, Handicap & Society, 7*(2), 177–188, https://doi.org/10.1080/02674649266780201

Sue, D. W. (2010). *Microaggressions in everyday life: Race, gender, and sexual orientation.* Hoboken, NJ: John Wiley & Sons.

Szymanski, D. M., Carr, E. R., & Moffitt, L. B. (2011). Sexual objectification of women: Clinical implications and training considerations. *Counseling Psychologist, 39*(1), 107–126. https://doi.org/10.1177/0011000010378450

Szymanski, D. M., & Lewis, J. A. (2016). Gendered racism, coping, identity centrality, and African American college women's psychological distress. *Psychology of Women Quarterly, 40*(2), 229–243. https://doi.org/10.1177/0361684315616113

Szymanski, D. M., & Stewart, D. N. (2010). Racism and sexism as correlates of African American women's psychological distress. *Sex Roles: A Journal of Research, 63*(3–4), 226–238.

Ward, E. C., Clark, L. O., & Heidrich, S. (2009). African American women's beliefs, coping behaviors, and barriers to seeking mental health services. *Qualitative Health Research, 19*(11), 1589–1601. https://doi.org/10.1177/1049732309350686

Watson, L. B., Lewis, J. A., & Moody, A. T. (2019). A sociocultural examination of body image among Black women. *Body Image, 31,* 280–287. https://doi.org/10.1016/j.bodyim.2019.03.008

Watson, L. B., Robinson, D., Dispenza, F., & Nazari, N. (2012). African American women's sexual objectification experiences: A qualitative study. *Psychology of Women Quarterly, 36*(4), 458–475. https://doi.org/10.1177/0361684312454724

Watson-Singleton, N. N. (2017). Strong Black Woman schema and psychological distress: The mediating role of perceived emotional support. *Journal of Black Psychology, 43*(8), 778–788. https://doi.org/10.1177/0095798417732414

West, C. M. (1995). Mammy, Sapphire, and Jezebel: Historical images of Black women and their implications for psychotherapy. *Psychotherapy: Theory, Research, Practice, Training, 32*(3), 458–466.

Woods-Giscombé, C. L. (2010). Superwoman schema: African American women's views on stress, strength, and health. *Qualitative Health Research, 20*(5), 668–683. https://doi.org/10.1177/1049732310361892

CHAPTER 2

Culturally Competent Counseling Practice with African American Women

Kimber Shelton

Mental health treatment utilization rates have risen for all ethnic and racial groups (Substance Abuse and Mental Health Services Administration [SAMHSA], 2015), and African American women's entrance into psychotherapy is higher than ever before (Agency for Healthcare Research and Quality [AHRQ], 2017). Passage of mental health parity law (Mental Health Parity and Addiction Equity Act of 2008) and the Affordable Care Act of 2010 have made mental health services accessible to a greater number of individuals. However, even with increased mental health legislation, across all racial and ethnic groups, cost of service and lack of insurance coverage continue to present as treatment barriers (SAMHSA, 2015). Beyond treatment cost and insurance limitations, African American women contend with additional barriers impacting their overall entry and continuance in treatment. Some of these treatment barriers are shared with their ethnic minority peers, while others are directly connected to the intersection of Blackness and womanness.

Culturally competent practice with African American women serves as a mitigator of systemic barriers impacting entrance into therapy and is inextricably tied to effective clinical treatment. This chapter presents a brief synopsis of the state of psychotherapy with African American women and details culturally competent practices for provision of affirming therapy with African American women.

STATE OF MENTAL HEALTH TREATMENT AND AFRICAN AMERICAN WOMEN

As previously stated, African American women are coming to psychotherapy (AHRQ, 2017). A 2015 SAMHSA study showed approximately 9 percent of Black Americans reported receiving mental health services, and approximately 7 percent reported taking psychiatric medications in the last year. With 10.3 percent of services being accessed by Black women and only approximately 7 percent of Black men accessing services, Black women make up the majority of Black Americans seeking treatment. Although entry into treatment increased, mental health service utilization for Black women is considerably less than for their White counterparts. Whereas 10.3 percent of Black women engage in mental health treatment, almost a quarter of White women reportedly engage in treatment. In comparison to White counterparts, Black Americans underutilize outpatient treatment options, yet Black men and women are overrepresented in inpatient care (1.4 percent of Black Americans vs. 0.07 percent of White Americans in inpatient care).

With approximately 17 percent of Black Americans reportedly having a mental illness (SAMHSA, 2015) and 3–3.5 percent reportedly having a serious mental illness (e.g., schizophrenia) (SAMHSA, 2015; 2017), counseling can serve as a primary treatment method in addressing the psychological needs of African American women. However, continued disparities in mental health care, cultural mistrust and stigma, and limited access to preferred service providers negatively impact African American women's ultimate use of mental health treatment.

Disparity

"A health disparity is a difference or inequality that occurs in health status or in the provision of and access to healthcare that is often linked with social, economic, and environmental disadvantage" (Manuel, 2018, 1407). Behavioral health disparities include, but are not limited to, no or inadequate access to mental health professionals, derisory treatment and mental health options, and use of culturally insensitive and pathologically based therapy methods. The wave of mental health legislation has been insufficient in resolving the disparities associated with the mental health care needs of African Americans. The 2018 National Healthcare Quality and Disparities Report (Agency for Healthcare Research and Quality [AHRQ], 2019), a Congress-mandated report to overview both quality care and disparities, showed Black individuals continue experiencing multiple health disparities in the priority areas of care coordination, effective treatment, healthy living, patient safety, and person-centered care. When care is accessed, African Americans receive lower-quality mental health care, do not have access to culturally competent care, obtain care inconsistent with treatment guidelines, and are more likely to obtain treatment from a general practitioner (U.S. Surgeon General, 2001).

Poverty and lack of insurance are commonly cited reasons why health disparities continue to prevail within the African American community (see Robinson & Finegold, 2012). Furthermore, the intersection of additional marginalized identities (e.g., sexual identity minority status or HIV-positive status) brings increased disparity for African American women (Calabrese et al., 2015; Geter, Sutton, & Hubbard, 2018). However, even when socioeconomic status is stable, access to care is available, and the need for help is recognized, Black women continue to report higher rates of serious psychological distress and their needs going unmet in comparison to Black men, and men and women of other races (CDC, 2016; Manuel, 2018; Primm & Lawson, 2010; SAMHSA, 2015).

Cultural Mistrust, Stigma, and Shame

Cultural Mistrust. African American women's mistrust of helping professionals is valid. The health-care field penalized, victimized, and pathologized African Americans' ancestors, and egregious behaviors continue today. Take maternal mortality rates of Black women and infants, for example. Enslaved Black women underwent unanesthetized experimental gynecological treatments, and investigational brain and bone procedures were performed on their infants (Washington, 2006). Post slavery, historical accounts detail African American mothers being treated in hospital basements and their newborns being placed in utility rooms where bedpans were emptied and needles were sterilized (Williams, 1999, as cited in Williamson, 2014). Today, as reported by the CDC, the pregnancy-related mortality rate of Black women is three to five times higher than that of White women (pregnancy-related mortality ratios increasing with mother's age) (Petersen et al., 2019), and Black newborns under the care of White physicians are three times more likely to die than when their pediatrician is Black (Greenwood et al., 2020). There is still much unknown about fertility, antepartum, and postpartum mental and physical health needs of African American women.

It bears repeating, African American women's mistrust of helping professionals is valid. Intergenerational messages to avoid mental and physical health care are founded in historical and present experiences of culturally incompetent and, at times, inhumane treatment. Attributing their health-care professional's racism to their unmet needs, Black women reported providers did not spend enough time with them, did not respect their intelligence, provided inadequate explanation, and broke trust (Nicolaidis et al., 2010). The presence of racism and sexism in mental health care undermines African American women's ability to seek and utilize this care.

Stigma and Shame. Stereotyping African American women as "strong," "superwomen," and "resilient" impedes their use of mental health treatment, for therapy may be seen as a sign of weakness (NAMI, 2020; Thompson, Bazile, & Akbar, 2004). The experience of gendered racism further stigmatizes counseling for African American women. Considering the pervasive sexism and racism African American women endure and overcome, concepts of mental wellness and self-care are made to feel trivial. Instead of viewing therapy as a useful tool in managing wellness, Black women might see it as a form of failure. For those who do enter treatment, building support can be a challenge as they may feel misunderstood and judged by family and friends who discover they are in treatment. African American women are exposed to comments such as, "Do you really need counseling?" or "I didn't know things were that bad," These comments serve to question the legitimacy of counseling and perpetuate the inaccurate belief that therapy is for people who are internally flawed or "crazy."

Additionally, some African American women may grow up in environments that protect privacy and secrecy (Williamson, 2014); where "you don't tell family business." Rightly so, the consequences of sharing environmental struggles have proven dangerous for African American families. Consider the fact that child protective services are more likely to remove ethnic minority children from their homes, even when their families have low abuse risk scores, than they are to remove White children from families with higher abuse risk scores (Child Welfare Information Gateway, 2016). In such cases, it can feel like seeking help creates more harm than not seeking help. Given this, African American women might find themselves prolonged in patterns and relationships that are detrimental to their mental wellness (e.g., intimate partner violence, sexual abuse, addiction).

Access to African American Female Therapists

It is unsurprising that the majority of this author's private practice caseload is comprised of African American women. During phone consultations and first appointments, many of these women express their desire to specifically work with an African American female therapist. In areas such as Atlanta, Dallas, and DC, African American women may have their pick of African American mental health professionals. However, outside major metropolitan areas (even 30 miles outside these locations), locating an African American therapist presents as a challenge. According to the National Alliance on Mental Illness (NAMI, 2009), only 2 percent of psychiatrists and 4 percent of social workers in the United States are African American. African American psychologists make up only 2 percent of the American Psychological Association (APA, 2014) and 4 percent of the total number of active psychologists (APA, 2019). That is approximately 3,500 Black female psychologists and 920 Black male psychologists, in comparison to approximately 57,200 White female psychologists and 25,500 White male psychologists (APA, 2019). On average, Black psychologists are generally younger and report regularly treating more African Americans than White psychologists (APA, 2019). Nearly 63 percent of active White psychologists reported never, rarely, or occasionally providing services to African American individuals (APA, 2019). Therefore, African American women may find themselves in treatment with a therapist who is older, White, and inexperienced in working with African American individuals. This reality may give African American women pause in seeking counseling.

Whether true or not, there is an assumed level of understanding and acceptance African American women believe they will receive from a therapist holding a shared racial and gender background. Although research shows cultural competence and the therapeutic alliance are greater determinants for therapy success than is the cultural match between client and therapist (Cabral & Smith, 2011; Owen et al., 2011; Swift et al., 2015), there is evidence supporting the importance of meeting clients' preferences (Cooper & Norcross, 2021). When a client's therapy preferences are met, including their desired therapist demographics, they experience improved therapy outcomes and are less likely to prematurely terminate therapy than when preferences are unmet (Swift et al., 2011; Swift, Callahan et al., 2013). Therefore, if so desired, having the autonomy and availability to choose to work with an African American female therapist will keep African American women engaged in therapy longer and yield improved therapy outcomes.

CULTURAL COMPETENCE AND MULTICULTURAL ORIENTATION

Every major psychological and counseling professional organization requires mental health professionals to engage in culturally competent counseling practice (see American Association of Marriage and Family Therapists, 2015; American Counseling Association, [ACA], 2014; APA, 2017a; National Association of Social Workers, 2017). Furthermore, many state licensure bodies require professional development hours in cultural diversity to retain a practicing license. Not without its faults, the *Diagnostic Statistical Manual-5* ([*DSM* 5] (American Psychiatric Association, 2013) also includes cultural provisions related to diagnosis. Additionally, numerous guidelines exist to support culturally competent practice (see APA Guidelines for Psychological Practice with Girls and Women, 2007; APA Multicultural Guidelines, 2017b). Cultural identity intersects with all aspects of counseling; as a result, ethical practice cannot exist without cultural competence (Arredondo & Toperek, 2004).

Traditionally defined, cultural competence encompasses awareness, knowledge, and skills—therapist awareness into their own cultural identity, holding knowledge and understanding of other cultural realties, and having skill in implementing culturally sound and sensitive interventions (Sue, Arredondo, & McDavis, 1992). Contemporarily, as well as attending to cultural competence, the mental health field is shifting to include a focus on a multicultural orientation. Whereas cultural competence focuses on how practitioners gain and utilize multicultural counseling competencies ("ways of doing"), multicultural orientation moves beyond knowledge and skill building, focusing instead on a practitioner's "cultural presence" or "ways of being" culturally oriented with a client (Hook et al., 2013; Owen et al., 2016). Further diverging from multicultural counseling competency's tendency to focus on the *therapist's* own self-reflection and assessment of cultural competence, multicultural orientation encompasses the *client's* perspective of their therapist's cultural humility and use of cultural opportunities (Shaw, 2017). Cultural humility is defined as the "ability to maintain an interpersonal stance that is other-oriented (or open to the other) in relation to aspects of cultural identity that are most important to the client" (Hook et al., 2013, 354). A therapist has intrapersonal understanding of their own identity and that their identity will always limit their perspective on others' cultural identities (Shaw, 2017). With this awareness, therapists remain open, respectful, considerate, humble, and interested in the client's cultural identity and experiences (Shaw, 2017).

Practitioners high in cultural humility engage in a therapeutic style that is collaborative and inviting of client cultural identity. Likely due to their "other orientation" and ability to acknowledge their mistakes and cultural transgressions, practitioners with cultural humility are less likely to bring biases into the therapy room and, when transgressions do occur, the impact of these biases is less intense (Hook et al., 2016). Cultural opportunities are moments when therapists effectively and appropriately attend to issues related to cultural identity (Shaw, 2017). Better therapy outcomes are reported when clients feel their therapist addressed salient cultural factors in treatment (Owen, 2016). Therefore, as well as building self-awareness, knowledge, and skill in working with African American women, a multiculturally oriented therapist owns limitations of their perspective based on their own understanding of their cultural self. They also remain interested and explorative into the client's perception of how their experiences are shaped by their cultural identities. The therapist both introduces and follows the client's lead in integrating cultural dialogues within the therapeutic environment. Finally, they invite feedback from the client on their ability to leave their African American client feeling heard, respected, and validated. Examples of multicultural orientation processing questions are provided below:

Cultural Humility

- How is my cultural identity limiting my understanding and connection with African American women?

- How am I remaining open and interested in continuing to learn about the experiences of African American women?
- How am I demonstrating my openness and respect for African American women?
- How do my personal worldview and values align with supporting the mental health and well-being of African American women?

Cultural Opportunities

- How am I inviting African American women to share salient parts of their cultural identity with me?
- To what nonverbal messages do I need to attend to better note a need to change gears, shift perspective, or stay focused on my client's cultural identity?
- How am I ensuring the therapeutic space is safe for clients to communicate to me that I committed a cultural misstep?
- What skills do I need to process negative feedback in the here and now and remain present and helpful in session?
- How do I apologize and repair cultural ruptures in a humble and helpful way?

CULTURALLY COMPETENT AND MULTICULTURALLY ORIENTED PRACTICE

Ethical care for African American women involves the provision of culturally competent and multiculturally oriented care throughout the therapeutic process, including pre-counseling contact, intake, rapport building, assessment, diagnosis and case conceptualization, interventions and treatment modalities, and termination and referral.

Pre-Counseling Contact

What is being done to attract African American women? How do African American women know the therapist's practice is culturally sensitive to their needs? Establishing a safe and trusting relationship with African American women begins prior to the initiation of therapy. Clients research therapists, especially those clients focused on locating a culturally competent practitioner. A therapist's platform (or absence thereof) provides African American women with an idea of who the therapist is and if they might feel comfortable working with that therapist. This platform includes the therapist's website, social media, blogs, videos, webinars, podcasts, professional articles, and books. When a client accesses professional information, they should get a sense of the therapist's inclusivity and understanding of intersectionality; ideally, leaving them feeling interested and motivated in working with the therapist.

In inviting African American women to counseling, and demystifying and destigmatizing the therapy process, practitioners need to clearly communicate their focused attention to aspects of diversity. An excerpt from this author's website:

> Your identity and background are important to me and the work that we do. I consider the culture of every individual I work with and have specialized training in providing competent care to ethnic minority and LGBTQ communities. In counseling with me, you will feel affirmed, supported, and respected.

Furthermore, when a client finds this author online and when entering her waiting room, they find a mission statement that addresses a personal and professional commitment to cultural competence and social justice. Additionally, in building a relationship with African American women, therapists demonstrate their commitment to cultural diversity through inclusion of images of African American individuals in marketing and psychoeducational materials, and consider inclusive aesthetics as related to office décor.

Culturally competent therapists must be accessible. Popular directories, such as Psychology Today, Good Therapy (gender only filter), and APA Psychologist Locator, provide filters for gender and ethnicity; however, most national therapy directories do not. Recognizing the needs of specific communities, there is a growing number of community-specific psychotherapy directories. To attract African American women, therapists might consider a professional listing on therapy directories specific to Black women. Table 2.1 provides a list of African American female–, African American–, and ethnic minority–focused directories.

Initial Consultation

First appointments with a new therapist can produce anxiety for clients, particularly those who bring cultural stigma into therapy, those for whom therapy is a novel experience, and those with previous negative therapy experiences. A culturally competent and humble approach to first appointments can help reduce anxieties African American women might experience early into treatment. Culturally competent intake paperwork allows for self-identification of race, ethnicity, sex, and gender. Even after clients indicate their demographic background on paperwork, during the clinical interview, practitioners verbally ask about ethnicity, gender identity, and sexual orientation, providing the client with multiple opportunities to share salient identities. For example, inquiring into ethnicity provides space to better learn how Black women identify (e.g., Black, African American, American, Haitian, African, Afro-Caribbean, Latina, Multiracial, etc.) and how that identity impacts their experiences.

Table 2.1
List of Therapist Referral Directories*

African American Women–Focused Directories	
Black Female Therapists	https://www.blackfemaletherapists.com/directory
Therapy for Black Girls	https://therapyforblackgirls.com/
African American–Focused Directories	
Association of Black Psychologists—Therapist Resource Directory	https://abpsi.site-ym.com
Black Doctor	https://blackdoctor.org/
Black Emotional and Mental Health Collective: Black Virtual Therapist Directory	https://www.beam.community/bvtn
Black Therapist Network	https://blacktherapistnetwork.com
Black Therapists Rock	https://www.blacktherapistsrock.com
Melanin & Mental Health	https://www.melaninandmentalhealth.com
Melanin Therapy	https://melanintherapy.com
Ourselves Black	https://ourselvesblack.com/home
Ethnic Minority–Focused Directories	
Ethnic Counselors	http://www.ethniccounselors.com
InnoPsych: Therapists of Color	https://www.innopsych.com
National Queer and Trans Therapists of Color Network	https://www.nqttcn.com/
POC Holistic Healers	https://www.pocdirectory.com/mental-health
Therapy for Queer People of Color	https://therapyforqpoc.com
Therapy in Color	https://www.therapyincolor.org/

*Note: Up to date as of July 2021.

First appointments also include coverage of informed consent and treatment procedures, confidentiality, and client/counselor responsibilities. Therapists advantage African American women in demystifying the therapeutic process through clarifying client and counselor expectations, and describing the counselor's therapy style. This author's informed consent paperwork addresses identity and attends to systemic issues: "I use an integrative approach to therapy which involves examining your thoughts, feelings and behaviors, recognizing how societal messages and cultural values influence you, and developing tailored solutions."

If working in an agency or group practice setting, where the intake clinician may not be the client's assigned therapist, it is important to ask for, and when possible, honor client preferences. As previously mentioned, meeting client gender and ethnicity preferences yields better treatment outcomes. Additionally, intakes should include questions about the client's desired treatment methods and outcomes. Considering the egregious treatment history of Black Americans, developing a collaborative and egalitarian relationship with African American women can help create a safe and trusting therapeutic relationship. Clients who feel their therapist's approach is clearly explained, and that they have consensually developed goals, are more likely to return after the intake, complete treatment, and experience increased treatment satisfaction (DeFife & Hilsenroth, 2011).

Rapport

Common Factors Theory. According to common factors theory (see Hubble, Duncan, & Miller, 1999), four factors account for change in therapy: client and extra therapeutic factors (40 percent), client/therapist relationship factors (30 percent), therapeutic model (15 percent), and hope and expectancy factors (15 percent). With 30 percent of change being attributed to the therapeutic relationship, adopting a common factors approach can help therapists develop and maintain a healthy alliance with African American women. As described by Laska and colleagues (2014, 469), the common factors model focuses on factors that are necessary and sufficient for change:

(a) an emotionally charged bond between the therapist and patient,
(b) a confiding healing setting in which therapy takes place,
(c) a therapist who provides a psychologically derived and culturally embedded explanation for emotional distress,
(d) an explanation that is adaptive (i.e., provides viable and believable options for overcoming specific difficulties) and is accepted by the patient, and
(e) a set of procedures or rituals engaged by the patient and therapist that leads the patient to enact something that is positive, helpful, or adaptive.

Specific to work with African American women, therapists are building rapport by showing sincere care for their client and her lived experiences; operating from a strength-based perspective as evidenced in language used with and conceptualization of client concerns; checking in with client for clarity, understanding, and agreement; providing room for disagreement and flexibility in approach; and showing comfort in introducing and connecting with client and clinician cultural variables.

Self-Disclosure. Generally, therapists are trained to limit their self-disclosures. Therapists refrain from self-disclosure to avoid shifting the focus of therapy off the client, placing the client in a position to do caretaking of the therapist, blur professional boundaries, or inadvertently project countertransference issues onto the client. However, the omission of self-disclosure, particularly in therapeutic models focused on egalitarianism and collaboration, can hurt the therapeutic alliance, particularly when addressing sensitive subjects. Clients find value in therapist self-disclosure as it provides a sense of connection and intimacy, builds trust, decreases alienation, leaves clients feeling cared about and understood, and provides a sense the therapist would hold themselves accountable for mistakes (Hanson, 2005). Particularly in cross-racial dyads, clients report wishing their therapist shared more about themselves (Chang & Berk, 2009).

African American women desire to feel understood and heard in therapy. Thoughtful and intentional therapist self-disclosure is one means of creating a connecting environment. The therapist is always considering how the disclosure might impact the client and the therapy relationship. At the end of this author's first session with African American women (and all other clients), clients are invited to converse on the therapeutic relationship and to ask questions about the therapist: "Are there any questions about myself, professionally or personally, that I can answer for you?" While maintaining autonomy over what and how much is shared, these limited therapist self-disclosures provide additional opportunity to demystify the counseling process and build an egalitarian relationship. Again, always targeted to the client's needs, this author feels comfortable sharing personal experiences of managing the duality of strength and vulnerability, issues related to professionalism and appearance, fears around targeted violence against Black bodies, and her affirmation of sexual orientation and gender identity diversity.

Assessment, Diagnosis, and Case Conceptualization

Assessment and Diagnosis. Cultural disparities in psychological and achievement testing are well documented (see Council of National Psychological Associations for the Advancement of Ethnic Minority Interests [CNPAAEMI], 2016; Helms & Ford, 2012). Assessment methods not normed with African American populations contribute to African Americans being misdiagnosed, underdiagnosed, and overdiagnosed (CNPAAEMI, 2016). Inaccurate assessment and diagnosis can impact the resulting psychological treatment, educational endeavors, employment standing, and/or forensic needs of African Americans. When possible, mental health practitioners are selecting assessment instruments normed with African Americans and that have high validity and reliability with African American individuals. See Benuto and Leany's *Guide to Psychological Assessment with African Americans* (2015) for specific procedures in psychological assessment with African Americans.

Diagnosing can be complicated. For one, each introduction of a new *DSM* brings with it diagnostic recategorization and change. Even with updates, diagnostic criteria do not fully account for cultural variance in the expression of mental illness. When determining diagnoses for African American women, practitioners are considerate of culturally sanctioned practices, functional impairment, and diagnostic biases. A practitioner also needs to consider the potential ramifications of sharing diagnoses with African American women. For some women, a diagnosis can provide a sense of relief. Instead of believing herself to be "crazy," a diagnosis of bipolar disorder means she can develop a wellness treatment plan. However, due to continued stigma and misinformation regarding mental illness, a diagnosis could detrimentally impact African American women's mental health. Whereas one woman might feel empowered having finally received a diagnosis and treatment plan, another woman might feel like a mental illness diagnosis is the end of her world. During assessment and before sharing a diagnosis, practitioners need to process cultural stigma related to diagnosis, provide clear understanding and rationale for the diagnosis(es), and help African American women integrate a diagnosis into their worldview. This is likely an ongoing conversation in which the clinician regularly intervenes to assess how the diagnosis impacts the client's identity and life.

Case Example: In going over the test results of a psychological assessment for differential diagnosis, this author shared a trauma-related diagnosis with her client. The author provided great detail on how they arrived at the specific diagnosis and spent considerable time discussing treatment options. In discussing assessment results, a detailed description on elevated Personality Assessment Inventory (PAI) (Morey, 2007) scales was provided. It was explained to the client an elevated schizophrenia scale suggested impairments in thinking and processing style, and feeling interpersonally disconnected; it did not mean she had schizophrenia. The client returned the next week expressing great stress and reduced functioning after being told she was "crazy" and "psychotic." During the session, she expressed she stopped listening to the assessment results after she heard "schizophrenia," as she was reminded of a family member with severely impaired functioning related to an untreated schizophrenia diagnosis. She imagined herself following on the same path as her family member. As a result, she never understood or processed the actual diagnosis provided. Fortunately, having a good relationship, she felt comfortable expressing this, which provided an additional opportunity to clarify the diagnosis and what it meant for her treatment and well-being. The dyad again processed mental illness stigma and its impact on the client's identity.

Culturally Competent Case Conceptualization. Formal and informal information gathered about client's background, presenting problems, family history, health history, alcohol and drug use, relationships, education and employment, safety and risks assessment, strengths, goals, and diagnosis are used to develop a clinical case conceptualization. A case conceptualization is a theory-driven hypothesis organizing and summarizing the etiology of a client's presenting concerns, how they fit together and how they are maintained, and how concerns are to be clinically treated (Osborn, Dean, & Petruzzi, 2004; Sperry & Sperry, 2012). It serves as a "snapshot" of who the client is, what is happening with them, why it is happening, and how these issues might be addressed. General case conceptualization skills focus on affect, basic counseling skills, rapport building, specific clinical interventions, and use of external resources (Osborn et al., 2004). However, general case conceptualization is insufficient in capturing the role cultural identity and sociocultural elements play in understanding the lived experiences and following mental health needs of African American women.

A complete and multicultural case conceptualization for African American women integrates cultural factors into the understanding of presenting concerns, their maintenance, and successful treatment. Sperry and Sperry (2012) describe case conceptualization as having four components: diagnostic, clinical, cultural, and treatment formulations. Cultural formulation is derived from elements of cultural identity, acculturation level and acculturative stress, cultural explanatory model, and the impact of cultural versus personality dynamics. It is used to answer the question "What role does culture play?" A multicultural case conceptualization focuses on culture, discrimination, use of culturally relevant clinical interventions, and use of external resources related to culture (Constantine, 2001). As well as accounting for the variables above, a multiculturally competent case conceptualization also asks, "What role does systemic oppression play in the development and maintenance of presenting concerns?" In exploring treatment options, a multicultural case conceptualization considers changes to systemic variables, which would aid in the mental wellness and recovery for African American women. A mock example using the character of Celie from the book *The Color Purple* (1985) is included below:

Generic Case Conceptualization of Celie
Celie is a 50-year-old woman. She presents with symptoms of sadness, despair, fatigue, and questions about her identity. She has a history of sexual, physical, and emotional abuse from her father and estranged husband. Additional traumas include her children and sister being forcibly removed from her life. These traumas contribute to her low self-esteem and sadness. Serving as the caregiver to others further exacerbates fatigue and difficulty with self-exploration. Celie currently lives with her same-sex partner and owns her own clothing store. Understanding her core beliefs and working to refute cognitive distortions and irrational thinking can help to resolve the symptoms, depression, and regret she currently experiences.

Multicultural Case Conceptualization of Celie

Celie is a 50-year-old Black woman raised and living in the rural South. She presents with symptoms of sadness, despair, fatigue, and questions about her identity. She was raised in a time period and geographic location where overt acts of discrimination and dehumanization of African Americans were socially accepted, and Eurocentric features were considered the beauty standard. These factors challenge Celie's ability to create and celebrate an affirming and secure identity. Acts of sexual, emotional, and physical violence foster feelings of inferiority and alter her cultural reality and sense of efficacy. She carries the guilt of stolen relationships with her sister and children, dynamics she was not responsible for and had no legal recourse in changing.

Despite little formal education and rampant heterosexism, Celie operates a successful clothing business honoring the sizes of all bodies. She is courageous in maneuvering through cultural and religiously based homophobia so she can live in an authentic and joyful relationship with her same-sex partner. Her social relationships are complex and demonstrate her capacity to forgive, heal, and love. At this point, Celie is focused on her self-care and recovery, while being aware that institutional practices of gendered racism and heterosexism will continue to challenge her well-being. Through reflection of sociocultural influences on core beliefs, identity development, and mental wellness, Celie can continue to dismantle narratives supporting inferiority and inadequacy, and continue to build her narrative of strength, resiliency, and self-acceptance. Integrating her spirituality and strong community support will help her recreate a cultural reality that respects the maintenance of her mental, physical, and spiritual well-being.

Interventions and Treatment Modalities

Culturally Specific and Culturally Adapted Treatment Interventions. Culturally specific clinical interventions and cultural adaptations of current models and practices (i.e., cognitive behavioral therapy, relational cultural theory) can be designed to meet the needs of African American women. Interventions meeting the needs of African American women create space to hold the dual reality in which many Black women reside. These interventions respect the collective experience of Blackness and womanness, while holding the unique identity of the individual, relationship, or family. Interventions with African American women build from the client's personal resilience and confront unhelpful intrapersonal dynamics, while naming and addressing systemic oppression impacting goal creation and attainment. Interventions honor self-expression, language, and voice, and create space for strengthening self-acceptance. Each chapter in this book provides culturally competent interventions in working with African American women.

Decolonizing Mental Health. In developing new interventions for African American women, practitioners are encouraged to explore decolonization and liberation psychology. Criticizing the impact colonialization had on the once French-occupied Algeria, psychiatrist Frantz Fanon wrote, "If psychiatry is the medical technique that aims to enable man no longer to be a stranger to his environment, I owe it to myself to affirm that the Arab, permanently alien [alie´ne´] in his own country, lives in a state of absolute depersonalization" (Fanon, 1967, as cited in Robcis, 2020, 303). Connecting the politics of colonialization to mental health, Robcis (2020) writes, "It could literally render someone mad by hijacking their person, their being, and their sense of self. The confiscation of freedom and the alienation brought about by colonialism and by racism were always simultaneously political and psychic" (304). These writers recognized politically sanctioned infiltration of another's country, body, and mind, and then pathologizing their existence to create an environment in which wellness cannot exist.

The history of colonialization of both Africa and the United States, post-colonization racism and sexism, and a psychological foundation that is both White and male subjugate African American women to a mental health system that may ultimately fail them. If African American women are to be healthy, the system treating them must first be healthy. Decolonizing mental health is defined as "putting a focus on how trauma from oppression and colonization plays a role in mental health and giving individuals the proper support they need" (Zapata, 2020). Decolonizing approaches to mental health for African American women include, but are not limited to:

- Voicing and mourning the disrespect, mistreatment, and abuse created by colonization
- Changing and healing systemic and political policies disempowering the health of African American women
- Embracing diversity within African American women
- Turning to African American women to define a cultural understanding of suffering and cultivate collectivist healing
- Addressing epigenetic impacts of trauma
- Embracing ancestral resilience and empowerment
- Rediscovery and recovery of self-identity prior to colonization
- Mind decolonization—"an emotional and personal process of reviewing our conditioning" and "unpacking our ancestral load and present-day patterns" (Mullen, 2020)

Liberation Psychology. Founded in principles of decolonization, liberation psychology emphasizes freeing psychology from oppression. Broadly speaking, across psychotherapy, research, and training, liberation psychology includes participatory practices (i.e., involvement of African

American women) and a continuous and fluid dialogue reflecting on and dismantling power, privilege, and oppression to transform psychology and advance social justice (Hocoy et al., 2020). Liberating psychology includes radical healing. Radical healing is operationalized as "the policies, actions, and practices, which aid individuals and their groups to live out their full potential in societies with a history of racial oppression" (Neville, 2017, 7). Building on existing frameworks rooted in liberation psychology, Black psychology, ethnopolitical psychology, and intersectionality theory, French and colleagues (2020) developed a psychological framework of radical healing in communities of color. Their paradigm for radical healing involves critical consciousness, radical hope, strength and resistance, cultural authenticity and self-knowledge, and collectivism. Specific to African American Women, Lewis and colleagues (2020) outline five steps for cultivating radical healing for Black women and gender-expansive folx:

1. Name and Identify Sources of Stress and Trauma—This includes intersectional oppression, microaggressions, systemic oppression, and intra- and interpersonal oppression.
2. Engage in Mind-Body Healing—Use of mind-body interventions such as yoga, meditation, and mindfulness.
3. Lean on Support Networks—Utilization of collective supports and reframing support as strength.
4. Envision Possibilities for Wellness, Freedom, and Dignity—Empowering healing through imagination of possible changes and explored narratives.
5. Stand for Social Justice and Take Action—Fostering individual healing through community involvement, connection and healing.

Termination and Referral

Termination. Ideally, therapy relationships end when a client meets their identified goals. Furthermore, if needed, the client recognizes that should she desire or need to, she can return to therapy in the future. Therapists should strive for African American women to end therapy relationships feeling empowered, having greater understanding of self and self in relation to the world, and motivated to continue to effect change within their lives and experiences.

Other than client and counselor-initiated termination, a host of additional circumstances can lead to therapy's end. Termination may be a forced choice due to planned or unplanned logistical issues (e.g., maternity leave, changes in employment or insurance). Or clients may prematurely drop out, ending therapy before therapeutic goals are met. A myriad of reasons exist why a client might prematurely end therapy—the client might not be ready to do the work of therapy, they feel better after the first meeting, they forget to come back, scheduling was not convenient for them. The client's perception of the therapist's cultural incompetence is an additional reason for premature termination (Vasquez, 2007; APA, 2015). When African American women feel misunderstood or invalidated and when dual alienation manifests itself (oppression from society and mental health field) (Harris & Licata, 2000), rightly so, they end therapy.

From a multiculturally oriented standpoint, therapists can follow up with African American women to better understand their reasons for discontinuing therapy. It is up to the client to respond; however, the culturally competent and multiculturally oriented therapist provides space to understand the needs of African American women and advance their own cultural competence. Of note, it is not the client's responsibility to educate their therapist, only to provide feedback on her experience of the therapist's cultural competence and sensitivity. This follow-up might take the form of a phone call or secure email that includes questions such as, "How well do you feel that your cultural identities were integrated into our work together?", or use of rating scales, "On a scale of 0–5, how well did your therapist respect your cultural identities?"

Referral. Therapists are ethically required to be competent in referral (ACA, 2014; APA, 2017). Referral for counseling services occur when the client's needs are outside of the practitioner's scope of competence, the client needs require a higher level of service (e.g., hospitalization), therapy services are coming to a premature ending (e.g., therapist no longer practicing), the client requests a referral, or the type of therapy provided is no longer effective. Broadly speaking, clients underutilize referrals. About 60 percent of clients of color do not utilize referrals (Owen, Devdas, & Rodolfa, 2007). This means, when providing a referral to an African American woman, chances are, she won't continue in therapy. It might have been challenging to seek help to begin with, and it could feel overwhelming to consider having to retell her story and start a relationship with a new person. Additionally, the referral may not work due to the referral source. A recent study by Kugelmass (2016) showed people of color are less likely to receive appointment callbacks from therapists than are White individuals.

To increase the likelihood of African American women using referrals, clinicians take ownership of their clinical limitations in assisting the client and are specific in the rationale for providing the referral. Psychoeducation is provided to reduce the client possibly internalizing the belief that she is somehow responsible for the current therapy relationship not working. Clinicians can empathize with and normalize the hardship created in having to build a new therapeutic relationship, while confirming a relationship with a different therapist is still the better option. Clinical time is spent in exploring the reasons why the client might be hesitant to use the referral, and the therapist engages in motivational interview strategies or other processes to increase motivation for change and use of the referral.

Clinicians need a well-developed referral network of culturally competent and multiculturally oriented therapists to refer African American women to. Although all African American women may not want to see an African American female therapist, many may; therefore, practitioners take steps to cultivate relationships with African American therapists. A well-developed referral network for African American women would also include referral sources for culturally competent psychiatric and medical care as well. Clinicians respect client autonomy; however, if desired by the client, they can attempt to contact the referral during the last therapy appointment. Finally, after the referral is made, the referring therapist may consider following up with the client to determine if the referral was used or if additional assistance is needed.

CONCLUSION

African American women are deserving of a therapy relationship that protects and enhances their mental wellness, empowers growth and healing, and accepts and honors their full identity. This can only be accomplished through culturally competent and multiculturally oriented practices and interventions. Ongoing self-reflection and culturally oriented training, developing strategies to decolonize and liberate therapy, and seeking explicit feedback from African American women are steps in creating a therapeutic practice well designed to meet the needs of African American women.

Black women—We are you. We hear you. We see you. We honor you. We do better for you.

REFERENCES

Agency for Healthcare Research and Quality (AHRQ). (2017). 2016 National Healthcare Quality and Disparities Report. *AHRQ Pub. No. 17-0001*. Rockville, MD: Author.

Agency for Healthcare Research and Quality (AHRQ). (2019). National Healthcare Quality and Disparities Report introduction and methods. *AHRQ Publication No. 19-0070-EF*. Rockville, MD: Author.

American Association of Marriage and Family Therapists. (2015). *Code of ethics.* https://www.aamft.org/Legal_Ethics/Code_of_Ethics.aspx

American Counseling Association (ACA). (2014). *Code of ethics.* https://www.counseling.org/resources/aca-code-of-ethics.pdf

American Psychiatric Association. (2013). *Diagnostic and statistical manual of mental disorders-5 (DSM-5;* 5th ed.). Washington, DC: Author.

American Psychological Association. (2007). Guidelines for psychological practice with girls and women. *American Psychologist, 62*(9), 949–979.

American Psychological Association. (2014). *Demographic characteristics of APA members by membership characteristics.* https://www.apa.org/workforce/publications/14-member/table-1.pdf

American Psychological Association (APA). (2017a). *Ethical principles of psychologists and code of conduct.* https://www.apa.org/ethics/code/ethics-code-2017.pdf

American Psychological Association. (2017b). *Multicultural guidelines: An ecological approach to context, identity, and intersectionality.* http://www.apa.org/about/policy/multicultural-guidelines.pdf

American Psychological Association. (2019). *CWS Data Tool: Demographics of the U.S. Psychology Workforce* [Interactive data tool]. https://www.apa.org/workforce/data-tools/demographics

American Psychological Association Presidential Task Force on Evidence-Based Practice. (2006). Evidence-based practice in psychology. *American Psychologist, 61,* 271–285.

Arredondo, P., & Toperek, R. (2004). Multicultural counseling competencies—Ethical practice. *Journal of Mental Health Counseling, 26*(1), 44–55.

Benuto, L. T., & Leany, B. D. (2015). *Guide to psychological assessment with African Americans.* New York, NY: Springer.

Cabral, R. R., & Smith, T. B. (2011). Racial/ethnic matching of clients and therapists in mental health services: A meta-analytic review of preferences, perceptions, and outcomes. *Journal of Counseling Psychology, 58,* 537–554.

Calabrese, S. K., Meyer, I. H., Overstreet, N. M., Haile, R., & Hansen, N. B. (2015). Exploring discrimination and mental health disparities faced by Black sexual minority women using a minority stress framework. *Psychology of Women Quarterly, 39*(3), 287–304.

Centers for Disease Control and Prevention. (2016). *Health, United States, 2015: In Brief.* www.cdc.gov/nchs/data/hus/hus15_inbrief.pdf

Chang, D. F., & Berk, A. (2009). Making cross-racial therapy work: A phenomenological study of clients' experiences of cross-racial therapy. *Journal of Counseling Psychology, 56*(4), 521–536.

Child Welfare Information Gateway. (2016). *Racial disproportionality and disparity in child welfare.* Washington, DC: U.S. Department of Health and Human Services, Children's Bureau.

Constantine, M. G. (2001). Multicultural training, theoretical orientation, empathy, and multicultural case conceptualization ability in counselors. *Journal of Mental Health Counseling, 23*(4), 357–372.

Cooper, M., & Norcross, J. (2021). Working with client preferences. *Therapy Today, 32*(3), 32–35.

Council of National Psychological Associations for the Advancement of Ethnic Minority Interests (CNPAAEMI). (2016). *Testing and assessment with persons & communities of color.* Washington, DC: American Psychological Association. https://www.apa.org/pi/oema/resources/testing-assessment-monograph.pdf

DeFife, J. A., & Hilsenroth, M. J. (2011). Starting off on the right foot: Common factor elements in early psychotherapy process. *Journal of Psychotherapy Integration, 21*(2), 172–191.

Fanon, F. (1967). *Toward the African revolution.* New York, NY: Grove Press.

French, B. H., Lewis, J. A., Mosley, D. V., Adames, H. Y., Chavez-Dueñas, N. Y., Chen, G. A., & Neville, H. A. (2020). Toward a psychological framework of radical healing in communities of color. *Counseling Psychologist, 48*(1), 14–46.

Geter, A., Sutton, M. Y., & Hubbard McCree, D. (2018). Social and structural determinants of HIV treatment and care among Black women living with HIV infection: A systematic review: 2005–2016. *AIDS Care, 30*(4), 409–416.

Greenwood, B. N., Hardeman, R. R., Huang, L., & Sojourner, A. (2020, August). Physician–patient racial concordance and disparities in birthing mortality for newborns. *Proceedings of the National Academy of Sciences, 117*(35), 21194–21200. https://www.pnas.org/content/early/2020/08/12/1913405117

Hanson, J. (2005). Should your lips be zipped? How therapist self-disclosure and non-disclosure affects clients. *Counselling & Psychotherapy Research, 5*(2), 96–104.

Harris, H. L., & Licata, F. (2000). From fragmentation to integration: Affirming the identities of culturally diverse, mentally ill lesbians and gay men. *Journal of Gay & Lesbian Social Services, 11*(4), 93–103.

Helms, J. E., & Ford, D. Y. (2012). Testing and assessing African Americans: "Unbiased" tests are still unfair. *Journal of Negro Education, 81*(3), 186–189.

Hocoy, D., Kipnis, A., Lorenz, H., & Watkins, M. (2020). *Liberation psychologies: An invitation to dialogue.* https://www.pacifica.edu/degree-program/community-liberation-ecopsychology/what-is-liberation-psychology/

Hook, J. N., Davis, D. E., Owen, J., Worthington, E. L., Jr., & Utsey, S. O. (2013). Cultural humility: Measuring openness to culturally diverse clients. *Journal of Counseling Psychology, 60*(3), 353–366.

Hook, J. N., Farrell, J. E., Davis, D. E., DeBlaere, C., Van Tongeren, D. R., & Utsey, S. O. (2016). Cultural humility and racial microaggressions in counseling. *Journal of Counseling Psychology, 63*(3), 269–277.

Hubble, M. A., Duncan, B. L., & Miller, S. D. (1999). *The heart and soul of change: What works in therapy?* Washington, DC: American Psychological Association.

Kugelmass, H. (2016). "Sorry, I'm not accepting new patients": An audit study of access to mental health care. *Journal of Health and Social Behavior, 57*(2), 168–183.

Laska, K. M., Gurman, A. S., & Wampold, B. E. (2014). Expanding the lens of evidence-based practice in psychotherapy: A common factors perspective. *Psychotherapy, 51*(4), 467–481.

Lewis, J. A., Neville, H. A., Mosley, D. V., French, B. H., Chavez-Dueñas, N. Y., Adames, H. Y., & Chen, G. A. (2020). #SayHerName: Radical healing for Black women and gender expansive folx. https://www.psychologytoday.com/us/blog/healing-through-social-justice/202005/sayhername

Manuel, J. I. (2018). Racial/Ethnic and gender disparities in health care use and access. *Health Services Research, 53*(3), 1407–1429.

Mental Health Parity and Addiction Equity Act of 2008, Pub. L. No. 110-343, Title V, Subtitle B of Division C, §§ 511–512 (2008).

Morey, L. C. (2007). *Personality Assessment Inventory professional manual (2nd ed.).* Lutz, FL: Psychological Assessment Resources.

Mullen, J. (2020, April). Decolonizing our minds: Unlearning colonial mentality. *Moon Times Digest.* https://us16.campaign-archive.com/?id=97f25034e9&u=974e8f3a912b4b321b971a99e

National Alliance on Mental Illness (NAMI). (2009). *African American community mental health fact sheet.* http://dbhds.virginia.gov/library/cultural%20and%20linguistic%20competence/provider%20material/diverse/africanamerican_mentalhealth_factsheet_2009.pdf

National Alliance on Mental Illness (NAMI). (2020). *Black/African American.* https://www.nami.org/Support-Education/Diverse-Communities/African-American-Mental-Health

National Association of Social Workers. (2017). *Code of ethics.* https://www.socialworkers.org/About/Ethics/Code-of-Ethics/Code-of-Ethics-English

Neville, H. A. (2017, February). The role of counseling centers in promoting well-being and social justice. Keynote address presented at the Big Ten Counseling Centers Conference, Champaign, IL.

Nicolaidis, C., Timmons, V., Thomas, M. J., Waters, A. S., Wahab, S., Mejia, A., & Mitchell, S. R. (2010). "You don't go tell white people nothing": African American women's perspectives on the influence of violence and race on depression and depression care. *American Journal of Public Health, 100*(8), 1470–1476.

Osborn, C. J., Dean, E. P., & Petruzzi, M. L. (2004). Use of simulated multidisciplinary treatment teams and client actors to teach case conceptualization and treatment planning skills. *Counselor Education & Supervision, 44*(2), 121–134.

Owen, J., Devdas, L., & Rodolfa, E. (2007). University counseling center off-campus referrals: An exploratory investigation. *Journal of College Student Psychotherapy, 22*(2), 13–29.

Owen, J., Imel, Z., Tao, K. W., Wampold, B., Smith, A., & Rodolfa, E. (2011). Cultural ruptures in short-term therapy: Working alliance as a mediator between clients' perceptions of microaggressions and therapy outcomes. *Counselling & Psychotherapy Research, 11*(3), 204–212.

Owen, J., Tao, K. W., Drinane, J. M., Hook, J., Davis, D. E., & Kune, N. F. (2016). Client perceptions of therapists' multicultural orientation: Cultural (missed) opportunities and cultural humility. *Professional Psychology: Research and Practice, 47*(1), 30–37.

Petersen, E. E., Davis, N. L., Goodman, D., et al. (2019). Racial/Ethnic disparities in pregnancy-related deaths—United States, 2007–2016. *Morbidity and Mortality Weekly Report, 68,* 762–765.

Primm, A., & Lawson, W. B. (2010). African Americans. In P. Ruiz & A. Primm (Eds.), *Disparities in psychiatric care: Clinical and cross-cultural perspectives* (pp. 19–29). Washington, DC: Lippincott, Williams &Wilkins.

Robcis, C. (2020). Frantz Fanon, institutional psychotherapy, and the decolonization of psychiatry. *Journal of the History of Ideas, 81*(2), 303–325.

Robinson, W., & Finegold, K. (2012). The affordable care act and African Americans. U.S. Department of Health and Human Services. https://aspe.hhs.gov/report/affordable-care-act-and-african-americans

Shaw, S. (2017). Practicing cultural humility. *Counseling Today, 59*(7), 42–48.

Sperry, L., & Sperry, J. (2012). *Case conceptualization: Mastering this competency with ease and confidence.* New York, NY: Routledge.

Substance Abuse and Mental Health Services Administration (SAMHSA). (2017). *Center for Behavioral Health Statistics and Quality, National survey on drug use and health, 2017.* Rockville, MD: Author.

Substance Abuse and Mental Health Services Administration (SAMHSA). (2015). Racial/Ethnic differences in mental health service use among adults. *HHS Publication No. SMA-15-4906.* Rockville, MD: Author.

Substance Abuse and Mental Health Services Administration (SAMHSA). (2019). Behavioral Health Barometer: United States, Volume 5: Indicators as measured through the 2017 National Survey on Drug Use and Health and the National Survey of Substance Abuse Treatment Services. *HHS Publication No. SMA–19–Baro-17-US*. Rockville, MD: Author.

Sue, D. W., Arredondo, P., & McDavis, R. J. (1992). Multicultural counseling competencies: A call to the profession. *Journal of Counseling & Development, 70*(4), 477–486.

Swift, J. K., Callahan, J. L., Ivanovic, M., & Kominiak, N. (2013). Further examination of the psychotherapy preference effect: A meta-regression analysis. *Journal of Psychotherapy Integration, 23*(2), 134–145.

Swift, J. K., Callahan, J. L., Tompkins, K. A., Connor, D. R., & Dunn, R. (2015). A delay-discounting measure of preference for racial/ethnic matching in psychotherapy. *Psychotherapy, 52*(3), 315–320.

Swift, J. K., Callahan, J. L., & Vollmer, B. M. (2011). Preferences. *Journal of Clinical Psychology, 67*(2), 155–165. https://doi.org/10.1002/jclp.20759

Thompson, V. L. S., Bazile, A., & Akbar, M. (2004). African Americans' perceptions of psychotherapy and psychotherapists. *Professional Psychology: Research and Practice, 35*(1), 19–26.

U.S. Surgeon General. (2001). *Mental health: Culture, races, and ethnicity—A supplement to Mental health: A report of the surgeon general.* Health & Human Services. https://pubmed.ncbi.nlm.nih.gov/20669516/

Vasquez, M. J. T. (2007). Cultural difference and the therapeutic alliance: An evidence-based analysis. *American Psychologist, 62*(8), 878–885.

Walker, A. (1982). *The color purple.* New York, NY: Houghton Mifflin Harcourt Publishing.

Washington, H. A. (2006). *Medical apartheid: The dark history of medical experimentation on Black Americans from colonial times to the present.* New York, NY: Harlem Moon.

Williams, M. (1999, August). Oral History *Interview with Mabel Williams: Interview K-0266.* Southern Oral History Program Collection (#4007) in the Southern Oral History Program Collection, Southern Historical Collection, Wilson Library, University of North Carolina at Chapel Hill. https://docsouth.unc.edu/sohp/html_use/K-0266.html

Williamson, M. E. (2014). The reluctance of African-Americans to engage in therapy. *Public Access Theses and Dissertations from the College of Education and Human Sciences.* 216. http://digitalcommons.unl.edu/cehsdiss/216

Zapata, K. (2020, February 27). Decolonizing mental health: The importance of an oppression-focused mental health system. *Calgary Journal.* https://www.calgaryjournal.ca/more/calgaryvoices/4982-decolonizing-mental-health-the-importance-of-an-oppression-focused-mental-health-system.html

CHAPTER 3

Depression and Anxiety in African American Women

Lauren Simone Harper
Courtney Williams

The National Institute of Mental Health (NIMH, 2019a) calculated the prevalence of major depression and anxiety disorders among the American population. Major depressive episodes were higher among adult female–identified individuals, at 8.7 percent, compared to male-identified persons at 5.3 percent. Moreover, African Americans had lower prevalence rates at 5.4 percent compared to European Americans (7.4 percent). NIMH also found that the prevalence rates for anxiety disorders was higher for those who identified as women (23.4 percent) compared to those who identified as men (14.3 percent). This survey did not account for race. It is challenging to gauge the usefulness of these findings for the treatment of anxiety and depression for African American women considering the survey's lack of cultural context. The prevalence of depression is surveyed specifically considering a major depressive episode, which requires meeting diagnostic criteria for clinical depression. On the contrary, the survey assessing anxiety is broader in its consideration of symptom presentation. Taken together, there is a dearth in the literature about the experiences of African American women regarding anxiety and depression.

What we do know, however, is that depression and anxiety are two of the most common contributors of mental distress among American women (NIMH, 2019a; NIMH, 2019b). Risk factors for clinical depression and anxiety among African American women include low-income, low-education level, and comorbid chronic illness (Wicks et al., 2007). While this literature provides some insight into African American women's experiences with depression and anxiety, there are additional factors to consider. This incomplete picture gives support to the need for specific understanding of, and treatment recommendations for, depression and anxiety among African American women.

Regarding diagnosis of anxiety and depression among African American women, it is important to note that misdiagnosing is common among this population, thus affecting the type of treatment African American women receive on these issues. There is also a lack of competency around treating anxiety and depression in transgender and gender non-conforming (TGNC) African American women who experience additional distress from racial-gendered oppression both outside and inside of the therapy room (Lefevor et al., 2019). Implications for misdiagnosis could be related to African American women's potential subclinical presentation, concerns that impact help-seeking, or access to treatment. Practitioners should consider diagnosis, treatment, and interventions for anxiety and depression among African American women from a bio-psycho-socio-cultural model as best practice (Rudski, Sperber, & Ibrahim, 2018). Therefore, the purpose of this chapter will be to discuss culturally specific symptom presentation, treatment considerations, treatment recommendations, and other factors to account for regarding accessibility, diagnosis, and intervention for African American women across the gender spectrum.

DEPRESSION AND ANXIETY SYMPTOM PRESENTATION IN AFRICAN AMERICAN WOMEN

Understanding the difference in symptom presentation for anxiety and depression in African American women is highly important for accurate diagnosis and treatment. African American women have been found to present with somatic or physical complaints that may or may not be a function of a physical health issue (Myers et al., 2002). Due to the nature of the complaint, it is more likely an African American woman may present to their health-care professional (i.e., primary care doctor, nurse practitioner, etc.) for their concerns rather than to a mental health professional. Therefore, guidelines for symptom presentation when diagnosing depression or anxiety in African American women are needed for both mental health and physical health practitioners. Myers et al. (2002) also suggested that considering level of education, employment status, and marital status is as important for diagnosing depression and anxiety among this population as those in their sample who were low-income, working-class women.

Perceived discrimination is directly related to mental and physical health issues. Specifically, discrimination leads to issues in affect, and subsequently increasing issues of anxiety and depression in African Americans (Gibbons et al., 2014). Gibbons et al. (2014) discuss that discrimination can have an immediate influence on mental health. Understanding the effects of discrimination on the mental health of African American women is crucial for culturally responsive assessment and treatment. Gibbons et al. (2014) found that African American women reacted to perceived racial discrimination through internalizing (increased anxiety and depression) and externalizing (through hostility and anger). Long-standing internalizing factors had impacts on physical health, while externalizing factors resulted in substance use problems. Additionally, TGNC African American women have higher initial anxiety and depression rates from racial-gendered discrimination, oppression, and violence in society, as well as in discrimination in health-care and therapy treatment settings due to practitioner stigma and bias (Lefevor et al., 2019). These findings are important for practitioners to remember during assessment to support appropriate diagnosis and treatment of African American women.

Treatment Considerations

Definitive studies for treating depression among African American women are sparse (Sohail, Kennedy Bailey, & Richie, 2014). A metanalysis conducted by van Loon and colleagues (2012) concluded the most effective treatment for depression and anxiety among African American women was treatment that is adapted to include a client's cultural values, beliefs, and presentation. Consistent with understanding an African American woman's presentation, and subsequently her mental health, we must first realize how African American women are viewed in this country (Neal-Barnett, 2018). There are three main archetypes of the African American woman: the Strong Black Woman, the Angry Black Woman, and the Jezebel/Video Vixen (Neal-Barnett, 2018).

Culturally, there are norms within the African American women community that have guided coping strategies around anxiety and depression. Holden et al. (2014) speak to the high resiliency among African American women. Watson and Hunter (2015) coined the term Strong Black Woman (SBW), a race-gender schema arguing that African American women use resiliency and silence in coping with distress versus accessing mental health services. More specifically, women may respond to mental distress by taking on more at work or home, experiencing irritability, functioning as a caretaker for others, and pushing through distress. The Strong Black Woman archetype is conceived from the continued narrative that Black women are the pillars of their community. All these coping strategies fulfill the SBW prophecy, and can produce burnout and physical illness, having implications for anxiety and depression (Wicks et al., 2007).

There are often projected, and assumed, expectations that African American women provide support to their loved ones (e.g., financially, emotionally, and physically). Mental health implications, such as depression and anxiety, arise when African American women do not experience reciprocity in the support they provide. Concurrently, African American women are socialized to believe that "strength" means minimizing their own problems and navigating issues independently. Thus, Stanton et al. (2017) argue that the internalization of this stereotype is both harmful and helpful. They argue that while embracing the Strong Black Woman schema can limit one's self-care, as African American women who endorse this archetype can perceive themselves as "superhuman" and dismiss their emotions and needs, the internalization of this archetype may also serve as a protective factor that enhances survival and self-efficacy.

Second, the Angry Black Woman archetype depicts a hostile, aggressive, and bitter image of African American women, which does not contextualize the historical, cultural, political, and economical factors that may contribute to an African American woman's lived experience. Ashley (2014) speaks to the "angry Black woman myth" that permeates our society, further oppressing African American women and stigmatizing their emotional expression. Considering the culturally specific factors that may impact a Black woman's presentation, especially related to the mental health and medical field, it is important for clinicians to be mindful of the mythology of the "Angry Black Woman" and how it impacts treatment (Ashley, 2014).

Third, Black women as Jezebels have been consistently publicized in popular media, depicted as promiscuous, hypersexual, and immoral. This archetype was developed from European Christian missionaries who thought Black women to be oversexualized and immoral beings; as well as the social construction of "Black femininity," a combination of the female Hottentot that represents the Black female in the nineteenth century, and the prostitute, which represents the sexualized woman (Gillman, 1992; Pleck, 1990). Mullings (1992) and Stasiulis (1990) observe that the sexualities of Black and White women became polarized during slavery, as they were based on a romanticized image of the ideal woman as pure, passive, and moral. It is an ideology that situated Black and White women on opposite ends of the spectrum, portraying European American women as fragile, meek, and sexually repressed and African American women as aggressive, resilient, and sexually immoral.

This literature provides insight into how stereotypes held about African American women can play a major role in their mental health. Moreover, it is important to consider the race- and gender-based trauma that comes along with being an African American woman in this country. Neal-Barnett (2018) speaks to the racism, sexism, and other contextual factors that African American women experience in America, as well as to the social anxiety experienced by African American women, particularly in school and professional settings. Many times, African American women are navigating predominantly White and heteronormative spaces, where they are the first and/or only African American woman in that setting. The acculturative stress that is associated with navigating spaces when no one looks or presents like you or trying to adapt to the majority culture brings about emotional labor and fatigue. Historically, messaging around being "twice as good, to go half as far" has communicated to African American women that we are not viewed as equals and the labor that we carry is twice as large as our European American counterparts (Neal-Barnett, 2018). To manage the cognitive dissonance accompanied by acculturative stress, African Americans have often adapted code-switching or "acting White" to navigate these systems.

A qualitative study by Waite and Killian (2008) was conducted in a group of African American women to explore health beliefs among this group, and beliefs about depression, as well as to gain insight regarding treatment decisions. Themes from the study included the following: perceived susceptibility to depression, perceived severity of depression, perceived benefits of treating depression, perceived barriers to treatment, and cues to action. A majority of participants in the study felt that one was more susceptible to depression when one had "weak mind, poor health, a troubled spirit, and lack of self-love." Additionally, participants varied in their responses to acceptable modes of treatment for depression—pastor, medication, psychotherapy, and nurse. Waite and Killian (2008) also explored important factors that lead African American women to seek help in the first place. Individuals from the study shared that they may be called to action due to "internal reminders" like physical symptoms, or "external reminders" such as media, family, and community. Ashley (2014) suggests that providers who misunderstand the disenfranchisement of Black women may also misinterpret their emotional experiences and responses to stress, thus impacting diagnosis, symptom assessment, and the overall provision of treatment.

Treatment Recommendations

Regarding cultural adaptations to treatment, Neal-Barnett (2018) argues that thorough and culturally sensitive assessment is necessary for a holistic case conceptualization when treating the (mental) health concerns of African American women. Additionally, she urges the consideration of the use of sister circles, an Indigenous form of healing, to provide community and support, understanding and normalcy, as well as catharsis and treatment. Neal-Barnett (2018) adds that relational cultural theory may be a great way to conceptualize and develop treatment interventions for African American women. Given the evidence-based practice (EBP) of cognitive-behavioral therapy (CBT) across varied treatment groups, it has been found that culturally adapting CBT to include musical cognitive restructuring can be a helpful treatment as well (Neal-Barnett, 2018). Sohail and colleagues (2014) also found cognitive therapy to be equally, if not more, effective than pharmacotherapy. According to their research, they found a significant symptom reduction after 12 sessions (Sohail et al., 2014). They also suggest that holistic therapies that integrate spirituality, physical health, social health, and so on can be an effective modality in treating anxiety and depression among this population. When treating TGNC African American women, it is recommended practitioners beware of minimizing or exaggerating gender and making blanket generalizations that deflect from the presenting concern and could inflict further trauma on the client (Lefevor et al., 2019). Because African American women often function as caretakers among their interpersonal relationships, Martin Richards (2018) highlights the importance of self-care. Treatment recommendations specific to this population may include physical activity, sleep hygiene, social connectedness, spiritual practice, and knowing limits.

We have discussed in this chapter that African American women are more likely to be diagnosed with anxiety and/or depression by their primary care provider before a mental health professional. It is recommended for best practice in diagnosing and treating African American women that providers move away from focusing primarily on symptom management and move toward improving our functioning and overall quality of life. This can be accomplished by an integrated and/or collaborative care model of physical and mental health care. Porcerelli and Jones (2017) discuss the limits to commonly used screening measures such as the Patient Health Questionnaire (PHQ-9) and Generalized Anxiety Disorder questionnaire (GAD-7), which give severity scores that can help with tracking symptom management but do not inquire of changes in level of functioning. The authors also note that screening tools should not be relied on for diagnosing anxiety and depression, but rather a comprehensive assessment of symptoms and functioning are necessary. Primary care physicians (PCPs) should work with African American women on addressing their symptoms, while using screening tools as a rationale to refer to a mental health provider to address functioning and quality of life. PCPs and mental health providers can improve their practice further by incorporating additional screening measures of functioning such as the Duke Health Questionnaire or conducting functional assessments like the Live, Love, Work, Play of the modality Functional Acceptance and Commitment Therapy (FACT) (Strosahl, Gustavsson, & Robinson, 2012). As we consider treatment recommendations for depression and anxiety among African American women, it is also important to discuss how disparities in the quality of mental health care impact treatment availability and accessibility among this group (Holden et al., 2014).

Treatment Availability and Accessibility

Treatment for anxiety and depression among African American women typically begins with the first entry point being the primary care physician's office. A large percentage of people receive mental health care in primary care settings (Holden et al., 2014). Research shows that African American women may seek treatment for somatic symptoms such as headaches, stomach issues, colds, and other physical complaints. Moreover, racial minorities are more likely to report depressive symptoms to their PCP (Holden et al., 2014).

Rudski, Sperber, and Ibrahim (2018) note that African American women are twice as likely to be diagnosed with depression, as well as given medication for treatment, compared to men. Primary care physicians and gynecologists can prescribe medications for the treatment of mental health (Martin Richards, 2018). Conversely, African American women are found to be underdiagnosed and undertreated for psychiatric disorders (U.S. Department of Health and Human Services, 2001). Reasons for this disparaging data are suggested to be related to recognition/diagnosis of disorder, access to mental health services, and attitudes toward mental health care and medication (Wang et al., 2005). Waite and Killian (2008) found that participants in a qualitative study held the following as perceived barriers to treatment for depression: (a) distrust of their healthcare providers, (b) denial that they had depression, (c) limited knowledge about the etiology of depression, (d) stigma associated with depression, and (e) lack of finances to continue professional therapy sessions.

Neighbors, Musick, and Williams (1998) argue that African American women are more likely to find refuge via religious outlets rather than mental health services. Moreover, there is a stigma among the African American community about receiving treatment for mental health concerns. Underdiagnoses and misdiagnoses for African American women were also found to be related to the high prevalence of somatization among this community (Zhang & Snowden, 1999). Moreover, research has repeatedly shown how accurate diagnosis is significantly impacted by the rapport of the relationship in both medical and mental health settings (Scarinci, Beech, & Watson, 2004). Additionally, continuity of care was found to have major implications for overall health outcomes among the African American women in this study.

Research shows that African Americans are underdiagnosed for affective disorders and overdiagnosed and overtreated for psychotic disorders (Holden et al., 2014). More specifically, O'Malley, Forrest, & Miranda (2003) found the following factors among lower-income African American women to improve their chances of accurately detecting and treating depression: providers who were perceived as respectful, women who had an ongoing relationship with their provider, and providers who implemented comprehensive care. This study found that when medical providers were able to fulfill an expansive amount of their patients' medical needs, they were more likely to provide care and attention to the patient's psychosocial needs.

The bio-psycho-socio-cultural model argues that a more comprehensive treatment for African American women, including psychotherapy, medication, and increased involvement in social change, can address inequities in diagnosis and treatment experiences. Sosulski and Woodard

(2013) explored help-seeking behaviors of African American women, finding that help was found through professional support (i.e., mental health treatment), informal supports (family, friends, and community members), or no support at all. The authors of the study attribute various reasons to African American women not seeking any support including subclinical experience, low-literacy levels, stigma of accessing help, low access to professional help and/or no desire to engage in said help, and no access to informal support. Lefevor et al. (2019) discuss for TGNC African American clients there is further anxiety, in addition to their presenting concern, that comes from having to find a TGNC-affirming therapist and having to educate the therapist on TGNC issues. Additionally, if African American women engage in medical treatment, cultural psychopharmacology considerations are needed. Jackson (2006) discussed the laborious process people must go through to find medication efficacy. The author charged providers to consider the racial-gendered response and metabolic response to antidepressants as African American women can chemically process medications differently due to genetics, body fat, and other factors. Literature on effective treatment argues that knowing family medical and psychiatric history is a very helpful way for current patients/clients to discover possible treatment modalities that will work for them. The authors of this chapter argue that recalling, or even reporting, familial treatment history comes with its own set of barriers in that due to the stigmatization of mental health among the Black community, it may be difficult to truly know if family members have sought mental health treatment themselves. Additionally, the authors consider the implication of the difficulty in tracing African American people's lineage and understanding family medical history.

McCall, Schwartz, and Khairat (2019) reported results from an exploratory, web-based study conducted by the University of North Carolina at Chapel Hill. This study found that Black women younger than 50 showed high acceptance rates for communicating with mental health professionals via video calls in order to manage their depression and anxiety. This implies promising results for the use of telemental health with Black women under the age of 50 for anxiety and depression. Sosulski et al. (2017) also considered the impact of social media on mental health, finding that increased endorsement of the SBW ideal and high social media use increased experiences of depression and anxiety in African American women. These findings are particularly important to explore with the increase in the importance of technology in millennials' lives.

Case Study of Jo

Jo presents to counseling after being referred by her primary care provider for complaints of headaches, "knots in stomach," difficulty sleeping, and chronic fatigue. Jo's PHQ-9 and GAD-7 scores were 12 and 10 respectively, both within the moderate range. Jo's PCP referred her to a mental health provider, as Jo preferred talk therapy to medication at the time. Jo shared her reservations about both therapy and medication, as she had never used either; however, because her friends had already recommended she try therapy, she thought this would be the best first step.

Jo presents to therapy with an African American, female-identified therapist, per her request. Jo is a 35-year-old, self-identified African American, bisexual, cisgender female. Jo's pronouns are she/her/hers. She considers herself middle class and works in the human resources department at a local university as a human resources manager. Jo is highly educated, holds a master's degree in human resources, and describes her job as "a good challenge."

Jo was born and raised in Louisville, Kentucky. She describes her social support network as follows: work colleagues (mainly outside of the department), college friends, local friends she's met through church, social and networking events, and her partner Asia. Jo was raised in a single-parent home by her father after her mother died when she was 16 years old. She has one older brother and one younger sister with whom she is close and is also extremely close with their father. More specifically, Jo shares everything with family, and they are fully in support of her. Jo identifies as Christian, nondenominational and states she was raised Christian, an active participant at an inclusive and affirming church home.

Over the course of her work with her mental health provider, Jo described experiencing fatigue, irritability, sleep issues, problems with concentration and memory, tightness in muscles, crying spells, and trouble getting out of bed. She reports she experiences these symptoms most days, and these problems started when she was a teenager. She never had any treatment for these symptoms and thought they were normal. Jo also reports that she has experienced discrimination from work colleagues. Though subtle, she is often on the receiving end of microaggressions regarding her race and sexuality.

Current coping mechanisms of Jo's are faith practices, talking and spending time with loved ones, and going to the gym. She notes, however, that she has little free time outside of work, volunteering, and community leadership roles. Jo consistently presents to therapy on a weekly basis and has collaborated with the therapist on treatment goals of boundary setting, knowing limits, and prioritizing taking care of herself.

Case Study Discussion Points

Conceptualizing clinical cases from a strengths-based perspective is a key factor in case conceptualization, treatment planning, and building and maintaining rapport with clients. It can be important for the therapist not only to identify and hold strengths for the cases they are treating, but also to invite clients to make meaning of the strengths about their own presenting concerns/lived experiences. Strength-based practice helps foster resiliency, highlight protective factors, and buffer against mental health crises. Regarding this particular case, Jo has many protective factors that provide her with support as she copes with symptoms of anxiety and depression including a strong network of supportive people and good health behaviors like exercising, her faith community, and engagement in the community.

It would be helpful to explore how Jo utilizes her support systems (e.g., for emotional support, financial support, etc.). If the therapist discovers that the client utilizes her social supports for emotional support, it may be helpful to unpack to what extent this emotional support is provided. Do loved ones know the full extent of Jo's concerns? Does Jo feel like there are some things she can discuss, but holds back others? She is resilient and has been successful professionally. Jo's positionality related to education and career place her in a particular social class that would allot her more resources and knowledge regarding health-related factors. She communicates her needs and sought help for her concerns through her PCP and then establishing with a therapist. Moreover, Jo presents as willing, open, and committed to therapy, as evidenced by her consistent attendance to therapy appointments, collaboration of therapeutic goals, and reflectiveness in historical considerations and present challenges.

There are several specific factors in Jo's case to consider as important in addressing her symptoms of depression and anxiety. First, it is important to consider Jo's history of experiencing the traumatic event of her mother's death. That history has impacted her functioning throughout the years by manifesting in both her physical and mental health. It is possible that Jo has been struggling with untreated grief that she has learned to push through by staying busy personally and professionally. It is also important to factor in the messages Jo has received around being a Black, queer woman that shape how she shows up in the world and among interpersonal spaces and relationships. More specifically, it would be important to explore Jo's experiences of microaggressions in the workplace and beyond. As a therapist, you are also assessing the duration, frequency, and severity of depression and anxiety symptoms present. Moreover, gathering data points to understand how symptoms may be impacting functioning and how they present across settings is important. This will give you the information needed to diagnose Jo's concerns accurately, determine the level of care needed, and co-construct with a culturally responsive treatment plan.

Jo may have taken on factors of the Superwoman schema including caretaking for others, committing to many projects, and minimizing her own needs (e.g., not attending to or acknowledging symptoms of depression and anxiety). While caring for others and volunteering may be helpful tools for Jo's functionality, harmful effects of the Superwoman schema can lead to mental and physical health implications as mentioned in this chapter. Jo's caretaking improves her mood when helping others; it can be a helpful distraction from addressing her own problems; and it's positively reinforcing to know you're needed by others and that you are an effective helper.

It can be helpful as a therapist to reflect the dialectal relationship of the Superwoman schema archetype. More specifically, the therapist may first provide psychoeducation about the Superwoman schema, particularly exploring how identity factors impact the client's presenting concerns, as well as their potential endorsement and embodiment of this archetype. The therapist may ask the client to discuss messaging that the client has heard throughout her life regarding this archetype. The therapist may also further use herself as a tool to incorporate self-disclosure about how the Superwoman schema has impacted the therapist's own lived experiences, as well as discussing with the client to reflect on how the embodiment/endorsement of this archetype may impact the therapeutic relationships, given the therapist-client variables. Lastly, therapists may engage the client in identifying the dialectic of the functionality of the Superwoman schema as well as the potential risk factors involved.

REFERENCES

Ashley, W. (2014). The Angry Black Woman: The impact of pejorative stereotypes on psychotherapy with Black women. *Social Work in Public Health*, 29(1), 27–34. https://doi.org/10.1080/19371918.2011.619449

Gibbons, F. X., Kingsbury, J. H., Weng, C.-Y., Gerrard, M., Cutrona, C., Wills, T. A., & Stock, M. (2014). Effects of perceived racial discrimination on health status and health behavior: A differential mediation hypothesis. *Health Psychology*, 33(1), 11–19.

Gillman, S. L. (1992). Black bodies, White bodies: Toward an iconography of female sexuality in late 19th century art, medicine and literature. In J. Donald & A. Rattansi (Eds.), *Race, culture and difference*. London, England: Open University Press.

Holden, K. B., Bradford, L. D., Hall, S. P., & Belton, A. S. (2014). Prevalence and correlates of depressive symptoms and resiliency among African American women in a community-based primary health care center. *Journal of Health Care for the Poor and Underserved*, 24(4 Suppl.), 79–93.

Jackson, A. P. (2006). The use of psychiatric medications to treat depressive disorders in African American women. *Journal of Clinical Psychology*, 62(7), 793–800.

Lefevor, G. T., Janis, R. A., Franklin, A., & Stone, W.-M. (2019). Distress and therapeutic outcomes among transgender and gender nonconforming people of color. *Counseling Psychologist* 47(1), 34–58.

Martin Richards, E. (2018). *Mental health among African American women*. Johns Hopkins Medicine. https://www.hopkinsmedicine.org/health/wellness-and-prevention/mental-health-among-african-american-women

McCall, T., Schwartz, T., & Khairat, S. (2019). Acceptability of telemedicine to help African American women manage anxiety and depression. *Studies in Health Technology and Informatics*, 264, 699–703.

Mullings, L. (1992). *Race, class and gender: Representations and reality*. Memphis, TN: Research Clearing House and Curriculum Integration Project, Centre for Research on Women.

Myers, H. F., Lesser, I., Rodriguez, N., Mira, C. B., Hwang, W.-C., Camp, C., & Wohl, M. (2002). Ethnic differences in clinical presentation of depression in adult women. *Cultural Diversity and Ethnic Minority Psychology, 8*(2), 138–156.

National Institute of Mental Health (2019a). *Prevalence of a major depressive episode among adults*. https://www.nimh.nih.gov/health/statistics/major-depression.shtml#part_155033

National Institute of Mental Health (2019b). *Prevalence of any anxiety disorder among adults*. https://www.nimh.nih.gov/health/statistics/any-anxiety-disorder.shtml

Neal-Barnett, A. (2018). *To be female, anxious, and Black*. Anxiety and Depression Association of America. https://adaa.org/learn-from-us/from-the-experts/blog-posts/consumer/be-female-anxious-and-black

Neighbors, H., Musick, M., & Williams, D. (1998). The African American minister as a source of help for serious personal crises: Bridge or barrier to mental health care? *Health Education & Behavior 6*(25), 759–777. http://hdl.handle.net/2027.42/67669

O'Malley, A. S., Forrest, C. B., & Miranda, J. (2003). Primary care attributes and care for depression among low-income African American women. *American Journal of Public Health, 93*(8), 1328–1334.

Pleck, E. (1990). *Rape and the politics of race, 1865–1910*. Wellesley, MA: Wellesley College, Centre for Research on Women.

Porcerelli, J. H., & Jones, J. R. (2017). Uses of psychological assessment in primary care settings. In M. E. Maruish (Ed.), *Handbook of psychological assessment in primary care settings*, 2nd ed. New York, NY: Routledge

Rudski, J. M., Sperber, J., & Ibrahim, D. (2018). Addressing depression through psychotherapy, medication, or social change: An empirical investigation. *Neuroethics, 11*(2), 129–141.

Scarinci, I. C., Beech, B. M., & Watson, J. M. (2004). Physician-patient interaction and depression among African-American women: a national study. *Ethnicity & Disease, 14*(4), 567–573.

Sohail, Z., Kennedy Bailey, R., & Richie, W. D. (2014). Misconceptions of depression in African Americans. *Frontiers in Psychiatry, 5*(65).

Sosulski, M. R., & Woodward, A. T. (2013). African American women living with mental disorders: Factors associated with help seeking from professional services and informal supports. *Social Work in Public Health, 28*(7), 660–671.

Stanton, A. G., Jerald, M. C., Ward, L. M., & Avery, L. R. (2017). Social media contributions to Strong Black Woman ideal endorsement and Black women's mental health. *Psychology of Women Quarterly, 41*(4), 465–478.

Stasiulis, D. K. (1990). Theorizing connections: Gender, race, ethnicity and class. In P. Li (Ed.), *Race and ethnic relations in Canada* (pp. 269–305). Toronto, ON: Oxford University Press Canada.

Strosahl, K., Gustavsson, T., & Robinson, P. A. (2012). *Brief interventions for radical change: Principles & practice of focused acceptance & commitment therapy*. New Harbinger Publications.

U.S. Department of Health and Human Services, Center for Mental Health Services. (2001). *Mental Health: Culture, Race, and Ethnicity*; A Supplement to

"Mental Health: A Report of the Surgeon General" Report. Washington, DC: U.S. Department of Health and Human Services.

van Loon, A., van Schaik, A., Dekker, J., & Beekman, A. (2013). Bridging the gap for ethnic minority adult outpatients with depression and anxiety disorders by culturally adapted treatments. *Journal of Affective Disorders, 147*(1–3), 9–16.

Waite, R., & Killian, P. (2008). Health beliefs about depression among African American women. *Perspectives in Psychiatric Care, 44*(3), 185–195.

Wang, P. S., Lane, M., Olfson, M., Pincus, H. A., Wells, K. B., & Kessler, R. C. (2005). Twelve-month use of mental health services in the United States: Results from the National Comorbidity Survey Replication. *Archives of General Psychiatry, 62*(6), 629–640.

Watson, N. N., & Hunter, C. D. (2015). Anxiety and depression among African American women: The costs of strength and negative attitudes toward psychological help-seeking. *Cultural Diversity and Ethnic Minority Psychology, 21*(4), 604–612.

Wicks, M. N., Bolden, L., Mynatt, S., Rice, M. C., & Acchiardo, S. R. (2007). INSIGHT potentially prevents and treats depressive and anxiety symptoms in Black women caring for chronic hemodialysis recipients. *Nephrology Nursing Journal, 34*(6), 623.

Zhang, A. Y., & Snowden, L. R. (1999). Ethnic characteristics of mental disorders in five U.S. communities. *Cultural Diversity and Ethnic Minority Psychology, 5*(2), 134–146. https://doi.org/10.1037/1099-9809.5.2.134

CHAPTER 4

Post-Traumatic Stress and Complex Trauma

Shavonne J. Moore-Lobban
Maria Espinola
Karen Powdrill

Post-traumatic stress disorder (PTSD) is a mental health disorder that can develop after exposure to trauma incidents, such as physical assault, rape, motor vehicle accidents, and combat exposure. The *Diagnostic and Statistical Manual of Mental Disorders* (*DSM-5*) (American Psychiatric Association, 2013) lists four PTSD symptom clusters: reexperiencing (e.g., nightmares, flashbacks, intrusive memories), avoidance (e.g., avoiding reminders of trauma), hypervigilance (e.g., exaggerated startle response, feeling on edge), and negative cognitions and mood (e.g., depressed mood, inappropriate guilt). Although many people experience acute stress responses after traumatic incidents, only 8.3 percent of people who face life-threatening, terrifying events meet lifetime DSM-5 criteria for PTSD (Kilpatrick et al., 2013). In fact, about 38 percent of people who report lasting symptoms, post a traumatic incident, meet the criteria for other disorders such as substance use, anxiety, or depressive disorder instead of PTSD (O'Donnell et al., 2004).

Outside of the DSM-5 definition of trauma, a large body of research suggests that exposure to severe and prolonged trauma (e.g., childhood sexual abuse, domestic violence, human trafficking) can lead to the development of a broad constellation of symptoms that significantly alter affect regulation, attention, self-control, attachment, and interpersonal functioning (Courtois & Ford, 2013; van der Kolk et al., 2005). These long-term sequelae of trauma symptomatology are known as complex post-traumatic stress disorder (CPTSD) (Courtois & Ford, 2013; Herman, 1997). This line of research suggests that focusing on post-traumatic stress disorder symptoms developed after single incidents of trauma (e.g., rape, robbery) cannot be used to fully explain the experiences of individuals subjected to severe and prolonged trauma.

CPTSD became a formal *International Statistical Classification of Diseases and Related Health Problems* (11th ed.) (ICD-11) diagnosis in 2019. Differing from the DSM-5 (APA, 2013) categorization of trauma and the above CPTSD definition, exposure to severe and prolonged trauma is not a requirement. The ICD-11 (2019) criteria emphasize symptom severity and impairment as opposed to the frequency of trauma incidents. For example, a person who has a genetic vulnerability to develop mental health disorders and experiences a particular heinous crime can potentially meet the CPTSD criteria (International Society for Traumatic Stress Studies, 2018).

TRAUMA IN THE LIVES OF AFRICAN AMERICANS

Trauma can easily be seen as an epidemic in our society as it affects countless individuals across all walks of life. Although trauma has the potential to affect anybody, some individuals may be more vulnerable to trauma and experience higher rates of it than others. For example, racial and ethnic minorities are more likely to be exposed to different types of trauma, including Adverse Childhood Experiences (ACEs) (Slack, Font, & Jones, 2018). ACEs include childhood neglect, physical abuse, sexual abuse, witnessing domestic violence, and living with a family member who has been incarcerated or is mentally ill. Over 33.8 percent of African Americans report four or more ACEs as opposed to 15.03 percent of Whites (Slack, Font, & Jones, 2018). The Centers for Disease Control and Prevention (CDC, 2019) reported that ACEs have a graded dose-response with over 40+ outcomes, including mental illness, suicide attempts, diabetes, sexually transmitted diseases, cancer, heart disease, stroke, broken bones, chronic obstructive pulmonary disease, and pregnancy outcomes. Furthermore, ACEs are known to increase health risk behaviors (alcohol abuse, drug abuse, and smoking), reduce academic achievement and graduation rates, and increase time lost from work (CDC, 2019; Kalmakis & Chandler, 2015).

Notably, there have been mixed findings regarding ethnic differences in the prevalence of PTSD; however, literature has shown evidence that African Americans have disproportionately higher rates of trauma and PTSD. For example, according to the National Crime Victimization Survey, African Americans experienced the highest rates of violent victimization toward them in 2017, and the second-highest rate in 2018 (Morgan & Oudekerk, 2019). Further, in a study that analyzed data from a National Epidemiologic Survey on Alcohol and Related Conditions, researchers found that African Americans had higher lifetime prevalence of PTSD (8.7 percent) compared to their Hispanic (7.0 percent), White (7.4 percent), and Asian (4.0 percent) counterparts (Roberts et al., 2011). This finding is consistent with other studies that have shown African Americans have higher rates of trauma exposure and a diagnosis of PTSD (Alegría et al., 2013; see Hall-Clark et al., 2016 for review).

Indeed, African Americans contend with traumatic experiences from early on in their lives, and unfortunately, the traumas continue into adulthood. In a study examining mental health disorders among African Americans, Caribbean Blacks, and non-Hispanic Whites, Himle and colleagues (2009) found that African Americans and Caribbean Blacks were at higher risk for developing PTSD in their teenage years and continuing to experience PTSD across their lifespan. Later in life, African Americans have been shown to have higher rates of traumatic exposure through interpersonal violence (Alegría et al., 2013; Alim, Charney, & Mellman, 2006) and traumatic military experiences (Coleman, 2016; Kulka et al., 1990).

The Unique Experience of African American Woman

Physical and sexual violence against African American women are long-standing within society. Stereotyping African American women as sexually promiscuous, blaming them for assaults where they are clearly the victim, and seeing them as subordinate because of their racial and gender identities contribute to the biased lens that African American women are viewed through, and the discriminatory practices that leave their experiences of trauma unattended to.

African American women specifically have experienced higher rates of violence against them through sexual and physical assault (Black et al., 2011), as well as being victims of intimate partner violence (Gillum, 2019; Taft et al., 2009). More so, throughout the United States, they are disproportionately victims of sex trafficking when compared to their White counterparts, and they are also criminalized for being trafficked (i.e., charged with prostitution even if being forced into the trade) at rates that are higher than any other racial group (Rights4Girls, 2019). Take, for example, Cyntoia Brown, who at age 16 began serving a life sentence after being convicted of killing a 43-year-old man who solicited her for sex (Allyn, 2019). Her case garnered national attention through celebrities and social media as society began to better understand the implications of her being a victim of sex trafficking. Her sentence was eventually commuted after she served 15 years.

African American women encounter a greater degree of disparity and oppression in various arenas given the intersection of their identities as African American and as women. Such experiences can be understood through the term *gendered racism,* coined by Essed (1991), which proposes that African American women are subjected to distinctive forms of oppression due to the unique intersection of gender and race. Studies have explored the intersection of race and gender to the experience of African American women and found cognitive attributions of stress (King, 2005) as well as overall chronic strain and psychological distress (Perry, Harp, & Oser, 2013). Lewis et al. (2016) indicated that the experience of gendered racism is entrenched in societal stereotypes that are meant to marginalize and trivialize African American women. For example, stereotypes include being highly maternal and self-sacrificing (e.g., Mammy stereotype), angry and domineering (e.g., Sapphire stereotype), and promiscuous (e.g., Jezebel stereotype) (Lewis et al., 2016; Miller-Harris, 2011). Each stereotype has the potential to induce stress in African American women based on the way the stereotype is internalized, which can include role strain, shame, expression, or repression.

Another stress in the lives of African American women are the traumatic experiences of unexpected and unjust killings of those whom they love. The *Los Angeles Times* (Khan, 2019) recently published an article that indicated death by police is a leading cause of death for young African American men in America. According to the article, about 1 in 1,000 African American men and boys in America can expect to die due to state-sanctioned violence. That means that African American men are 2.5 times more likely than White men and boys to die during a police encounter. The same analysis showed that African American women and girls are also killed by police at higher rates than their White counterparts. For African American mothers—those who biologically and communally care for African American children—these statistics are particularly scary, especially when anti-Black violence is palpable. The reality of these statistics is experienced through these mothers' exposure to and witnessing of such trauma. This witnessing can also trigger vicarious trauma for them or other African Americans who identify with, or are personally connected to, these forms of violence (McCluney et al., 2017). African American women protecting their children from racism and state-sanctioned violence is stressful, and, one could argue, also traumatic.

Indeed, African American women experience the trauma of burying their children all too often, and such trauma can be especially wounding given that it exists within a system where their safety should be expected. Take, for example, Trayvon Martin, who was killed as a consequence of a system that supports devaluing Black boys and men, sees them as threats, and legally gives others the right to use lethal violence to "stand their ground" against such perceived threats. Unfortunately, there are also others such as Sandra Bland, who died in police custody, which is a place that should symbolize protection; Tamir Rice, a 12-year-old child whose death is an example of implicit bias (vs. safe community policing) as police officers saw him alone with a toy gun in a park and, within seconds of arriving, shot him to death; and Atatiana Jefferson, who is another example of implicit bias where instead of assuming a Black woman was not armed or harmful, police immediately perceived her as a threat to their safety and killed her while she was doing nothing in her own home (to learn more about these and other cases, see Almukhtar et al., 2018, and Hafner, 2018).

As the typical leaders within their family, African American women are put in a position to protect themselves, their children, and their entire family from unexpected and unimaginable situations. It is reasonable to see where these women, and their communities, might live in traumatized states of constant fear, hypervigilance, negative emotions and thoughts, and additional trauma responses. Notably, this state of contending with continued violence and trauma against them is not new in the lives of African American women.

Impact of Historical Trauma

The impact of historical trauma, which is defined as the lasting impact of oppression of Indigenous people and the suppression of their culture that is inherent in colonialization (Kirmayer, Gone, & Moses, 2014), is both deeply rooted and ever present in the lives of African Americans. Beginning with the Atlantic Slave Trade in the sixteenth century, Africans were ripped from their homes, forced onto cramped boats in unlivable conditions, beaten, starved, and forced to watch friends and family die right before their eyes, all while being chained to each other (DeGruy Leary, 2005). African American women were sexually assaulted (Bryant-Davis et al., 2010) and used as inanimate objects by White men who stripped them naked, put them on a block for display, and sold them to the highest bidder. These same traumas transferred from sea to land as the enslavement, violent assaults, and killings of African Americans continued. DeGruy Leary (2005) has noted how African American families were torn apart as family members were sold to different White families for servitude. African American women continued to be raped by slave owners and their slave owner's friends, and forced to carry children who resulted from such assaults. This created generations of children who were products of their mothers being raped. Indeed, slavery has profoundly affected African Americans, leaving a residual of psychological effects (Wilkins et al., 2013).

Even after three centuries of legalized enslavement and trauma toward African Americans were declared "over," overt and covert forms of racism continued to drive systemic policies and laws aimed at oppressing African Americans. Take, for example, legalized segregation, redlining and Jim Crow. Consider the civil rights movement of the mid-1960s when African Americans had fire hoses turned on them, their buses set on fire, and were dragged from restaurant counters while being told they didn't belong. Here again, African American women were tasked with protecting themselves, their husbands, children, and other community members from this violence. It is true that trauma experiences can build grit and result in resilience. Some even discuss this phenomenon as "post-traumatic growth" (Calhoun & Tedeschi, 2014). While there may be strength and resilience after everything that African American women have suffered, there is also hurt, pain, grief, loss, and vulnerability for more trauma. Unfortunately, the long-term implications of such trauma, rooted in racism, sexism, and discrimination, continue to persist within society today and are passed down from generation to generation.

Epigenetics is one way that historical and generational trauma are understood today, and may be a more present-day framework to better understand the association and impact of trauma in the lives of African Americans. Epigenetics studies the process that alters gene activity without changing the DNA sequence (Weinhold, 2006). It demonstrates how transgenerational trauma can manifest physiologically, and illustrates how it can have significant effects on the biological constitution of human beings that are not just limited to the specific person experiencing trauma, but can also extend to their offspring (Sullivan, 2013). The experience of multigenerational trauma resulting from centuries of slavery and current experiences of oppression can be passed down through the mother to her offspring, eliciting a predisposition for trauma symptoms on that offspring. See Francis (2011) and Sullivan (2013) for a fuller account of epigenetics.

TRAUMA IMPACT ON PHYSICAL AND MENTAL HEALTH

Despite recent improvements in racial minority access to health care, African Americans continue to be severely impacted by health disparities, including higher mortality rates than all other ethnic and racial groups for 8 of the top 10 causes of death (Kelly, 2015). The CDC reported that African American women are 20 times more likely to become infected with HIV (2016a), two times more likely to develop diabetes (2016b), and four times more likely to die due to pregnancy complications than White women (2016c). Although African American women are less likely to develop breast cancer than White women, they are 40 percent more likely to die from this condition (Kelly, 2015). Health disparities disproportionally impact African Americans of low socioeconomic status (National Center for Health Statistics, 2015), even when health-care access is available (Kelly, 2015). Research indicates that both trauma and discrimination increase health disparities among African American women.

Having an extensive trauma history is associated with higher rates of cardiovascular disease, chronic lung disease, and autoimmune disease (Kalmakis & Chandler, 2015). See Table 4.1. Research indicates these health disparities can be attributed to different factors, including a link between severe chronic stress, biological changes (e.g., allostatic overload), and disease (Tomasdottir et al., 2015). Additionally, studies suggest survivors often engage in behaviors that increase their risk of developing illnesses (Ford et al., 2011). In this realm, it has been noted that trauma-related symptoms (e.g., hyperarousal, irritability, dissociation, self-harming

Table 4.1
Summary of Physical and Mental Health-Related Implications of Trauma

Mental Health Consequences	Physical Consequences
Hyperarousal	Cardiovascular disease
Irritability	Chronic lung disease
Dissociation	Autoimmune disease
Self-harming behaviors	Allostatic overload
Treatment-interfering behaviors	Shorten life span
Negative changes in mood and cognitions	Infectious disease
Avoidance	

urges) can lead individuals to engage in treatment-interfering behaviors (e.g., missing or canceling appointments, not communicating clearly, not cooperating during procedures) (Linehan, 1993). As a result, physicians can identify survivors as "difficult patients" and respond with behaviors that can further impair survivors' access to quality health care (Bala, 1994).

Research indicates that both trauma and discrimination increase health disparities among African American women. Unfortunately for many African Americans, both experiences may be a daily reality. According to the Stress in America Survey conducted in 2015, people who endorsed experiences of discrimination rated their stress levels higher, on average, than those who had not endorsed experiences of discrimination (APA, 2016). Given that persistent stress is associated with various health disparities such as obesity, high blood pressure, disordered eating, depression, anxiety, and substance abuse (APA, 2016; Watson, Black, & Hunter, 2016), understanding the relationship between the experience of discrimination and persistent stress or trauma is vital. In fact, around 60 percent of African Americans have reported that their lives have been at least a little more difficult due to perceived experiences of discrimination (APA, 2016). Most concerning for health disparities is life expectancy. Although life expectancy in the United States reached a record high in 2014, African Americans continue to experience disproportionately lower life expectancy rates. According to Murphy et al. (2015), the average life expectancy for the United States for all races was 78.6 years. More specifically, the life expectancy for White Americans was 78.8 years, while the life expectancy for African Americans was 75.3 years (Murphy et al., 2015).

In general, experiences of racial discrimination have been identified as potentially traumatic due to their relationship with post-traumatic stress responses, including avoidance, hyperarousal, negative changes in mood and cognitions (Carter, 2007; Carter and Forsyth, 2010), and dissociation (Polanco-Roman, Danies, & Anglin, 2016). Although most studies have focused on the impact of racial and ethnic discrimination, there is evidence that highlights the negative effects of discrimination on the basis of other factors, including homelessness, mental illness, substance abuse history (Skosireva et al., 2014; Underhill et al., 2015), and LGBT identification (House et al., 2011). Further, people who report being exposed to greater frequency of discriminatory actions (Kessler, Mickelson, & Williams, 1999) and discrimination on the basis of multiple factors have worse outcomes (House et al., 2011).

African American women who are marginalized on the basis of multiple factors report both disproportionate levels of exposure to stressors and higher levels of trauma symptomatology (Speirs, Johnson, & Jirojwong, 2013). Homeless women are particularly vulnerable to be impacted by trauma due to multiple levels of marginalization, such as mental illness, substance abuse, and sex work (Bowen et al., 2015). Further, studies have indicated that homelessness among women is often precipitated and/or perpetuated by a history of severe interpersonal trauma, including childhood sexual abuse (Stermac & Paradis, 2001), intimate partner violence (Roschelle, 2008), and sexual exploitation (Chohaney, 2015). In terms of health disparities, homeless individuals show higher prevalence rates of infectious diseases and chronic medical conditions, including HIV/AIDS, tuberculosis, pneumonia, chronic obstructive lung disease, and cardiovascular disease (Schanzer et al., 2007).

TREATMENT AND INTERVENTION CONSIDERATIONS

Barriers to Treatment

Studies have shown that African Americans are more likely than Whites to be diagnosed with severe mental illnesses (rates ranging from 9 percent to 32 percent; DeCoux Hampton, 2007), they are underrepresented in outpatient settings, and they are overrepresented in inpatient settings. It is believed that stigma, misdiagnosis, and lack of access to outpatient care lead African Americans to be seen during crisis (vs. noncrisis) situations (Marrast, Himmelstein, & Woolhandler, 2016).

African Americans are 50 percent less likely to receive outpatient mental health services than their White peers (McGuire & Miranda, 2008). Numerous factors contribute to the underutilization of mental health services among African Americans, including cultural factors, mental health stigma, financial constraints (Marrast, Himmelstein, & Woolhandler, 2016), and racism (Kugelmass, 2016). In 2016, Kugelmass conducted a phone-based research experiment to determine whether or not therapists would discriminate against prospective patients based on race and class. The author found that patients of middle-class backgrounds are offered appointments three times more often than patients of lower-class backgrounds and that only 8 percent of Black working-class people receive callbacks from therapists.

As previously mentioned in this chapter, African Americans have been severely oppressed by slavery, segregation, police brutality, and widespread racism. Historical and current oppression can prevent African Americans from trusting mental health care providers. Mistrust can stop African Americans from seeking care or cause delays in treatment. It can also hurt the therapeutic relationship and diminish the quality of the care received. It is well established that therapists hold a position of power over their clients. This power differential can get intensified by race, gender, and socioeconomic status. For example, a low-income Black woman may have difficulty developing trust and feeling safe in a room with a wealthy, doctoral-level clinician who is White and male.

African Americans also have a tendency to keep information within the family and avoid "airing dirty laundry." One of the beliefs that reinforces this tendency is the idea that those who cannot resolve their problems by praying and leaning on family members are weak (Matthews et al., 2006). This belief not only keeps individuals from seeking services but can also intensify feelings of shame.

When African Americans are able to overcome the aforementioned barriers and finally access outpatient mental health services, they have received poorer quality of care, were less satisfied with professional mental health services, and had higher rates of dropout than White patients (Shim et al., 2017). A recent study indicated the importance of trust and comfort, the incorporation of spiritual beliefs, decreasing structural barriers, and effectively targeting racial disparities in mental health to reduce stigma (Gaston et al., 2016). Research indicates a high demand for African American or ethnic minority therapists (Thompson-Sanders, Bazile, & Akbar, 2004), as well as for therapists who are training in areas of cultural competence that might allow them to better understand the experiences of African American clients (Kohn-Wood & Hooper, 2014). Unfortunately, there is often a lack of racially diverse therapists available (Thompson-Sanders et al., 2004), and in general, many therapists report a lack of cultural diversity–related training within graduate programs (Green et al., 2009). As such, it is critically important to increase the presence of African American and culturally competent mental health workers.

Unique Symptom Presentation

African American women's symptom presentation is influenced by their history of oppression, current circumstances, and cultural factors. As previously mentioned, their experiences of racism and oppression can intensify the severity of their trauma-related symptoms. In addition, socioeconomic conditions and physical symptoms can add significant complexity to their cases. Due to the health and socioeconomic disparities faced by Black women, mental health providers have to be prepared to consider how to address these issues in treatment. For example, the therapeutic treatment of a low-income Black woman who has breast cancer and lacks transportation should include collaboration with her physicians as well as a case manager or patient navigator.

African Americans' symptomatology may also be shaped by the need to wear a "mask" to appear strong or the tendency to minimize symptoms (Donovan & West, 2015). This need can be fueled by the belief that strength is part of the Black woman identity and also by current stressors (e.g., being the breadwinner in the family). African American women may also feel that their current circumstances are not as difficult when compared to everything they have been through in their lives.

African American women's symptom presentation can also leave them more vulnerable to revictimization. For example, African American women who struggle with symptoms of dissociation might be unable to identify threats and respond to dangerous situations with appropriate emotional responses. This impaired emotional response could then hinder their ability to heal (e.g., a woman who couldn't recognize the danger of dating a man with a history of violence might blame herself for his attacks against her in the future). In addition, exhibiting symptoms of hypoarousal can leave Black women vulnerable to being judged as cold, distant, and emotionally unavailable.

Evidence-Based Treatments

Clinicians seeing patients who have experienced trauma should conduct accurate assessments before deciding the appropriate course of action and treatment. As mentioned at the beginning of this chapter, only 8.3 percent of people who face life-threatening, terrifying events meet lifetime DSM-5 criteria for PTSD (Kilpatrick et al., 2013). Besides PTSD, traumatized patients must be assessed for other common diagnoses (e.g., major depressive disorder, anxiety disorders, substance abuse) and safety concerns (e.g., suicide risk, self-harming behaviors, current living with an abusive partner).

There are different guides that offer treatment recommendations for individuals who meet the DSM-5 criteria for PTSD. In 2017, the American Psychological Association published a practice guideline for PTSD treatment that strongly recommends the use of prolonged exposure therapy (PE) (Foa, Hembree, & Rothbaum, 2007), cognitive processing therapy (CPT) (Resick, Monson, & Chard, 2016) or cognitive behavioral therapy (CBT). That same year, the Veteran Affairs/Department of Defense (VA/DOD) released a different guideline that specifically indicates manualized trauma-focused treatment (TFT), such as EMDR (Shapiro, 2001), CPT (Resick et al., 2016), and PE (Foa et al., 2007) for the treatment of PTSD. Both guidelines say that PTSD can be addressed with the aforementioned treatments alone or in combination with pharmacological interventions. The VA/DOD guide states that psychotherapy is more effective for trauma treatment than pharmacological interventions. For those interested in pharmacological interventions, the APA and the VA/DOD recommend the following medications: fluoxetine, paroxetine, sertraline, and venlafaxine.

Cultural adaptations have been proposed to ensure that evidence-based treatments can properly meet the needs of African Americans. For example, Williams et al. (2014) focused on developing a culturally adapted PE intervention by offering more sessions to develop trust and establish rapport, using assessment tools that capture race-related issues, and openly discussing the individuals' experiences of discrimination. Williams et al. (2014) also emphasized the need to discuss with clients who in their social network can provide support and strength during the treatment process. Importantly, she endorsed an Afrocentric approach that "emphasized resiliency, optimism, faith, and family support."

In her book *Cultural Competence in Trauma Therapy*, Laura Brown (2013) recommends adaptations to treatment based not only on phenotype but also on the intersections of gender, age, sexual orientation, disability, and migration. Brown emphasizes self-awareness and the importance of understanding cultural competency as a journey of constant learning, rather than a destination.

Importantly, researchers disagree on whether trauma-focused treatments developed for PTSD should be used for individuals who have complex PTSD. Judith Herman originally proposed a phase-based model for the treatment of complex PTSD in 1992. A phase-based model has been endorsed by a large number of researchers and clinicians since then (Green & Myrick, 2014). Phase-based models focus on increasing patients' safety and improving patients' ability to regulate emotions and social skills before exploring their trauma history (Cloitre et al., 2012). Table 4.2 provides a list of clinical guidelines inclusive of the needs of African American women.

Table 4.2
Treatment Guidelines Inclusive of African American Women Needs

Increased number of sessions to develop trust and establish rapport

Use of assessment tools that capture race-related issues

Open discussion of the client's experiences of discrimination

Focus on strengths, relationships, and self-care

Emphasis on resiliency, optimism, faith, and family support

Recognition of intersectionality issues

Need for therapists to increase their self-awareness and to understand cultural competency as a journey, not a destination

Exploration of generational survival strategies

Understanding of African American women's legacy of strength, resilience, activism, connection, and support

Use of creative expression (e.g., poetry, art)

Interventions focused on spiritual histories, gifts, and creation of a spiritual recovery action plan

Use of body movements as a form of healing (e.g., dance, yoga)

Recommendations: A Womanist Approach to Treatment

A womanist view can be a very powerful approach to helping African American women who have survived (and who continue to survive) trauma. First coined by Alice Walker (1983), *womanist* theory was birthed during a time where Black women were not in the majority group, scholarly theories and social movements were not centrally focused on them and their needs, and feminist theory that focused on understanding the unique experiences of women did not fully capture the complexity of Black women, their identity, and their experiences. Over the past three decades, it has continued to be developed by Black women for Black women. It has roots in multicultural feminist psychology "wherein the core of the [theory] is not just a form of feminism but goes beyond that to attend to culturally emergent, culturally shaped, and culturally immersed ways of being, knowing, relating, and healing" (Bryant-Davis & Moore-Lobban, 2019, 18). Indeed, a womanist approach to working with Black women is quite holistically focused. It seeks to understand the nature of navigating identity through racism, sexism, and classism in a nonhierarchical way that explores the collective wholeness of each 'ism as central to understanding the experience on all sides. In that way, the oppression and resilience of African American women are seen through an intersectional reality of their experiences.

Womanist theory encapsulates ways of helping African American women resist internalized negative cultural messages, through exploring the inherent contextual roots of such messages (Williams, 2000). Therapists who use a womanist approach work to understand and celebrate the many positive aspects of African American women's identity. In that way, the therapeutic process encourages dialogue, space to speak about one's own experiences, self-care, and spirituality as means of solving real-life problems. As a step past exploring generational trauma, African American women are further encouraged to explore generational survival strategies they have learned through socialization within their families and overall cultures. For example, Williams (2005) notes that helping African American women understand their legacy of strength, resilience, activism, connection, and support is critically important to the therapeutic process of working with them. Understanding the generational ways in which African American women have continued to thrive (more than simply survive) is at the heart of a womanist approach to counseling them.

In this way, a womanist approach to counseling is strength-based and relational, which is of most importance for working with trauma survivors. The strength-based approach has been mentioned already, in terms of understanding the resilience, endurance, and strength that have echoed in the African American community despite centuries of oppression. The relational component involves building a trusting and safe therapeutic relationship where African American women can explore their own narratives around life and trauma, in ways that are honest and genuine to them. In these ways, therapy should be an empowering space where the wholeness of a person is welcomed and not separated from the context of their identities. Bryant-Davis (2005) put it well when she noted that "for trauma recovery to be effective, clients must be able to explore and reflect on the self in relation to the world around them, and this must include issues of race, religion/spirituality, and sexuality, among other factors" (413).

Additionally, African American women may benefit from the freedom to try other means of healing within therapy, outside of the standard evidence-based practices above. For example, there are many forms of dance that can be utilized as an intervention to treating trauma. One such form is ritualized dance. Ritualized forms of dance offer the chance to process coping with a traumatic experience by linking it with familiar situations (Hanna, 1968). Hanna (1968), who has researched African dance extensively, indicated that components of rituals and cultural traditions utilize dance, song, and other spiritual practices in preparation for threatening experiences. Through these ritualized practices, people gain a sense of mastery over overpowering emotions, which promotes resiliency and the ability to address and work through traumatic experiences. Dance/ movement therapy (DMT) is also considered an effective treatment for people who have experienced trauma and for people with a strong connection to traditional culture (Dunphy, Elton, & Jordan, 2014).

Additional effective trauma interventions include poetry, music, art, and spoken word. Poetry is a genre of writing in which succinct, vivid, and intense language is given to feelings, images, and ideas (Raab, 2019). Many people find poetry a healing experience, and finding words to convey a traumatic experience can bring healing (Carroll, 2005). In general, these forms of expression can create an environment that feels culturally congruent and open for African American women and may serve as a catalyst for change in a variety of ways.

Spirituality is another component of a womanist approach toward holistically understanding the client and their means of coping. Spirituality and religion are often considered means of coping among African American women exposed to trauma, and they incorporate dealing with stressful occurrences through beliefs and practices based around their own identified religious affiliation (Johnson, Williams, & Pickard, 2016). Pickard et al. (2011) found that African American women with a greater level of social support from fellow worshipers are increasingly likely to seek aid when challenged with an emotional problem. Bowland, Edmond, and Fallot (2012) studied spiritual intervention in African American women and found that intervention focusing on spiritual histories, gifts, and creation of a spiritual recovery action plan had a degree of success in trauma-related symptom reduction.

Notably, there are many programs throughout the United States that emphasize healing through arts and mind-body connections; therapists may find exploring information from these programs helpful for their own work with trauma survivors. For example, the BodyWise Foundation, based in Baltimore, offers trauma-informed yoga programs that can assist in providing healing to people dealing with trauma, as well as tools to cope with its residual effects while boosting their physical well-being. In addition to body-movement healing techniques, visual and performing arts organizations also advocate for and participate in events that spotlight trauma and healing. Violence Transformed is a visual and performing arts event that celebrates artists and art-making to challenge, confront, and mediate violence. Violence Transformed occurs annually, and includes art exhibits, music, dance, and theatrical performances featuring a host of artists and venues from various locations. Additionally, these events have included artist-led workshops for health-care providers and provider-led, trauma-informed workshops for artists, activists, and other providers working with those impacted by violence. These are two of many organizations that utilize body movement and the arts as forms of healing and provide cost-efficient and creative ways to enhance trauma-informed care. Such approaches may be helpful for African American women as they explore their unique experiences of trauma in non-traditional ways that respect the complexity of their needs.

CASE STUDY

Dana is a 35-year-old African American heterosexual woman who describes herself as someone who had to "raise herself" and "just survive" throughout her life. Dana has experienced so much trauma that she has difficulty ever remembering the feeling of calm. She has always been "on edge, waiting for the next bad thing to happen," or waiting to see who else is going to hurt her. For the first three sessions, Dana struggled to sit still in the room, maintain eye contact, and share her story. From a trauma-informed model, before exploration of her history of abuse, it was important to build safety and trust in the therapy relationship and understand the conditions she grew up in.

Dana was born and raised in the Midwest, in one of the most segregated cities in the United States. She has always lived in a neighborhood where 92 percent of the residents are Black and the median income is $13,000. The racial disparities in her area are so profound that Black babies are three times more likely to die than White babies. Those who make it through infancy face a shortened life span. Dana feels the weight of "being a second-class citizen" every day and has felt the racism in almost every encounter with Whites. Dana has also been the target of colorism by family members and others in the community who harassed and abused her "for being too dark-skinned."

Dana's mother was 15 years old when she had her. Dana says that her mother "just didn't know what to do with her." Dana's father "disappeared" during the pregnancy and never contacted Dana's mother again.

Dana explained that her mother began using drugs and "hanging out with the wrong crowd." She would leave Dana alone at home or with men who abused her. Dana cannot remember how old she was the first time she was molested, but she believes it must have happened when she was an infant. Having her body being violated by men is a consistent memory in her life.

Dana said that when she was four years old, she and her mother moved in with her mother's boyfriend, Derek. She said that Derek treated her well at the beginning. She remembers seeing her mother happy for the first time and feeling hopeful that things were finally going to change for them. Dana says that she would have done anything to keep her mother happy. Derek began molesting Dana a few months after they had moved in with him. He would wait for Dana's mother to go to work to go to Dana's room and "play." Dana dreaded those moments but learned to "keep (her) mind away." She said that thinking about her mother being happy helped her survive the abuse for three years. When Dana's mother found out about the abuse, she blamed Dana for it and yelled at her. Dana's mother became "resentful and hateful" toward her. Dana also blamed herself for the molestation and assumed that she must somehow deserve to be treated the way she was treated. Derek left her mother three years later, but her mother's hateful attitude toward her continued.

When she turned 14, Dana met a boy she liked. His name was Eric. He was popular in school and made her laugh. One day, while hanging out, he began to touch her sexually. She agreed to have sex to keep him happy. In many ways, she felt that was going to be the only way someone would want to be with her. The next time they hung out he brought five other boys who had all heard that she had sex with Eric. They told her to drink alcohol and smoke marijuana with them and she did. The next thing she remembered was "being passed around, them taking turns to rape (her)." They then told "everybody at the school," who would make cruel jokes about her for the next two years. Dana would get physically sick at school with disgust, anger, and profound sadness.

At age 16, Dana attempted suicide for the first time and was hospitalized for a few days. Following the attempt, she began to abuse alcohol and drugs as a way to manage her symptoms. Eventually, she became addicted, dropped out of school, and began using sex as a way to obtain drugs, alcohol, and money. Subsequently, Dana faced numerous arrests and assaults. She went on to spend almost 15 years "on the streets." During this time, she had two children (ages 10 and 12) by two different men. Both children were removed from her custody seven years ago after they were found wandering one night when she was too intoxicated to care for them. Her children were placed with one of her cousins. The fathers of her children are now dead; one was stabbed while serving time in prison for drug trafficking five years ago, and the other one died of an overdose a year ago. Dana identifies this last death as a "breaking point" for her. She said that it led her to reflect on how many people she has seen die due to addiction and how close she has been to dying over the years. When she entered treatment, Dana said that a desire to get sober, get reunited with her children, and live independently led her to seek help.

Dana's treatment consisted of 25 individual therapy sessions. Culturally adapted PE therapy was utilized. The focus of the first sessions were on developing a warm, trusting, and egalitarian relationship with Dana. Her case conceptualization and therapeutic approach were discussed openly. Dana's symptoms were viewed as specialized coping behaviors rather than manifestations of pathology. Dana was reassured that the therapeutic approach used was nonjudgmental and centered in compassion and empowerment. Her feelings of helplessness, anger, disgust, and mistrust were validated.

Issues regarding Dana's gender socialization, cultural background, and experiences of racism, colorism, and oppression were explored. Dana was invited to look at how these issues have influenced her life experiences and her current worldview. She shared that the messages she received from society had become part of her internal dialogue. Therapy then focused on increasing her ability to engage in self-compassion and self-validation. These techniques helped Dana find greater inner peace, and unconditionally appreciate who she is and who can she become.

Dana's need for maintaining the image of a "Strong Black Woman" was discussed. She shared that accepting mental health care meant that she was not strong enough. She also disclosed feeling guilty over spending time in treatment when she "should be taking care of (her) children." During therapy, she was able to explore how seeking help when in need can be in itself a sign of strength as well as a necessary step before caring for others. Dana was reassured that she will be connected with an attorney before ending treatment.

Prior to starting the exposure sessions, Dana was asked to think about activities outside of therapy that she found therapeutic. Completing PE therapy can generate a high level of stress, so these activities were meant to help her lower her discomfort. Dana identified spending time with one of her girlfriends, nieces, going to Church, singing, and drawing as therapeutic. She also spoke about the benefit of attending Narcotics Anonymous (NA) meetings. She explained at the beginning of treatment that she had been sober for two years and that attending NA meetings was fundamental in her recovery.

Dana completed a total of 10 imaginary and in-vivo exposure sessions. During the imaginary sessions, she described her traumatic experiences of being sexually assaulted by different perpetrators. During the in-vivo sessions, she engaged in safe activities that she had avoided due to painful reminders (e.g., sleeping with the door open). Describing her experiences multiple times over the course of therapy allowed her to fully recognize that these experiences were in the past and that she was finally in a safe environment. Engaging in safe activities that she had avoided allowed her to feel empowered, as past experiences were no longer determining what she was capable of doing.

Once Dana began to feel a significant reduction in her symptoms, she was referred to an attorney as well as a program for women with histories of sexual exploitation. The program focused on helping Dana maintain the progress she made in treatment while also teaching her skills to secure employment, obtain safe housing, maintain her sobriety, improve her physical health, further her education, and get reunited with her children.

During the termination sessions, Dana was encouraged to concentrate on the strengths that allowed her to survive many challenges throughout her life. She was asked to recognize and use her sense of personal power to overcome her current struggles. By reducing her PTSD and complex trauma symptoms, Dana was able to improve her ability to regulate emotions, tolerate distress, and increase her self-confidence. She decided to finish high school and pursue a career in counseling "to help other women like (her)." Dana said she wanted to dedicate more time to the relationship she learned to have with herself during therapy, one in which she could love herself unconditionally, independently of societal norms, standards, or expectations.

Note: This case was inspired by the lives of 20 different women. All identifying information has been altered to protect their confidentiality.

REFERENCES

Alegría, M., Fortuna, L. R., Lin, J. Y., Norris, L. F., Gao, S., Takeuchi, D. T., . . . & Valentine, A. (2013). Prevalence, risk, and correlates of posttraumatic stress disorder across ethnic and racial minority groups in the United States. *Medical care*, *51*(12), 1114–1123.

Alim, T. N., Charney, D. S., & Mellman, T. A. (2006). An overview of posttraumatic stress disorder in African Americans. *Journal of Clinical Psychology*, *62*(7), 801–813.

Allyn, B. (2019, August 7). Cyntoia Brown released after 15 years in prison for murder. *NPR News*. https://www.npr.org/2019/08/07/749025458/cyntoia -brown-released-after-15-years-in-prison-for-murder

Almukhtar, S., Benzaquen, M., Cave, D., Chinoy, S., Davis, K., Keller, J., Lai, K. K., Lee, J. C., Oliver, R., Park, H., & Royal, D. C. (2018, April 9). Black lives upended by policing: The raw videos sparking outrage. *New York Times*. https://www .nytimes.com/interactive/2017/08/19/us/police-videos-race.html

American Psychiatric Association. (2013). *Diagnostic and statistical manual of mental disorders: DSM-5*, 5th ed. Arlington, VA: American Psychiatric Association.

American Psychological Association (APA). (2016). *Stress in America: The impact of discrimination*. Stress in America Survey. Washington, DC: American Psychological Association.

Bala, M. (1994). Caring for adult survivors of sexual abuse: Issues for family physicians. *Canadian Family Physician*, *40*, 925–931.

Black, M. C., Basile, K. C., Breiding, M. J., Smith, S. G., Walters, M. L., Merrick, M. T., . . . & Stevens, M. R. (2011). *The National Intimate Partner and Sexual Violence Survey (NISVS): 2010 Summary Report*. Atlanta, GA: National Center for Injury Prevention and Control, Centers for Disease Control and Prevention.

Bowen, E., Canfield, J., Trostle, A., & Harley, D. (2015). Predictors of stable housing for homeless women leaving a sex work-exiting program. *Journal of Contemporary Social Services, 96*(4), 268–276.

Bowland, S., Edmond, T., & Fallot, R. D. (2012). Evaluation of a spiritually focused intervention with older trauma survivors. *Social Work, 57*(1), 73–82.

Brown, L. (2013). *Cultural competence in trauma therapy.* Washington, DC: American Psychological Association.

Bryant-Davis, T. (2005). Coping strategies of African American adult survivors of childhood violence. *Professional Psychology: Research and Practice, 36*(4), 409–414.

Bryant-Davis, T., & Moore-Lobban, S. J. (2019). A foundation for multicultural feminist therapy with adolescent girls of color. In T. Bryant-Davis (Ed.), *Multicultural feminist therapy: Heling adolescent girls of color to thrive.* (pp. 15–41). Washington, DC: American Psychological Association.

Bryant-Davis, T., Ullman, S. E., Tsong, Y., Tillman, S., & Smith, K. (2010). Struggling to survive: Sexual assault, poverty, and mental health outcomes of African American women. *American Journal of Orthopsychiatry, 80*(1), 61–70.

Calhoun, L. G., & Tedeschi, R. G. (Eds.). (2014). *Handbook of posttraumatic growth: Research and practice.* New York, NY: Psychology Press.

Carroll R. (2005). Finding the words to say it: The healing power of poetry. *Evidence-Based Complementary and Alternative Medicine: eCAM, 2*(2), 161–172. https://doi.org/10.1093/ecam/neh096

Carter, R. T. (2007). Racism and psychological and emotional injury: Recognizing and assessing race-based traumatic stress. *Counseling Psychologist, 35*(1), 13–105.

Carter, R. T., & Forsyth, J. (2010). Reactions to racial discrimination: Emotional stress and help-seeking behaviors. *Psychological Trauma: Theory, Research, Practice, and Policy, 2*(3), 183–191.

Centers for Disease Control and Prevention (CDC). (2016a). *CDC Fact Sheet: HIV among African Americans.* https://www.cdc.gov/nchhstp/newsroom/docs/factsheets/cdc-hiv-aa-508.pdf

Centers for Disease Control and Prevention (CDC). (2016b). *National Diabetes Surveillance System.* http://www.cdc.gov/diabetes/statistics/prevalence_national.htm

Centers for Disease Control and Prevention (CDC). (2016c). *Pregnancy Mortality Surveillance System.* http://www.cdc.gov/reproductivehealth/maternalinfanthealth/pmss.html

Centers for Disease Control and Prevention (CDC) (2019). Preventing Adverse Childhood Experiences (ACEs): Leveraging the best available evidence. https://www.cdc.gov/violenceprevention/pdf/preventingACES.pdf

Chohaney, M. L. (2015). Minor and adult domestic trafficking risk factors in Ohio. *Journal of the Society for Social Work and Research, 7*(1), 117–141.

Cloitre M., Courtois, C. A., Ford, J. D., Green, B. L., Alexander, P., Briere, J., . . . & Van der Hart, O. (2012). The ISTSS expert consensus treatment guidelines for complex PTSD in adults. https://www.istss.org/ISTSS_Main/media/Documents/ISTSS-Expert-Concesnsus-Guidelines-for-Complex-PTSD-Updated-060315.pdf

Coleman, J. A. (2016). Racial differences in posttraumatic stress disorder in military personnel: Intergenerational transmission of trauma as a theoretical lens. *Journal of Aggression, Maltreatment & Trauma, 25*(6), 561–579.

Courtois, C., & Ford, J. D. (Eds.). (2013). *Treating complex traumatic stress disorders (adults): Scientific foundations and therapeutic models.* New York, NY: Guilford Press.

Courtois, C. A., Sonis, J., Fairbank, J. A., Friedman, M., Jones, R., Roberts, J., & Schulz, P. (2017). *Clinical practice guideline for the treatment of posttraumatic stress disorder (PTSD) in adults.* Washington DC: American Psychological Association.

DeCoux Hampton, M. (2007). The role of treatment setting and high acuity in the overdiagnosis of schizophrenia in African Americans. *Archives of Psychiatric Nursing, 21*(6), 327–335.

DeGruy Leary, J. (2005). *Post traumatic slavery syndrome.* Milwaukie, OR: Uptone Press.

Donovan, R. A., & West, L. M. (2015). Stress and mental health: Moderating role of the Strong Black Woman stereotype. *Journal of Black Psychology, 41*(4), 384–396.

Dunphy, K., Elton, M., & Jordan, A. (2014). Exploring dance/movement therapy in post-conflict Timor-Leste. *American Journal of Dance Therapy, 36*(2), 189–208.

Essed, P. (1991). *Understanding everyday racism: An interdisciplinary theory.* Thousand Oaks, CA: Sage.

Francis, R. C. (2011). *Epigenetics: The ultimate mystery of inheritance.* New York: W. W. Norton.

Foa, E. B., Hembree, E. A., & Rothbaum, B. O. (2007). *Prolonged exposure therapy for PTSD: emotional processing of traumatic experiences.* New York, NY: Oxford University Press.

Ford, E., Anda, R., Edwards, V., Perry, G., Zhao, G., Li, C., & Croft, J. (2011). Adverse childhood experiences and smoking status in five states. *Preventive Medicine, 53*(3), 188–193.

Gaston, G. B., Earl, T. R., Nisanci, A., & Glomb, B. (2016). Perception of mental health services among Black Americans. *Social Work in Mental Health, 14*(6), 676–695.

Gillum, T. L. (2019). African American survivors of intimate partner violence: Lived experience and future directions for research. *Journal of Aggression, Maltreatment, & Trauma, 0,* 1–18. https://doi.org/10.1080/10926771.2019.1607962

Green, D., Callands, T. A., Radcliffe, A. M., Leubbe, A. M., & Klonoff, E. A. (2009). Clinical psychology students' perceptions of diversity training: A study of exposure and satisfaction. *Journal of Clinical Psychology, 65*(10), 1056–1070.

Green, E., & Myrick, A. (2014). Treating complex trauma in adolescents: A phase-based, integrative approach for play therapists. *International Journal of Play Therapy, 23*(3), 131–145.

Hafner, J. (2018, March 29). Police killings of Black men in the U.S. and what happened to the officers. *USA Today.* https://www.usatoday.com/story/news/nation-now/2018/03/29/police-killings-black-men-us-and-what-happened-officers/469467002/

Hall-Clark, B., Sawyer, B., Golik, A., & Asnaani, A. (2016). Racial/ethnic differences in symptoms of posttraumatic stress disorder. *Current Psychiatry Reviews, 12*(2), 124–138.

Hanna, J. L. (1968). Field research in African dance: Opportunities and utilities. *Ethnomusicology, 12*(1), 101–106.

Herman, J. (1997). *Trauma and recovery: The aftermath of violence: From domestic abuse to political terror.* New York, NY: Basic Books.

Himle, J. A., Baser, R. E., Taylor, R. J., Campbell, R. D., & Jackson, J. S. (2009). Anxiety disorders among African Americans, Blacks of Caribbean descent, and non-Hispanic Whites in the United States. *Journal of Anxiety Disorders, 23*(5), 578–590.

House, A., Van Horn, E., Coppeans, C., & Stepleman, L. (2011). Interpersonal trauma and discriminatory events as predictors of suicidal and nonsuicidal self-injury in gay, lesbian, bisexual, and transgender persons. *Traumatology, 17*(2), 75–85.

Institute of Medicine (2003). *Unequal treatment: Confronting racial and ethnic disparities in health care.* Washington, DC: National Academies Press.

International Society for Traumatic Stress Studies (2018). *ISTSS guidelines position paper on complex PTSD in adults.* https://istss.org/getattachment/Treating-Trauma/New-ISTSS-Prevention-and-Treatment-Guidelines/ISTSS_CPTSD-Position-Paper-(Adults)_FNL.pdf.aspx

Johnson, S. D., Williams, S. L., & Pickard, J. G. (2016). Trauma, religion, and social support among African American women. *Social Work & Christianity, 43*(1), 60–73.

Kalmakis, K., & Chandler, G. (2015). Health consequences of adverse childhood experiences: A systematic review. *Journal of the American Association of Nurse Practitioners, 27*(8), 457–465.

Kelly, R. (2015). *Kelly Report 2015: Health disparities in America.* CBC Health Braintrust. https://www.lupus.org/s3fs-public/Doc%20-%20PDF/2015%20Kelly%20Report%20on%20Health%20Disparities%20in%20America.pdf

Kessler, R. C., Mickelson, K. D., & Williams, D. R. (1999). The prevalence, distribution, and mental health correlates of perceived discrimination in the United States. *Journal of Health and Social Behavior, 40*(3), 208–230.

Khan, A. (2019, August 26). Getting killed by police is a leading cause of death for young black men in America. *Los Angeles Times.* https://www.latimes.com/science/story/2019-08-15/police-shootings-are-a-leading-cause-of-death-for-black-men

Kilpatrick, D. G., Resnick, H. S., Milanak, M. E., Miller, M. W., Keyes, K. M., & Friedman, M. J. (2013). National estimates of exposure to traumatic events and PTSD prevalence using DSM-IV and DSM-5 criteria. *Journal of Traumatic Stress, 26*(5), 537–547. http://dx.doi.org/10.1002/jts.21848

King, K. R. (2005). Why is discrimination stressful? The mediating role of cognitive appraisal. *Cultural Diversity & Ethnic Minority Psychology, 11*, 202–212.

Kirmayer, L. J., Gone, J. P., & Moses, J. (2014). Rethinking historical trauma. *Transcultural Psychiatry, 51*(3), 299–319.

Kohn-Wood, L. P., & Hooper, L. M. (2014). Cultural competency, culturally tailored care, and the primary care setting: Possible solutions to reduce racial/ethnic disparities in mental health care. *Journal of Mental Health Counseling, 36*(2), 173–188.

Kugelmass, H. (2016). "Sorry, I'm not accepting new patients": An audit study of access to mental health care. *Journal of Health and Social Behavior, 57*(2), 168–183.

Kulka, R. A., Schlenger, W. E., Fairbank, J. A., Hough, R. L., Jordan, B. K., Marmar, C. R., & Weiss, D. S. (1990). *Trauma and the Vietnam War generation: Report of findings from the National Vietnam Veterans Readjustment Study.* New York: Brunner/Mazel.

Lewis, J. A., Mendenhall, R., Harwood, S. A., & Browne Huntt, M. (2016). "Ain't I a Woman?": Perceived gendered racial microaggressions experienced by Black women. *Counseling Psychologist, 44*(5), 758–780.

Linehan, M. (1993). *Cognitive-behavioral treatment of borderline personality disorder.* New York, NY: Guilford Press.

Marrast, L., Himmelstein, D. U., & Woolhandler, S. (2016). Racial and ethnic disparities in mental health care for children and young adults: A national study. *International Journal of Health Services: Planning, Administration, Evaluation, 46*(4), 810–824.

Matthews, A. K., Corrigan, P. W., Smith, B. M., & Aranda, F. (2006). A qualitative exploration of African-Americans' attitudes toward mental illness and mental illness treatment seeking. *Rehabilitation Education, 20*(4), 253–268.

McCluney, C. L., Bryant, C. M., King, D. D., & Ali, A. A. (2017). Calling in Black: A dynamic model of racially traumatic events, resourcing, and safety. *Equality, Diversity and Inclusion: An International Journal, 36*(8), 767–786.

McGuire, T. G., & Miranda, J. (2008). New evidence regarding racial and ethnic disparities in mental health: Policy implications. *Health Affairs, 27*(2), 393–403.

Miller-Harris, M. V. (2011). *Sister citizen: Shame, stereotypes, and Black women in America.* New Haven, CT: Yale University Press.

Morgan, R. E., & Oudekerk, B. A. (2019). Criminal victimization, 2018. Bureau of Justice Statistics. NCJ, 253043.

Murphy, S. L., Kochanek, K. D., Xu, J. Q., & Arias, E. (2015). Mortality in the United States, 2014. (NCHS data brief, no 229). Hyattsville, MD: National Center for Health Statistics. https://www.cdc.gov/nchs/data/databriefs/db229.pdf

National Center for Health Statistics (2015). Health, United States: With special feature on racial and ethnic health disparities. Hyattsville, MD: National Center for Health Statistics.

O'Donnell, M. L., Creamer, M., Pattison, P., & Atkin, C. (2004). Psychiatric morbidity following injury. *American Journal of Psychiatry, 161*(3), 507–514. http://dx.doi.org/10.1176/appi.ajp.161.3.507

Perry, B. L., Harp, K. L. H., & Oser, C. B. (2013). Racial and gender discrimination in the stress process: Implications for African American women's health and well-being. *Sociological Perspectives, 56*(1), 25–48.

Pickard, J. G., Inoue, M., Chadiha, L., & Johnson, S. (2011). The relationship of social support to African American caregivers' help-seeking for emotional problems. *Social Service Review, 85*(2), 1–20.

Polanco-Roman, L., Danies, A., & Anglin, D. (2016). Racial discrimination as race-based trauma, coping strategies, and dissociative symptoms among emerging adults. *Psychological Trauma, 8*(5), 609–617.

Raab, D. (2019, April 11). How poetry can heal: Psychologists and writers understand the healing power of writing. Here's how. *Psychology Today.* https://www.psychologytoday.com/us/blog/the-empowerment-diary/201904/how-poetry-can-heal

Resick, P. A., Monson, C. M., & Chard, K. M. (2016). *Cognitive processing therapy for PTSD: A comprehensive manual.* New York, NY: Guilford Press.

Rights4Girls. (2019). *Racial and gender disparities in the sex trade.* http://rights4girls.org/wp-content/uploads/r4g/2019/05/Racial-Disparity-fact-sheet-May-2019-1.pdf

Roberts, A. L., Gilman, S. E., Breslau, J., Breslau, N., & Koenen, K. C. (2011). Race/ethnic differences in exposure to traumatic events, development of post-traumatic stress disorder, and treatment-seeking for post-traumatic stress disorder in the United States. *Psychological medicine, 41*(1), 71–83.

Roschelle, A. (2008). Welfare indignities: Homeless women, domestic violence, and welfare reform in San Francisco. *Gender Issues, 25*(3), 193–209.

Schanzer, B., Dominguez, B., Shrout, P., & Caton, C. (2007). Homelessness, health status, and health care use. *American Journal of Public Health, 97*(3), 464–469.

Shapiro, F. (2001). Eye movement desensitization and reprocessing: Basic principles, protocols, and procedures. New York, NY: Guilford Press.

Shim, R. S., Compton, M. T., Zhang, S., Roberts, K., Rust, G., & Druss, B. G. (2017). Predictors of mental health treatment seeking and engagement in a community mental health center. *Community Mental Health Journal, 53*(5), 510–514.

Skosireva, A., O'Campo, P., Zerger, S., Chambers, C., Gapka, S., & Stergiopoulos, V. (2014). Different faces of discrimination: Perceived discrimination among homeless adults with mental illness in health care settings. *BMC Health Services Research, 14*(376), 1–11.

Slack, K. S., Font, S. A., & Jones, J. (2018). The complex interplay of adverse childhood experiences, race, and income. *Health & Social Work, 42*(1), 24–31.

Smith, C. (2016). Facing the dragon: Black mother, sequelae, and gendered necropolitics in the Americas. *Transforming Anthropology, 24*(1), 31–48.

Speirs, V., Johnson, M., & Jirojwong, S. (2013). A systematic review of interventions for homeless women. *Journal of Clinical Nursing, 22*(7/8), 1080–1093.

Stermac, L. & Paradis, E. (2001). Homeless women and victimization: Abuse and mental health history among homeless rape survivors. *Resources for Feminist Research, 28*(3–4), 65–80.

Sullivan, S. (2013). Inheriting racist disparities in health: Epigenetics and the transgenerational effects of white racism. *Critical Philosophy of Race, 1*(2), 190–218.

Taft, C. T., Bryant-Davis, T., Woodward, H. E., Tillman, S., & Torres, S. E. (2009). Intimate partner violence against African American women: An examination of the socio-cultural context. *Aggression and Violent Behavior, 14*(1), 50–58.

Thompson, V. L. S., Bazile, A., & Akbar, M. (2004). African Americans' perceptions of psychotherapy and psychotherapists. *Professional Psychology: Research and Practice, 35*(1), 19–26.

Tomasdottir, Sigurdsson, J., Petursson, H., Kirkengen, A., Krokstad, S., McEwen, B., . . . & Getz, L. (2015). Self-reported childhood difficulties, adult multimorbidity and allostatic load: A cross-sectional analysis of the Norwegian HUNT study. *PLos One, 10*(6), e0130591.

Underhill, K., Morrow, K., Colleran, C., Holcomb, R., Calabrese, S., Operario, D., Galárraga, O., & Mayer, K. (2015). A qualitative study of medical mistrust, perceived discrimination, and risk behavior disclosure to clinicians by U.S. male sex workers and other men who have sex with men: Implications for biomedical HIV prevention. *Journal of Urban Health, 92*(4), 667–686.

van der Kolk, B. A., Roth, S., Pelcovitz, D., Sunday, S., & Spinazzola, J. (2005). Disorders of extreme stress: The empirical foundation of a complex adaptation to trauma. *Journal of Traumatic Stress, 18*(5), 389–399.

van Ryn, M., Burgess, D., Malat, J., & Griffin, J. (2006). Physicians' perceptions of patients' social and behavioral characteristics and race disparities in treatment recommendations for men with coronary artery disease. *American Journal of Public Health, 96*(2), 351–357.

Walker, A. (1983). *In search of our mothers' gardens.* New York, NY: Harcourt, Brace, Jovanovich.

Watson, N. N., Black, A. R., & Hunter, C. D. (2016). African American women's perceptions of mindfulness meditation training and gendered race-related stress. *Mindfulness, 7*(5), 1034–1043.

Weinhold, B. (2006). Epigenetics: The science of change. *Environmental Health Perspectives, 114*(3), 160–167.

Wilkins, E. J., Whiting, J. B., Watson, M. F., Russon, J. M., & Moncrief, A. M. (2013). Residual effects of slavery: What clinicians need to know. *Contemporary Family Therapy, 35*(1), 14–28.

Williams, C. B. (2000). African American women, Afrocentrism and feminism: Implications for therapy. *Women & Therapy, 22*(4), 1–16.

Williams, C. B. (2005). Counseling African American women: Multiple identities—multiple constraints. *Journal of Counseling & Development, 83*(3), 278–283.

Williams, M., Malcoun, E., Sawyer, B., Davis, D., Nouri, L., & Bruce, S. (2014). Cultural adaptations of prolonged exposure therapy for treatment and prevention of posttraumatic stress disorder in African Americans. *Behavioral Sciences, 4*(2), 102–124. https://doi.org/10.3390/bs4020102

World Health Organization (2019). *International Statistical Classification of Diseases and Related Health Problems* (11th ed.). https://www.who.int/standards/classifications/classification-of-diseases

CHAPTER 5

African American Women and Chronic Mental Illnesses

Natalie D. Haslem

The *Diagnostic and Statistical Manual of Mental Disorders 5* (5th ed.) (DSM-5) (American Psychiatric Association, 2013) covers nearly 300 disorders in multiple categories. With treatment, many DSM-5-listed disorders could be considered temporary health concerns (e.g., acute trauma disorder, adjustment disorder), and many disorders may be responsive to brief treatment models (i.e., brief solution-focused therapy, brief psychodynamic therapy). Furthermore, with some diagnoses, psychotherapy alone may be the treatment of choice over psychopharmacological intervention. For example, psychotherapy only has been found to be an effective treatment for anxiety disorders; the introduction of medication showed little improvement in anxiety with combined psychotherapy (American Psychological Association, 2017). However, a number of DSM-5 diagnoses have significant acuity and chronicity, requiring long-term care and in many cases, medication (APA, 2017). A select few of these diagnoses will be explored in this chapter—schizophrenia, bipolar disorders, and personality disorders. Furthermore, to best respond to the mental health needs of Black women, this chapter operationalizes diagnostic and treatment issues from a social determinant model.

DIAGNOSES

Schizophrenia

Schizophrenia is a genetically linked disorder that typically begins in late adolescence to early adulthood (Belbasis et al., 2017). Schizophrenia often results in the progressive loss of self-care and social functioning (Chien et al., 2013). Not an inclusive list, symptoms of the disorder include one or a combination of positive psychotic symptoms of hallucinations (auditory and visual being most common) and delusions, positive disorganized symptoms including disorganized speech and/or thought, loosening of associations, and disorganized behavior, and negative symptoms including alogia (poverty of speech), flat affect, avolition, and anhedonia. The DSM-5 (APA, 2013) describes five types of schizophrenia—paranoid (which African Americans are most likely to be diagnosed with, Schwartz & Blankenship, 2014), disorganized, catatonic, undifferentiated, and residual.

Schizophrenia significantly affects social functioning. The limitations posed by the symptoms of schizophrenia result in a downward social drift or limited upward social mobility (Ebert, Leckman, & Petrakis, 2019). Such social skills deficits present a substantial challenge to leading a fulfilling and productive life (Chio et al., 2018). Individuals with schizophrenia also face challenges in learning, working, and maintaining interpersonal relationships (Chio et al., 2018). The progression of the disease leads to frequent hospital readmissions, high medical care costs, drug noncompliance, and lack of insight into the illness by the patient. Given the severe and long-standing nature of the effects of schizophrenia, the effective diagnosis and treatment of African American women with the disease is paramount given their often marginalized status. Although not fully detailed in this chapter, it is worth noting additional psychotic-related disorders listed within the DSM-5 (APA, 2013)—schizophreniform disorder, schizoaffective disorder, delusional disorder, brief psychotic disorder, psychotic disorder due to another medical condition, substance/medication-induced psychotic disorder, unspecified schizophrenia spectrum disorder and other psychotic disorder, and other specified schizophrenia spectrum and other psychotic disorder.

Cultural Considerations. According to Holden and colleagues (2013), African American women (and men) are more likely to be overdiagnosed and overtreated for psychotic disorders in general. Compared with Whites with the same symptoms, African Americans are more frequently diagnosed with schizophrenia and less frequently diagnosed with mood disorders (Bell, Jackson, & Bell, 2015). Similarly, Husaini et al. (2002) reported African Americans have significantly higher rates of diagnosis for dementia, organic psychosis, and schizophrenia, whereas Whites have significantly higher rates for mood and anxiety disorders.

Discrepancies in diagnosing can be explained by biases and lack of cultural awareness by clinicians (Anglin & Malaspina, 2008; Williams et al., 2019). Lack of awareness into differences in how African American women convey symptoms of emotional distress may lead to misdiagnosis or at least contribute to the over pathologizing (Bell, Jackson, & Bell, 2015). African American women display behavioral, emotional, or cognitive problems when responding to emotional distress. Behavioral symptoms include irrational, bizarre, violent, and suicidal behaviors (Ward & Heidrich, 2009). Behavioral problems also include sleep problems and difficulty keeping a job. Emotional symptoms include excessive crying, extreme reactions to events and situations, emotional instability, and signs of depression and post-traumatic stress disorder, according to Ward and Heidrich (2009). Furthermore, cognitive problems were described as distorting reality, mental disturbance, and difficulty solving problems and making decisions. Emotional distress and how it is expressed, in essence, can catapult the perception or misperception of mental illness.

The incidence of schizophrenia ranges from 8 to 43 new cases per 100,000 population (Ebert, Leckman, & Petrakis, 2019). Most recent data suggest the age of onset is bimodal in women with two peaks: one in the twenties and the second after the age of 45 (Ebert et al., 2019). Onset before age 10 or after age 45 is rare. Iniesta, Ochoa, & Usall (2012) found that there were several gender differences in the presentation of schizophrenia, specifically premorbid and social functioning is better in women, and comorbid substance abuse is lower in women than men. In terms of the disease process, women have lower relapse rates and better remission rates than men (Iniesta et al., 2012). There are studies on cognitive functioning, but data is inconclusive on the neuropsychological profile between men and women.

Bipolar Disorders

Bipolar disorders are divided into three classes: (1) bipolar I disorder, consisting of episodes of mania cycling with depressive episodes; (2) bipolar II disorder, which consists of episodes of hypomania cycling with depressive episodes; and (3) cyclothymic disorder, which consists of hypomania and less severe episodes of depression (Ebert, Leckman, & Petrakis, 2019). In bipolar I disorder, mania is preceded or followed by a depressive episode. Bipolar II disorder is characterized by recurrent episodes of hypomania and major depression. Manic episodes may include increased motor activity, decreased sleep, racing thoughts, restlessness, impulsivity, anger, grandiosity, and/or changes in spending, gambling, or sexual habits. Hypomanic episodes are similar to mania episodes but generally do not last more than four days and are less intense and do not cause social impairment. Hypomania, as in cyclothymic disorder, does not present with severe racing thoughts or marked psychomotor agitation as found in mania (Ebert et al., 2019). Of note, bipolar patients have a two to three times higher risk for suicide compared to the general population (Ebert et al., 2019).

Cultural Considerations. Rapid-cycling bipolar criteria include the experience of four or more affective episodes per year. Only about 10–15 percent of patients experience rapid cycling (Sadock et al., 2015).

Of this percentage, women are represented disproportionately. Women make up 80–95 percent of rapid-cycling patients. A variety of factors can cause an individual with bipolar disorder to experience rapid cycling including treatment with antidepressants and variable neurotransmitter levels (Ebert et al., 2019).

The exact cause of bipolar disorder is unknown, but consensus rests on multiple factors that include genetic, biochemical, and socioenvironmental factors (Sadock et al., 2015). Breslau and others (2006) reported higher prevalence of lifetime bipolar disorders among Black individuals than among White individuals. Erving, Thomas, and Frazier (2018) found the prevalence of bipolar disorder lower in Black women than men, but higher among Black women than White women. It is unclear whether stressful life events (i.e., poverty, incarceration, role strain) often experienced more by Black women precede the onset of bipolar disorder or whether the disruptive nature of mood cycling actually causes one to experience more negative life events. Erving et al. (2018) also found Black women with lower SES experience higher rates; however Black women overall experienced lower incidence of psychiatric disorders than White women. Erving et al. (2018) attributed Black women's views on self-sufficiency and inner strength as protective factors against mental illness such as bipolar disorder.

Personality Disorders

The DSM-5 (APA, 2013) describes personality disorders as "an enduring pattern of inner experience and behavior that deviates markedly from the expectations of the individual's culture, is pervasive and inflexible, has an onset in adolescence or early adulthood, is stable over time, and leads to distress or impairment" (645). According to the DSM-5, there are 10 personality disorders grouped into three major categories or clusters. Cluster A is composed of individuals who are generally eccentric or odd. The disorders in Cluster A are paranoid, schizoid, and schizotypal personality disorders. Cluster B personality disorders consist of individuals with dramatic and emotionally dysregulated behavior. Antisocial personality, borderline, histrionic, and narcissistic personality disorders are included in Cluster B. Cluster C disorders are marked prominently by anxiety and avoidance behaviors. These are avoidant, dependent, and obsessive-compulsive personality disorders. DSM-5 also includes criteria for three other personality disorder diagnoses that include personality change due to another medical condition, other specified personality disorder, and unspecified personality disorder. Coverage of every personality disorder is beyond the scope of this chapter; however, paranoid personality disorder (Cluster A) and borderline personality disorder (Cluster B) are discussed due to prior research and information relevant to African American women.

Cultural Considerations. The prevalence of diagnosable personality disorders in the general population is estimated to be between 10 and 20 percent (Sadock et al., 2015), yet the prevalence of personality disorders by ethnicity and gender is unclear. McGilloway et al. (2010) conducted a metanalysis of prevalence studies that indicated African Americans have a lower prevalence of personality disorders than non-Hispanic whites and Hispanics. In contrast, the National Epidemiological Survey on Alcohol and Related Conditions revealed that African Americans are diagnosed with higher rates of personality disorders than non-Hispanic Whites and Hispanics, with 12-month prevalence rates of 16.6 percent for Blacks, 14.6 percent for non-Hispanic Whites, and 14.0 percent for Hispanics (Hasin & Grant, 2015).

These contrasting results suggest the influence of race and ethnicity on perception and behavior is not clear-cut as there is a great deal of variability within and between racial and ethnic groups. Second, environmental factors such as socioeconomic status, level of gender discrimination and racism encountered, peer support, and acculturation affect behavior and thus presentation of personality disorders (Baca et al., 2014). For example, self-reported psychological and physical health problems between African Americans and non-Hispanic Whites are significantly reduced after taking into account income and, to a lesser extent, education (Williams et al., 1997). Krieger (1999) further explains that the differences in presentation of personality disorders may be due to race and ethnicity influences on well-being via factors such as personal experience of discrimination and neighborhood resources.

Finally, gender differences have been observed in patterns of risky sexual behavior (those typically used to diagnosis personality disorders), among individuals struggling with psychiatric and/or substance use disorders (Sadock et al., 2015). A similar gender difference was observed in adults with personality disorders. In 2014, Baca et al. found the prevalence rate of personality disorders among women veterans who had also been diagnosed with post-traumatic stress disorder ranged from 45 to 79 percent. This study also analyzed ethnic differences and found the adjusted odds ratio for having a Cluster A personality disorder was almost three times higher for African American women than Hispanic and White women. The results potentially reflect an adaptive response to racial discrimination (Baca et al., 2014). Considering race and gender, these studies again assert that African American women are subjected to more stressful experiences and therefore experience more psychological symptoms than other groups, including those consistent with personality disorders.

Paranoid Personality Disorder. The prevalence of paranoid personality disorder (PPD) is estimated to be between 0.5 and 4.5 percent of the general population (Sadock et al., 2015). The cardinal feature of paranoid personality disorder is the presence of generalized distrust or suspiciousness

(Sadock et al., 2015). Symptoms of PPD are characterized by maladaptive suspiciousness and distrust in the absence of psychotic symptoms, which affects role impairment, substance abuse, and poor social functioning (Iacovino, Jackson, & Oltmanns, 2014). These individuals may feel that they are being treated unfairly, are resentful of the perceived maltreatment, and bear long-lasting grudges against the perceived offender. Researchers hypothesize that PPD symptoms are strongly related to cultural and environmental influences that foster feelings of victimization, alienation, and lack of control (Whaley, 1997; 1998). Environments that support feelings of victimization, alienation, and lack of control are theorized to contribute to the occurrence of paranoid symptoms (Whaley, 1998). Evidence points out that African Americans are more likely to experience victimization and report interpersonal mistrust and cultural mistrust in the dominant White culture than other groups (Roberts et al., 2011).

Iacovino et al. (2014) found that socioeconomic status and childhood trauma occur more frequently among Black Americans compared with White Americans and are the two types of disadvantages most associated with PPD symptoms that may explain racial differences in PPD symptoms. These disadvantages create a feeling of powerlessness and lead the affected race to view the dominant culture as threatening and hostile. This in turn leads to appropriate mistrust and paranoia, disproportionately in African Americans as members of the nondominant culture. Furthermore, African Americans often place a high value on autonomy and may react with hostility if they perceive those from the dominant cultural as controlling (Whaley, 1998). African American women have been similarly more affected by trauma and low SES due to double minority status and may in turn be mistrustful and paranoid to the degree of a diagnosable PPD. Similar to delusional disorder, it is important for a clinician to distinguish healthy paranoia and cultural mistrust from significant deviations that may lead to serious impairment.

Borderline Personality Disorder. The prevalence of borderline personality disorder is 1 to 2 percent in the general population (Sadock et al., 2015). Borderline personality disorder (BPD) occurs more often in families of patients with the disorder, and there is some evidence that bipolar disorder and/or major depressive disorder occurs more often in families with borderline personality disorders. The pervasive feature of borderline personality patients is a pattern of dysregulated mood associated with unstable interpersonal relationships (Sadock et al., 2015). It is not uncommon for the borderline patient to exhibit impulsivity, inappropriate or intense anger, recurrent suicidal threats and gestures, and self-mutilating behavior. Other personality disorders may be confused with borderline personality disorder because they have certain features in common. For example, histrionic personality disorder is characterized by attention seeking, manipulative behavior, and rapidly shifting emotions, whereas borderline personality disorder is distinguished by self-destructiveness, angry disruptions in close relationships, and chronic feelings of emptiness and loneliness (APA, 2013).

Data from the Epidemiological Catchment Area study showed that higher rates of BPD occurred in non-White individuals but was not statistically significant (De Genna & Feske, 2013). McGilloway et al. (2010) reviewed 14 studies done in the United States and United Kingdom and concluded that there was evidence that BPD was less prevalent in Blacks compared to Whites. As a whole, the lack of statistical power due to the small sample size of most studies does not allow for identification of BPD prevalence differences among race, ethnicity, and sex.

Borderline personality disorder is often thought of as an illness of White women. However, research indicating similar prevalence rates across race and gender indicates that there is no significant difference (Newhill, Eack, & Conner, 2009). Other studies suggest there may be more subtle cultural differences in how BPD presents. African American women experience greater affective intensity and emotional dysfunction, fewer self-harming behaviors, and more thoughts of interpersonal aggression than their White counterparts (Newhill et al., 2009). Yet in African American women, BPD often co-occurs with depressive or bipolar disorders (De Genna & Feske, 2013). De Genna and Feske (2013) conclude that African American women present with more symptoms suggestive of a lack of anger control and fewer suicidal behaviors than White women and thus may be misdiagnosed and receive treatments that are not suitable for BPD. Furthermore, such personality change can be due to a medical condition, substance abuse, or identity problems (De Genna & Feske, 2013).

Paranoia can also be present in borderline personality disorder, but is transient, interpersonally reactive, and responsive to external structuring in borderline personality disorder (APA, 2013). Yet in paranoid personality disorder, the paranoia is enduring, beginning in early adulthood and present in a variety of contexts. In De Genna and Feske's (2013) study, the researchers identified that African American women also met criteria for such personality disorders as antisocial and narcissistic personality disorders. Therefore, other personality disorders, medical conditions, as well as mood disorders may be differential diagnoses for BPD.

SOCIAL DETERMINANTS AND GENETIC FACTORS AFFECTING MENTAL HEALTH

Social Determinants

Working with African American women, it is important for readers to contextualize the sequalae of mental health needs with consideration of social determinants. The Centers for Disease Control and Prevention (CDC, 2020) assert that biological, socioeconomic, psychosocial, behavioral, and social influences determine the health of a population. While genetics and nature play a role in the inheritance of mental illness, nurture may be a bigger factor. Factors that nurture mental illnesses are commonly referred to as social determinants, that is, the conditions in which people are born, grow, live, work, and age, including the healthcare system (CDC, 2020). Discrimination based on race and gender, poverty, incarceration, and role strain are only a few examples of many social determinants impacting the development and proliferation of chronic and severe mental illness for African American women (Watson, Roberts, & Saunders, 2012). According to the United States Department of Health and Human Services (2020), other social determinants include exposure to crime, violence, social disorder, language and literacy, and culture. These factors are highly associated with, and thus social determinants of, the onset of severe and chronic mental illnesses such as schizophrenia, bipolar disorder, and personality disorders (Schneider et al., 2000).

Discrimination and Poverty. African American women are affected by both racism and sexism (gendered racism), which lowers their educational attainment, personal and household income, occupational status, wealth accumulation, and chances of socioeconomic advancement (Keith & Brown, 2017. In recent years, meta-analytic reviews (Russell et al., 2018) show significant associations between experiences of discrimination and psychological distress. This includes a link between experiences of racial discrimination and major depressive disorder in African Americans (Molewyk Doornbos, De Groot, & Zandee, 2013; Russell et al., 2018) and anxiety in African American women (Molewyk Doornbos et al., 2013).

Gendered racism affects socioeconomic status and creates a system where African American women are twice devalued as compared to White females or Black males. The twofold devaluation of African American women is reflected in their income. The median annual income for African American women in 2018 was $38,036 in comparison to $48,390 for White women, $44,386 for Black men, and $61,576 for White men (U.S. Census Bureau, 2019). Also, African American women without college degrees earn less than their White counterparts (Alon & Haberfeld, 2007). Even in retirement, African American women as a group have lower retirement incomes than African American men and Whites (Hogan & Perrucci, 2007).

Poverty is considered one of the most consistent predictors of mental distress among women, particularly African American women (Keith & Brown, 2017). Poverty among African American women contributes to daily worries such as financial troubles, relationship problems, poor health, and unemployment, which can contribute to the onset of depression. Impoverished women are overrepresented in the depression and anxiety statistics, and even more so for women of color (Molewyk Doornbos et al., 2013). Furthermore, in 2016, more than one-quarter (25.74 percent) of African American women lived in poverty compared to 11.7 percent of

White women, 9.1 percent of White men, and 20.4 percent of Black men (U.S. Department of Commerce, 2014). These statistics suggest the risk of depression and anxiety for African American women with low-income status is almost double that of their wealthier counterparts.

Mass Incarceration. Mass incarceration in U.S. jails and prisons is a major public health concern in the African American community. In 2009, African American women were imprisoned at a rate of roughly three times that of their White counterparts (Cox, 2012). Incarcerated women experience disproportionately high rates of mental health issues, and most incarcerated women are mothers of minor children (Mumola, 2000). Mothers of minor children who leave jails and prisons with mental health issues face increased risks of experiencing substance use, risky behaviors, homelessness, and recidivism. Instead of treatment, African American women with mental health conditions, particularly schizophrenia, bipolar disorders, and other psychoses, are more likely to be incarcerated than people of other races (U.S. Department of Justice, 2016).

Multiple Role Strain. Role overload, which is defined as stressors resulting from the triangulation of racism, sexism, and low socioeconomic status (Brown & Keith, 2003), is another aggregate of social, cultural, and psychological factors negatively affecting the well-being of African American women. In relation to role overload, African American women may operate from the Superwoman schema (SWS), which is a persona to face social, cultural, and psychological stressors in their lives and to preserve self, the African American community, and the Black family (Woods-Giscombe et al., 2016). Significant role strain in African American women leads to particular stressful life circumstances and conflicts such as balancing employment and parenthood (Brown & Keith, 2003). Specific stressors of African American women often include being in a demanding work position; being a single mother; holding multiple caregiving roles to grandchildren; and caring for elderly parents, adult children, and other kin who may be unemployed, ill, or disabled (Brown & Keith, 2003). Furthermore, as well as the above-mentioned responsibilities, physical illness, especially if chronic or terminal, compounds the effects of social, cultural and psychological factors weighing on the well-being of African American women, and thus contributes to the development or exacerbation of mental illness.

Genetics

Given the evidence of genetic links, it is important to gather a thorough family history of African American women presenting with severe and chronic mental illness. The percentage that offspring will inherit schizophrenia from a parent is 80 percent (Chou et al., 2017). First-degree relatives of schizophrenic probands (the first family member with the disease) were at increased risk of inheriting schizophrenia. Half-siblings had a significantly increased risk of schizophrenia in maternal half-siblings, slightly less risk of schizophrenia for paternal half-siblings, but substantially lower than that of the full siblings. Recent work has revealed substantial epidemiological overlap between schizophrenia and bipolar disorder (Lichtenstein et al., 2009), as well as shared associations within genomic regions. When relatives of probands with bipolar disorder were studied, researchers found that there was an increased risk for schizophrenia in all relationships, including adopted children to biological parents with bipolar disorder (Lichtenstein et al., 2009). Heritability for schizophrenia and bipolar disorder was 64 percent in the genetic study (Lichtenstein et al, 2009). Dean and Murray (2005) reported shared environmental effects were uncommon in general but substantial for those with schizophrenia. Shared environmental factors proposed to have a causal relationship with schizophrenia include obstetric complications, adverse child-rearing, drug abuse, season of birth (specifically winter and spring), child abuse, migration, ethnicity, prenatal or postnatal infection, head injury, urbanization, maternal malnutrition, social adversity, maternal stress, and major life events (Dean & Murray, 2005). Genetic factors are clearly important in the expression and inheritability of schizophrenia, but the environment in which an individual's genes find expression contributes to the development of the disease as well.

Twin and family studies provide a strong link for a genetic component in bipolar disorders. In monozygotic twins, the concordance rate is 80 percent for bipolar disorder, whereas the rate for unipolar disorder is only 54 percent (Ebert, Leckman, & Petrakis, 2019). In dizygotic twins, concordance rates are 24 percent for bipolar disorder and only 19 percent for unipolar disorder. Adoption studies show that even when children are not reared by biological-affected parents, they show an increase for developing a mood disorder. Also, first-degree relatives of individuals with bipolar disorder have an elevated rate of having bipolar disorder (Ebert et al., 2019).

Genetic factors are also influential in the etiology of personality disorders, yet a combination of biologic, temperamental, and social influences are typically involved. For example, family, twin, and adoption studies provide evidence that schizotypal personality disorder is linked to a family history of schizophrenia (Sadock et al., 2015). There is a similar link in genetic relationships in antisocial and borderline personality disorders (De Genna & Feske, 2013). Given the complexity of social determinants and the prevalence of some disorders in families, collateral sources may be used to gather family history of African American women.

TREATMENT OPTIONS AND RECOMMENDATIONS

Regarding treatment options, clinicians must consider the significance of receiving a diagnosis for a severe and chronic mental illness. African American women, placed in polarized positions of strength or vulnerability, may grapple with a chronic mental illness diagnosis. Black women operating from the SWS may feel devastated in learning they have a chronic mental illness. Holding an identity of strength, resiliency, and achievement may feel compromised upon a mental illness diagnosis. The later onset of some chronic mental illnesses can also bring confusion and pain. For example, consider a college student who has been academically strong and career driven who develops symptoms of schizophrenia during her senior year. This woman had years of high functioning and achievement, which depending on severity of symptoms and without proper treatment, could be severely compromised. By contrast, African American women experiencing poverty and negative environment influences may have limited resources for diagnosis or treatment of a chronic mental illness. Given this, by the time treatment is sought, they may have already experienced significant impairments to functioning and stability. The diagnosis becomes another form of marginalization. Considering this, clinicians must account for the ramifications of a chronic mental illness diagnosis, and the impact this will have on the lives of African American women.

There is little scientific evidence that pervasive and chronic mental illness can be cured; however, with proper treatment, many individuals with pervasive and chronic mental illness live fulfilling and healthy lives. The goal of modern treatment is to reduce the symptoms and maximize functioning in those diagnosed with schizophrenia and other chronic mental illnesses. This is typically accomplished through a combination of medication and psychotherapy. Medications used to treat chronic and pervasive mental illness include antipsychotics, antidepressants, and mood stabilizers. The information covered on medication is intended to be a quick reference for nonprescribing clinicians. Similarly, the psychotherapies discussed in the sections below are commonly used treatments for severe and chronic mental disorders including individual counseling, group and/or family counseling, and community interventions. More extensive coverage of these psychotherapy modalities and inpatient treatment may be found in Chapters 8, 9, 10 and 11 of this handbook.

Medications

Antipsychotics. Antipsychotic medications are used for the treatment of schizophrenia, schizoaffective disorder, bipolar disorder, delusional disorder, BPD, and PPD. There are first-generation antipsychotic drugs known as "typical" or "conventional" drugs that were on the market before 1990. These typical antipsychotics produce more negative side effects in the form of acute extrapyramidal symptoms (EPS) (e.g., tremors, drooling) and tardive dyskinesia (TD) (involuntary body movements) and include drugs such as haloperidol, fluphenazine, and perphenazine. Second-generation antipsychotics (SGAs), or atypical antipsychotic drugs, produce less acute EPS and TD. Atypical antipsychotics include

risperidone, olanzapine, quetiapine, ziprasidone, iloperidone, and pali-
peridone. Table 5.1 includes a list of SGAs and their effects and side effects.

With schizophrenia, antipsychotic medications aim to minimize positive
symptoms, negative symptoms, conceptual disorganization, neurocognitive deficits, anxiety, and depressive symptoms including suicidality (Ebert,
Leckman, & Petrakis, 2019). Generally, antipsychotic drug treatment works
well to bring about a reduction in positive symptoms such as hallucinations and delusions, as well as disorganized speech and behavior and psychotic agitation. Positive symptoms are quite distressing, but do not appear
to correlate significantly with long-term functioning. Negative symptoms,
on the other hand, such as anhedonia, affective flattening, alogia, avolition,
and social withdrawal are more difficult to treat pharmacologically and are
robust predictors of long-term functional incapacity (Ebert et al., 2019).

All atypical antipsychotics appear to have acute antimanic effects and can
be used to treat bipolar disorders. Additionally, first- and second-generation
antipsychotics have been shown to reduce paranoid and other psychotic ideation, impulsive aggression, and depression (Sadock et al., 2015).

Antidepressants. Antidepressant drugs are used for the treatment of
major depression. There are many types of antidepressants including selective serotonin reuptake inhibitors (SSRIs), serotonin and norepinephrine
reuptake inhibitors (SNRIs), and older antidepressant medications such
as tricyclics. SSRIs are the most popular type of antidepressant and are
included on Table 5.1 (National Institute of Mental Health, 2016). Of note,
in treating bipolar disorder, tricyclic antidepressants should be avoided in
depressive episodes due to the potential of induction of mania, mixed state,
or rapid cycling (Goldberg & Ernst, 2019). Antidepressants may be used in
combination with medications in other classes for a combined treatment
effect. For example, olanzapine (antipsychotic) combined with fluoxetine
(antidepressant) has been shown to be efficacious in the treatment of bipolar disorder. Similarly, mood-stabilizing agents such as lithium, carbamaze-
pine, or divalproex may be required adjunctively for the treatment of mood
cycling. Lastly, if delusional symptoms or agitation is present, antipsychotics or benzodiazepines need to be added (Ebert, Leckman, & Petrakis, 2019).
Often treatments will need to be combined for optimal stabilization.

Mood Stabilizers. Mood stabilizers, such as lithium and divalproex,
are frequently used to treat bipolar disorder and BPD. Mood stabilizers
can help in diminishing anger, irritability, and self-mutilation (Ebert,
Leckman, & Petrakis, 2019). Acute manic episodes can be managed with
lithium, divalproex, or an atypical antipsychotic. Research showing
lamotrigine may be effective in treatment of bipolar depression is promising (Ebert et al., 2019) but the effectiveness of lamotrigine as an adjunctive
antidepressant or mood stabilizer in African American women specifically is unknown. See Table 5.1 for additional mood stabilizers.

Table 5.1
Overview of Common Medications Used to Treat Severe and Chronic Mental Health Conditions

	Names	Diagnoses Treated	Treatment Effects	Potential Side Effects
Antipsychotics (SGAs)	• Olanzapine • Quetiapine • Risperidone • Ziprasidone • Paliperidone • Lurasidone • Aripiprazole	• Schizophrenia • Bipolar disorder • Psychosis • Severe depression • Eating disorders • Post-traumatic stress disorder (PTSD) • Obsessive-compulsive disorder (OCD) • Generalized anxiety disorder	• Decrease positive symptoms • Decrease negative symptoms • Stabilize mood	• Drowsiness • Dizziness • Restlessness • Weight gain (the risk is higher with some atypical antipsychotic medicines) • Dry mouth • Constipation • Nausea • Vomiting • Blurred vision
Antipsychotics (FGAs)	• Chlorpromazine • Haloperidol • Perphenazine • Fluphenazine	• Same as above		Rigidity • Persistent muscle spasms • Tremors • Restlessness • Tardive dyskinesia (TD)
Antidepressants (SSRIs)	• Fluoxetine • Sertraline • Escitalopram • Paroxetine	• Depression • Social phobia • Generalized anxiety disorder • Eating disorders • Obsessive-compulsive Disorders (OCD)	• Reduce anxiety • Reduce panic attacks	• Weight gain • Headaches • Nausea • Vomiting • Sexual dysfunction • Suicidality

| Mood Stabilizers | • Carbamazepine
• Lamotrigine
• Oxcarbazepine
• Valproic Acid
• Lithium | • Depression (along with antidepressant)
• Disorders of impulse control
• Certain mental illnesses in children
• Schizoaffective disorder | • Stabilize moods | • Itching, rash
• Excessive thirst
• Frequent urination
• Tremor (shakiness) of the hands
• Nausea and vomiting
• Slurred speech
• Fast, slow, irregular, or pounding heartbeat
• Blackouts
• Changes in vision
• Seizures |

Source: Adapted from: Mental Health Medications, https://www.nimh.nih.gov/health/topics/mental-health-medications/index.shtml.

Psychotherapy

Individual Counseling. The major forms of psychotherapeutic interventions for schizophrenia are cognitive behavioral therapy (CBT), social skills training, cognitive therapy, cognitive remediation, psychoeducation, acceptance and commitment therapy (ACT), and supportive psychotherapy (Ebert, Leckman, & Petrakis, 2019). The goals of CBT in the treatment of schizophrenia include belief modification, reattribution, and normalizing of psychotic experiences. CBT has been identified as an effective treatment modality for African American women in both individual and group settings (Carter et al., 2003; Hofmann et al., 2012). Social skills training improves interpersonal communication and social interaction to counteract the loss in social functioning due to negative symptoms (Chio et al., 2018). A variation of CBT is ACT, whose goal is to help the individual recognize and accept their thoughts and feelings. Gaudiano and Herbert (2006) found that ACT was effective in an 80 percent African American inpatient population in a public mental hospital for improving overt psychotic behavior.

Clinicians should consider the adaptability of CBT, ACT, and other therapies with African American women with severe and chronic mental illness. For example, dialectical behavior therapy (DBT) was designed as an intervention with women with BPD and is used to teach mindfulness skills and awareness of emotional states (Mercado & Hinojosa, 2017). The three focus areas include affect regulation, healthy self-soothing, and enhancement of interpersonal relationships. Mercado and Hinojosa (2017) asserted DBT can be adapted for work with diverse groups based on their literature review. Specifically, a culturally adapted approach for DBT must include a culturally competent therapist who recognizes clients' culturally influenced behavior and clarifies to clients why the recommended interventions are culturally appropriate (McFarr et al., 2014, as cited in Mercado & Hinojosa, 2017). Other cultural adaptations for all individual treatment should incorporate family education and support given the importance of family in African American culture.

Family Counseling. Diagnosis of a severe and chronic mental illness not only impacts the individual; it impacts her entire family. Family members may be impacted by their loved one's frequent and long hospitalizations, loss of income, or treatment needs. As previously noted, chronic mental illness shows high comorbidity with substance use and other high-risk behaviors, which can impact stability and family functioning. Additionally, family members may feel afraid of or for their family member (particularly during a psychotic or manic episode), may feel hurt or shamed by their actions and behaviors (e.g., infidelity during a manic episode, child embarrassed by a mother's disorganized speaking), or confused and sad (e.g., loved one's expression of suicidality or delusions). There may also be identity and role shifts that occur. For example, an African American woman operating from the SWS may need more sleep due to medication side effects. This may mean that others in the home must take on more household and/or financial responsibilities. Given genetic predispositions, family members may feel concern for their own mental health. There also remain great misconceptions about mental illness, which can impact how the individual and her family process a new diagnosis. Ackerman (2020) asserts that family therapy can be used to help the family transition through a difficult period or cope with behavioral or mental problems in family members. Family counseling may include psychoeducation on mental illness, its sequelae and treatment. Understanding the diagnosis may help family members support their loved one's individual treatment and medication compliance. Family counseling provides support to changes and adjustments needed to reestablish and/or maintain the family's wellness. Family counseling can also identify social determinants impacting mental health and develop familial patterns to counter said determinants.

Group Counseling. Group therapy is a common therapeutic modality in settings where severe and chronic mental illness is treated such as inpatient units and intensive outpatient programs. However, research on the efficacy of group therapy for African American women in this diagnostic category is limited. In general, group therapy is considered appropriate for patients with a variety of mental disorders including schizophrenia, PTSD, depression, bipolar, and personality disorders (Novotney, 2019). Mashinter (2020) proposes that group counseling is both cost-effective and therapeutically effective. Mashinter (2020) also proposes that the power of group therapy lies in the reinforcement of social support. It also helps the patients to normalize their feelings by sharing their stories with others in a group setting, which for African American women who value collectivism may be particularly beneficial. Severe and chronic mental illness limits social function and thus may lead to social isolation, which group therapy can remedy in a confidential and safe place. In addition, group therapy for African American women with chronic mental illness can help diminish stigma to seeking treatment and normalize and reinforce help-seeking behaviors. As previously mentioned, CBT, DBT, and ACT have been deemed effective with this population in the form of manualized treatment often administered in structured groups. One study (Pankowski et al., 2017) found that a manualized ACT group treatment was effective with patients with bipolar disorder and associated anxiety in lowering depression and anxiety symptoms, improving quality of life, and increasing psychological flexibility.

Community Intervention. Community interventions to promote mental health in individuals with severe and chronic mental illness are vital to recovery. Community interventions are those that involve multi-sector partnerships, emphasize community members as integral to the intervention, and/or deliver services in community settings (Castillo et al., 2019). Castillo and others (2019) focused on seven topic areas: collaborative care, early psychosis, school-based interventions, homelessness, criminal justice, global mental health, and mental health promotion/prevention. They noted that many collaborative care studies have concentrated on incorporating mental health services to varying degrees within primary care settings. For example, women with depression can receive medication from their primary care physicians or mid-level providers. Services for early psychosis consisted of a treatment team composed of psychiatrists, therapists, social workers, nurses, and vocational therapists to reduce the dosage of antipsychotic therapy needed to control positive and negative symptoms in a patient suffering from mental illness. Homelessness services were provided to secure permanent housing for homeless individuals without the requirement of preplacement sobriety (Castillo et al., 2019).

Specifically, community intervention for African American women with severe and chronic mental illness must address social determinants of mental illness. Optimally, the programs address discrimination, poverty, role strain, and mass incarceration by providing job training, education, employment services, housing assistance, and childcare. Other comprehensive community-based services would assist with access to affordable health care including psychiatry and substance abuse treatment. Adaptive to African American communities, churches and spiritual groups can assist impacted families by housing support groups and psychoeducational programs that include religious and spiritual values (see Dalencour et al., 2017; Weisman de Mamani et al., 2014).

For incarcerated women, these services are even more essential for minimizing the "revolving door" in and out of the prison system. Criminal justice facilities attempt to connect repeat offenders to programs in the community to link them with services providing medical and mental health care, housing, insurance, employment, and transportation (Castillo et al., 2019). The author of this chapter works in a criminal justice facility where community services are coordinated for individuals in need of mental health care. The community interventions highlight the promise to promote mental health and broader outcomes at all social-ecological levels: individual, interpersonal/family, organizational/institutional, and community.

CASE EXAMPLE

Identification: Brittany is a 32-year-old, single, unemployed African American woman who was involuntarily admitted to an inpatient psychiatric unit. She has a history of more than 15 arrests for theft and fraud.

Chief Complaint: "I used to practice my signature because I always thought I would be a movie star."

History of Chief Complaint: Brittany described her dreams of being a star actress but has no education in the theatrical fields of drama or acting. She had been signing her autograph for strangers. A neighbor convinced her to seek professional help. Brittany presented with heightened confidence, impaired judgment, pressured speech, and decreased need for sleep (three hours a night). In the past, she had feelings of hopelessness, social withdrawal, sadness, crying spells, fatigue, anhedonia, increased appetite, and suicidal ideation. Brittany was hospitalized for several days, prescribed several medications, and diagnosed with bipolar disorder type I after presenting initially to a mental health crisis center.

Mental Status Examination upon hospitalization: Brittany appears her stated age. She is eccentric and wearing flashy clothing with large-size earrings and noticeable makeup and lipstick. She is cooperative with interviewer and makes appropriate eye contact. Her mood is elated with expansive affect. She behaves in an overly animated way. She is alert and oriented to time, place, person, and situation. She was able to recall events in her life with exact dates. Her concentration and attention are poor, and she is redirected frequently. Responses indicate that she can understand concepts and generalizations, and she is estimated to be above average in intelligence. Her speech and language are pressured and spontaneous. She denies auditory or visual hallucinations. Her thought content is abnormal given grandiose ideas, sexual preoccupation, and inflated self-confidence. She denies suicidal and homicidal ideations but has had several hospitalizations in the past for suicidality. Impulse control is impaired given excessive spending and shoplifting. Judgment is impaired but insight into illness is fair as she realizes the need for medication and treatment.

Personal and Family History: Brittany's father has bipolar disorder. The father's illness was not well managed, and Brittany witnessed domestic violence between her parents. Brittany did not have a close relationship with her father and was raised solely by her mother after age 7. She had no identified problems until the age of 12 when she was unsupervised often due to her mother working long hours and became known for sexual activity with boys in her neighborhood. Labeled as "fast" by her mother and others in her community, she began confiding in a school counselor who convinced her mother to seek treatment for Brittany. She started counseling and psychiatric treatment and was on and off medication. Despite her mental health problems, she managed to do well academically throughout school and went to college. After college, she was accepted into a master's program, yet she eventually dropped out due to several manic episodes, facing jail time, and multiple unsuccessful relationships resulting in two children with different men.

Medical History: Brittany has no known drug allergies. She has current medical illnesses including obesity, hypertension, and sleep apnea. She is of normal height and obese, with stable vital signs. Brittany says she began drinking alcohol at age 19. She considers herself a social drinker, only drinking at parties or special occasions and does not use illicit substances.

Treatment: Brittany did not continue with treatment in the past because of internalized SWS and limited family support (i.e., family members would say, "That's just Brittany" when she displayed impulsive and reckless behaviors), yet she continued to experience manic and depressive episodes and legal problems. Brittany has had trials of Haldol, bupropion, Celexa, Klonopin, Hydroxyzine, Lithium, and Gabapentin. After this most recent inpatient admission, she continued in an intensive outpatient program for indigent populations, learning how to recognize and manage her symptoms in group therapy that incorporated tenets of CBT and ACT. With the support of her neighbor, who Brittany later learned had also battled serious mental illness, she followed through with ongoing individual counseling and psychiatric treatment at the community service board. After being stabilized on Lithium, Latuda, and Paxil, she applied for and received social security benefits. She obtained legal assistance and began the process of regaining custody of her children. Brittany was proud of being the first college graduate in her family but felt a great deal of shame having to abruptly end her studies. In therapy, she discussed returning to school once she accomplished goals such as maintaining stable housing and being reunited with her children.

Conceptualization: The case example highlights the importance of appropriate diagnosis and treatment, continuity of care, social support, community resources, and assistance with contextual factors impacting mental health for African American women with severe and chronic illness.

REFERENCES

Ackerman, C. E. (2020). *What is family therapy? +6 techniques and interventions.* https://positivepsychology.com/family-therapy/ Alon, S., & Haberfeld, Y. (2007). Labor force attachment and the evolving wage gap between White, Black, and Hispanic young women. *Work and Occupations, 34*(4), 369–398. https://doi.org/10.1177/0730888407307247

American Psychiatric Association (APA). (2013). *Diagnostic and statistical manual of mental disorders,* 5th ed. https://doi.org/10.1176/appi.books.9780890425596

American Psychological Association (APA). (2017). *How do I choose between medication and therapy?* https://www.apa.org/ptsd-guideline/patients-and -families/medication-or-therapy

Anglin, D. M., & Malaspina, D. (2008). Ethnicity effects on clinical diagnoses in patients with psychosis: Comparisons to best estimate research diagnoses. *Journal of Clinical Psychiatry, 69*(6), 941–945.

Baca, J. C., Castillo, D., Mackaronis, J., & Qualls, C. (2014). Ethnic differences in personality disorder patterns among women veterans diagnosed with PTSD. *Behavioral Sciences, 4*(1), 72–86. https://doi.org/10.3390/bs4010072

Belbasis, L., Köhler, C. A., Stefanis, N., Stubbs, B., van Os, J., Vieta, E., . . . & Evangelou, E. (2018). Risk factors and peripheral biomarkers for schizophrenia spectrum disorders: An umbrella review of meta-analyses. *Acta Psychiatrica Scandinavica, 137*(2), 88–97. doi:10.1111/acps.12847

Bell, C. C., Jackson, W. M., & Bell, B. H. (2015). Misdiagnosis of African-Americans with psychiatric issues—Part II. *Journal of National Medical Association, 107*(3), 35–41.

Breslau, J., Aguilar-Gaxiola, S., Kendler, K. S. et al. (2006). Specifying race-ethnic differences in risk for psychiatric disorder in a USA national sample. *Psychological Medicine, 36*(1), 57–68.

Brown, D., & Keith, V. (2003*). In and out of our right minds: The mental health of African American women*. New York, NY: Columbia University Press.

Carter, M. M., Sbrocco, T., Gore, K. L., Marin, N. W., & Lewis, E. L. (2003). Cognitive-behavioral therapy versus a wait-list control in the treatment of African American women with panic disorder. *Cognitive Therapy and Research, 27*(5), 505–518.

Castillo, E. G., Shadravan, R., Moore, E., Mensah, M. O., Docherty, M., Nunez, M. G. A., . . . & Wells, K. B. (2019). Community interventions to promote mental health and social equity. *Current Psychiatry Reports, 21*(5): 35. https://doi.org/10.1007/s11920-019-1017-0

Centers for Disease Control and Prevention (CDC). (2020, August). *Social determinants of health: Know what affects health*. https://www.cdc.gov/socialdeterminants/index.htm

Chien, W. T., Leung, S. F., Yeung, F. K., & Wong, W. K. (2013). Current approaches to treatments for schizophrenia spectrum disorders, part II: Psychosocial interventions and patient-focused perspectives in psychiatric care. *Neuropsychiatric Disease and Treatment, 9*, 1463–1481.

Chio, F. H. N., Mak, W. W. S., Chan, R. C. H., & Tong, A. C. Y. (2018). Unraveling the insight paradox: One-year longitudinal study on the relationships between insight, self-stigma, and life satisfaction among people with schizophrenia spectrum disorders. *Schizophrenia Research, 197*, 124–130. https://doi.org/10.1016/j.schres.2018.01.014

Chou, I. J., Kou, C. F., Huang, Y. S., Grainge, M. J., Valdes, A. M., See, L. C., Yu, K. H., Lou, S. F., Huang, L. S., Tseng, W. Y., Zhange, W., & Doherty, M. (2017). Familial aggregation and heritability of schizophrenia and co-aggregation of psychiatric illnesses in affected families. *Schizophrenia Bulletin. 43*(5), 1070–1078.

Cox, R. J. A. (2012). The impact of mass incarceration on the lives of African American women. *Review of Black Political Economy, 39*(2), 203–212. https://doi.org/10.1007/s12114-011-9114-2

Dalencour, M., Wong, E. C., Lingqi, T., Dixon, E., Lucas-Wright, A., Wells, K., & Miranda, J. (2017). The role of faith-based organizations in the depression care of African Americans and Hispanics in Los Angeles. *Psychiatric Services, 68*(4), 368–374.

Dean, K., & Murray, R. M. (2005). Environmental risk factors for psychosis. *Dialogues in Clinical Neuroscience, 7*(1), 69–80.

De Genna, N. M., & Feske, U. (2013). Phenomenology of borderline personality disorder. *Journal of Nervous and Mental Disease, 201*(12), 1027–1034. https://doi.org/10.1097/NMD.0000000000000053

Ebert, M. H., Leckman, J. F., & Petrakis, I. (2019). *Current diagnosis & treatment*. New York, NY: McGraw-Hill Education.

Erving, C. L., Thomas, C. S., & Frazier, C. (2018). Is the Black-White mental health paradox consistent across gender and psychiatric disorders? *American Journal of Epidemiology, 188*(2), 314–322.

Gaudiano, B. A., & Herbert, J. D. (2006). Acute treatment of inpatients with psychotic symptoms using acceptance and commitment therapy. *Behaviour Research and Therapy, 44*(3), 415–437.

Goldberg, J. F., & Ernst, C. L. (2019). Managing the side effects of psychotropic medications, 2nd ed. New York, NY: American Psychiatric Association Publishing.

Hasin, D. S., & Grant, B. F. (2015). National Epidemiological Survey on Alcohol and Related Conditions (NESARC) Waves 1 and 2: Review and summary of findings. *Social Psychiatry Epidemiology 50*(11), 1609–1640. https://doi.org/10.1007/s00127-015-1088-0.

Hofmann, S. G., Asnaani, A., Vonk, I. J., Sawyer, A. T., & Fang, A. (2012). The efficacy of cognitive behavioral therapy: A review of meta-analyses. *Cognitive Therapy and Research, 36*(5), 427–440. https://doi.org/10.1007/s10608-012-9476-1

Hogan, R., & Perrucci, C. C. (2007). Black women: Truly disadvantaged in the transition from employment to retirement income. *Social Science Research, 36*(3), 1184–1199. https://doi.org/10.1016/j.ssresearch.2006.07.002

Holden, K. B., Bradford, L. D., Hall, S. P., & Belton, A. S. (2013). Prevalence and correlates of depressive symptoms and resiliency among African American women in community-based primary health care center. *Journal of Health Care for the Poor and Underserved, 24*(4), 79–93.

Husaini, B. A., Sherkat, D. E., Levine, R., Bragg, R., Holzer, C., Anderson, K., Cain, V., & Moten, C. (2002). Race, gender, and health care service utilization and costs among Medicare elderly with psychiatric diagnoses. *Journal of Aging and Health, 14*(1), 79–95.

Iacovino, J. M., Jackson, J. J., & Oltmanns, T. F. (2014). The relative impact of socioeconomic status and childhood trauma on Black-White differences in paranoid personality disorder symptoms. *Journal of Abnormal Psychology, 123*(1), 225–230.

Iniesta, R., Ochoa, S., & Usall, J. (2012). Gender differences in service use in a sample of people with schizophrenia and other psychoses. *Schizophrenia Research and Treatment, 2012*, 1–6. https://doi.org/10.1155/2012/365452

Keith, V., & Brown, D. (2017). African American women and mental well-being: The intersection of race, gender, and socioeconomic status. In T. Scheid & E. Wright (Eds.), *A handbook for the study of mental health: social contexts, theories, and systems* (3rd ed., pp. 304–321). Cambridge, UK: Cambridge University Press. https://doi.org/10.1017/9781316471289.019

Krieger, N. (1999). Embodying inequality: A review of concepts, measures, and methods for studying health consequences of discrimination. *International Journal of Health Services, 29*, 295–352. https://doi.org/10.2190/M11W-VWXE-KQM9-G97Q

Lewine, R., Burbach, D., & Meltzer, H. Y. (1984). Effect of diagnostic criteria on the ratio of male to female schizophrenic patients. *American Journal of Psychiatry, 141*(1), 84–87.

Lichtenstein, P., Yip, B. H., Bjork, C., Pawitan, Y., Cannon, T. D., Sullivan, P. F., & Hultman, C. M. (2009). Common genetic determinants of schizophrenia and bipolar disorder in Swedish families: A population-based study. *Lancet, 373* (9659), 234–239.

Mashinter, P. (2020). Is group therapy effective? *BU Journal of Graduate Studies in Education, 12*(2), 33–36.

McFarr, L., Gaona, L., Barr, N., Ramirez, U., Henriquez, S., Farias, A., & Flores, D. (2014). Cultural considerations in dialectical behavior therapy. In A.

Masuda (Ed.), Mindfulness and acceptance in multicultural competency: A contextual approach to sociocultural diversity in theory and practice (pp. 75–92). Oakland, CA: Context Press/New Harbinger Publications.

McGilloway, A., Hall, R. E., Lee, T., & Bhui, K. S. (2010). A systematic review of personality disorder, race and ethnicity: Prevalence, etiology and treatment. *BMC Psychiatry, 11*, 10–33.

Mental Health American. (2020). *Black and African American communities and mental health.* https://www.mhanational.org/issues/black-and-african-american -communities-and-mental-health

Mercado, A., & Hinojosa, Y. (2017). Culturally adapted dialectical behavior therapy in an underserved community mental health setting: A Latina adult case study. *Practice Innovations, 2*(2), 80–93. https://doi.org/10.1037 /pri0000045

Minsky, S., Vega., W., Miskimen, T., Gara, M., & Escobar, J. (2003). Diagnostic patterns in Latino, African American, and European American psychiatric patients. *Archives of General Psychiatry, 60*(6), 634–637.

Molewyk Doornbos, M., DeGroot, J., & Zandee, G. L. (2013, October 22). Social determinants of women's mental health and barriers to help-seeking in three ethnically diverse, impoverished, and underserved communities. https://sigma.nursingrepository.org/bitstream/handle/10755/304224 /Molewyk_SocialDeterminantsofWomens.pdf?sequence=1&isAllowed=y

Mumola, C. J. (2000). Incarcerated parents and their children. *PsycEXTRA Dataset.* https://doi.org/10.1037/e378362004-001

National Institute of Mental Health. (2016, October). *Mental health medications.* https://www.nimh.nih.gov/health/topics/mental-health-medications/index .shtml#part_149855

Newhill, C. E., Eack, S. M., & Conner, K. O. (2009). Racial differences between African and White Americans in the presentation of borderline personality disorder. *Race and Social Problems, 1*(2), 87–96.

Novotney, A. (2019). Keys to great group therapy. *Monitor on Psychology, 50*(4), 66. https://www.apa.org/monitor/2019/04/group-therapy

Pankowski, S., Adler, M., Andersson, G., Lindefors, N., & Svanborg, C. (2017). Group acceptance and commitment therapy (ACT) for bipolar disorder and co-existing anxiety—an open pilot study. *Cognitive Behaviour Therapy, 46*(2), 114–128. http://dx.doi.org/10.1080/16506073.2016.1231218

Piccinelli, M., & Homen, F. G. (1997). Gender differences in the epidemiology of affective disorders and schizophrenia. Geneva, Switzerland: World Health Organization.

Primm, A. B., & Lawsom, W. B. (2010). African Americans. In P. Ruiz & A. B. Primm (Eds.), *Disparities in psychiatric care* (pp. 19–29). Washington, DC: Lippincott, Williams & Wilkins.

Roberts, A. L., Gilman, S. E., Breslau, J., Breslau, N., & Koenen, K. C. (2011). Race/ ethnic differences in exposure to traumatic events, development of post-traumatic stress disorder, and treatment-seeking for post-traumatic stress disorder in the United States. *Psychological Medicine, 41*(1), 71–83. https://doi .org/10.1017/S0033291710000401

Russell, D. W., Clavél, F. D., Cutrona, C. E, Abrahams, W. T., & Burzette, R. (2018). Neighborhood racial discrimination and the development of major depression. *Journal of Abnormal Psychology, 127*(2), 150–159.

Sadock, B. J., Sadock, V. A., Ruiz, P., & Kaplan, H. I. (2015). *Kaplan & Sadock's synopsis of psychiatry: Behavioral sciences/clinical psychiatry*. Philadelphia, PA: Wolters Kluwer.

Schneider, B., Weber, B., Frensch, A., Stein, J., & Fritze, J. (2000). Vitamin D in schizophrenia, major depression and alcoholism. *Journal of Neural Transmission, 107*, 839–842. https://doi.org/10.1007/s007020070063

Schwartz, R. C., & Blankenship, D. M. (2014). Racial disparities in psychotic disorder diagnosis: A review of empirical literature. *World Journal of Psychiatry, 4*(4), 133–140. https://doi.org/10.5498/wjp.v4.i4.133

United States Department of Health and Human Services (U.S. DHHS). (2010). *Healthy People 2020*. https://www.healthypeople.gov

U.S. Census Bureau, Current Population Survey. (2019). PINC-05. *Work experience—people 15 years old and over, by total money earnings, age, race, Hispanic origin, sex, and disability status*. https://www.census.gov/data/tables/time-series/demo/income-poverty/cps-pinc/pinc-05.html

U.S. Department of Commerce. Economics and Statistics Administration, Census Bureau. (2014). *Age and sex of all people, family members and unrelated individuals iterated by income-to-poverty ratio and race*. http://www.census.gov/hhes/www/cpstables/032014/pov/pov01_100.htm

U.S. Department of Justice. (2016). Prisoners in 2015. NCJ 250229. *Bureau of Justice Statistics Bulletin*. https://www.bjs.gov/content/pub/pdf/p15.pdf

Ward, E. & Heidrich, S. M. (2009). African American women's beliefs about mental illness, stigma, and preferred coping behaviors. *Research Nursing Health, 32*(5), 480–492. https://doi.org/10.1002/nur.20344

Watson, K. T., Roberts, N. M., & Saunders, M. R. (2012). Factors associated with anxiety and depression among African-American and White women. *International Scholarly Research Network*, 1–8. https://doi.org/5402/2012/432321

Weisman de Mamani, A., Weintraub, M. J., Gurak, K., & Maura, J. (2014). A randomized clinical trial to test the efficacy of a family-focused culturally informed therapy for schizophrenia. *Journal of Family Psychology, 28*(6), 800–810. https://doi.org/10.1037/fam0000021

Whaley, A. L. (1997). Ethnicity/race, paranoia, and psychiatric diagnoses: Clinician bias versus sociocultural differences. *Journal of Psychopathology and Behavioral Assessment, 19*(1), 1–20. https://doi.org/10.1007/BF02263226

Whaley, A. L. (1998). Cross-cultural perspective on paranoia: A focus on the Black American experience. *Psychiatric Quarterly, 69*(4), 325–343. https://doi.org/10.1022134231763

Williams, D. R., Yu, Y., Jackson, J. S., & Anderson, N. B. (1997). Racial differences in physical and mental health: Socioeconomic status, stress, and discrimination. *Journal of Health Psychology, 2*(3), 335–351. https://doi.org/10.1177/135910539700200305

Williams, M. T., Rosen, D. C., & Kanter, J. W. (2019). *Eliminating race-based mental health disparities: Promoting equity and culturally responsive care across settings*. Oakland, CA: Context Press.

Woods-Giscombe, C., Robinson, M. N., Carthon, D., Devane-Johnson, S., & Corbie-Smith, G. (2016). Superwoman schema, stigma, spirituality, and culturally sensitive providers: Factors influencing African American women's use of mental health services. *Research, Education, and Policy, 9*(1), 1124–1144.

World Health Organization. (1998). *Gender disparities in mental health, 1998*. Executive summary. Geneva, Switzerland: World Health Organization.

CHAPTER 6

Substance Use and Dependence

Gemari Evans
Kimber Shelton

There are many factors that contribute to the introduction, maintenance, and treatment of alcohol and drug use, as well as the impact substance use has on the individual, their family, and the greater society. The confounding factors of gender and race create unique issues related to use patterns and treatment; yet much of the literature on alcohol and drug use does not emphasize the issues specific to African American women. This chapter explores unique substance use–related issues and treatment considerations for African American women.

DEFINITIONS

The *Diagnostic and Statistical Manual of Mental Disorders 5* (DSM 5; APA, 2013) provides diagnostic criteria for substance use disorders and substance-induced disorders. Substance use disorders range from mild to severe, classifying a pattern of substance use that continues despite negative consequences. Substance-induced disorders are psychological disorders that are resultant of substance use (i.e., substance-induced bipolar disorder). Additional commonly used substance-related terms include:

Abuse: Harmful or hazardous use of psychoactive substances, including alcohol and illicit drugs (World Health Organization, WHO, 2010).
Addiction: The repeated use of a substance to the extent that the user is "periodically or chronically intoxicated, shows a compulsion to take the preferred substance (or substances), has great difficulty in voluntarily ceasing or modifying substance use, and exhibits determination to obtain psychoactive substances by almost any means" (WHO, 2010).

Dependence: Physiological dependence on a substance(s) typically characterized by symptoms of tolerance and withdrawal (APA, 2013).

Illicit Drug: A substance that is prohibited, in terms of the use, production, and sale, by the Controlled Substance Act of 1970.

Misuse: The use of a substance for the purpose that is inconsistent with the medical and legal guidelines (WHO, 2010).

Substance: General term that refers to alcohol, cannabis, prescription drugs, heroin, and other drugs that are ingested, smoked, snorted, or injected and affect mental and physical processes.

RACISM AND AMERICA'S WAR ON DRUGS

Before authors discuss prevalence rates, addiction patterns, and treatment options, we believe it important to contextualize substance use through a lens of systemic racism. Black Americans' drug use has been criminalized and pathologized by a system that medicalizes and humanizes drug use of White Americans. For example, although "pharmacologically identical" (The Sentencing Project, n.d.), federal sentencing guidelines stipulate longer sentences for crack cocaine offenses than for powder cocaine offenses. Black Americans are more likely to use crack cocaine, while White Americans are more likely to use powder cocaine (Substance Abuse and Mental Health Services Administration, SAMHSA, 2020b); as such, federal sentencing guidelines fuel incarceration at higher rates for Black drug users and the consequential disruption of Black families (i.e., incarceration of Black parents). In 2010, under the Obama administration, the Fair Sentencing Act reduced the cocaine sentencing quantity disparity from 100-to-1 to 18-to-1 and increased the quantity of cocaine possession needed to trigger a minimum mandatory sentence; however, although the disparity between low-level rock and powder cocaine was reduced, the disparity remains (The Sentencing Project, n.d.). To bring this further into perspective, a SAMHSA (2020a) report stated "in 2017, though Black/African Americans represented 12 percent of the U.S. adult population, they made up a third of the sentenced prison population . . . in 2012, they accounted for 39 percent of the population incarcerated for drug-related offenses." Additionally, during the 1980s, the "crack baby" label became popular in describing children born with crack dependence. Again, with Black Americans' higher use of crack cocaine, the term crack baby was stereotyped to African American women and their children. Although the use of crack cocaine can compromise the health and development of a fetus, the effects were found to be similar to the negative effects found in the use of other drugs and alcohol, poor prenatal care, and poor maternal nutrition (U.S. Sentencing Commission, USSC, 2007).

Similar themes exist for marijuana and opioid use. Terms such as "marijuana mommies" and popular blogs like "Stoner Mom" normalize White women's recreational and medicinal use of marijuana. All the while, in all

50 states, Black Americans are arrested at higher rates than White Americans for marijuana-related offenses (American Civil Liberties Union, ACLU, 2020). For example, of the 2000 federally sentenced marijuana offenders in 2018, about 84 percent were people of color (USSC, 2018). Similarly, America is currently facing an "opioid epidemic," which began when use and overdose rates among White Americans grew following a surge in prescribing pain medication drugs. Despite Black Americans having the highest increase in opioid overdose death rates from 2011 to 2016 compared to other populations, most of the focus of the epidemic has been on White suburban and rural communities (SAMHSA, 2020a).

Black women's substance use rates are similar to their peers of different races and in some accounts lower. The ACLU (2020) routinely reports that each year, more Black Americans than White Americans report never using marijuana, and Black women's overall drug use is lower than that of other women and men (Stevens-Watkins et al. 2012). Drug use and dependence stigmatizes and criminalizes Black women; detainment on drug offenses impacts Black women's families (many of the Black women arrested are mothers); and future employment opportunities, and cultural mistrust and health professionals' cultural incompetence, negatively impact substance use care and treatment outcomes. Given these variables, mental health professionals need to pay special attention to the needs of Black women.

SUBSTANCE USE

Prevalence and Statistics

African Americans, like their peers of different ethnicities, report alcohol, tobacco, prescription medications, and illicit drug use. According to the National Survey on Drug Use and Health (NSDUH) (SAMHSA, 2020b) 7.3 percent of African Americans aged 18 years and older had a substance use disorder, and within this group 47.1 percent used illicit drugs, 67.6 percent used alcohol, and 14.8 percent used both alcohol and illicit drugs. Furthermore, 5.6 percent of Black individuals between 18 and 25 years old met criteria for alcohol use disorder in the past year, in comparison to 10.1 percent of the overall U.S. population of this same age group. There was a consistent decline in alcohol use disorder among Black youth and young adults during 2015–2018. Binge drinking is slightly less common among African Americans (23 percent), in comparison to White (25.7 percent) and Hispanic Americans (24.6 percent). In regard to heavy drinking, the rate is less common among African Americans (4.3 percent) than White Americans (7.2 percent) and the general population (6.1 percent) (SAMHSA, 2020b). The NSDUH (SAMHSA, 2020b) portrayed cannabis as the most popular illicit drug in 2018, with 17.8 percent of African American individuals over 12 years old using the substance; 15.9 percent of the overall U.S. population over 12 years old use cannabis.

In regard to opioid prescriptions, 8.8 percent of Black individuals over 12 years old that were prescribed hydrocodone misused the substance in the past year, in comparison to 11.5 percent of the overall U.S. population. Similar trends were displayed with tramadol and morphine prescriptions where Black individuals misused the prescriptions at lower rates than the overall U.S. population within the past year (SAMHSA, 2020b). African American individuals reported lower lifetime use of cocaine (8.5 percent), compared to White and Hispanic Americans, 17.6 percent and 11.1 percent, respectively (SAMHSA, 2020b). Although this statistic demonstrates less powder and crack cocaine use by African Americans in the country, a recent study stated that African Americans are more likely to use crack than other ethnic groups (Kaliszewski, 2020). In comparison to African American women who do not report illicit drug use, the women that do report drug use are likely to be single, separated, or divorced; have fewer social support resources; report alcohol and tobacco use along with the illicit drugs; and have not yet obtained a high school diploma or GED (Turner & Wallace, 2003).

According to NSDUH (SAMHSA, 2020b), there were significant increases in major depressive episodes with severe impairment among Black female young adults. Additionally, the report found significant increases in suicidal thoughts in Black individuals between 18 and 25 years old. Furthermore, there was a significant increase in serious mental illness among Black young adults aged 18–25 during 2015–2018 and among Black adults over 50 years old during 2008–2018 (SAMHSA, 2020b). These findings are important because use of one substance (alcohol or illicit substance) among Black individuals is "strongly correlated with polysubstance use and with major depressive episode and serious mental illness underscoring the need to screen for all substances as well as mental disorders when evaluating a person identifying a substance problem or mental health issue, and to treat all co-occurring disorders" (SAMHSA, 2020b, 56).

Variables Impacting Substance Use and Dependence

Many of the variables that impact African American women's substance use and/or dependence are the same as those of substance users in general and of all women who use. Like their peers, African American women's substance use can be related to biological predisposition, a comorbid mental illness, traumatic events and stress, a desire to feel better or different, and curiosity (National Institute on Drug Abuse, NIDA, 2020). Differing from their peers, African American women's experiences of racism and sexism are additional entryways to substance use and dependence. Curtis-Boles and Jenkins-Monroe (2000) state that African American women are often victimized by gender, race, and socioeconomic oppression, which urges them to use substances to escape from economic and social marginalization, and from feelings of alienation and powerlessness. In fact, racial discrimination is associated with problematic alcohol use and more alcohol-related issues with Black Americans. Continued stress from experiencing discrimination heightens psychological stress and depletes coping tools, which results in increased participation in maladaptive coping mechanisms, such as alcohol use (Desalu, Goodhines, & Park, 2019).

In addition, African American children, youth, and families have greater exposure and vulnerability to a plethora of social problems, including substance abuse. In comparison to White individuals, Black Americans are more likely to experience poverty, grow up in single-parent households, be unemployed, lack health care, and live in a crowded urban environment (Turner & Wallace, 2003).

Impact of Substance Use

Individual—Physical, Psychological, and Environmental Impact. African Americans typically experience more serious health and psychosocial issues as related to alcohol and drug use, including exposure to violence, alcohol-related illnesses (e.g., liver disease, heart disease, pancreatitis), legal repercussions, substance-related accidents, high-risk sexual behavior, and exposure to HIV/AIDS than their peers (American Addictions Centers, 2020; Turner & Wallace, 2003). Although use is generally lower than with White peers, Black Americans experience greater health consequences related to adverse smoking-related diseases and have high comorbidity between cannabis and tobacco use (Montgomery et al., 2017). Table 6.1 provides a list of common drugs used by Black women and the short- and long-term consequences of use.

Psychological and psychosocial factors related to substance use with African American women include anxiety, depression, suicidal behaviors, relationship conflicts, workplace problems, and self-esteem issues (Montgomery et al., 2017; Turner & Wallace, 2003). Psychological concerns may have been present before substance use began, or may be induced or exacerbated through substance use. Engagement in "drug culture" also increases susceptibility to incarceration, death, and child welfare involvement, all of which may negatively impact family cohesion and socioeconomic well-being in African American communities (Stevens-Watkins et al., 2012). Instability in family and marriages, pregnancy, truncated educational pursuits, diminished educational achievement, limited access to employment opportunities, poor occupational role performance, and restricted social engagement are all potential negative outcomes of substance use in women. Shame and embarrassment associated with addiction may hinder Black women from reaching out for support and keep them isolated within drug communities.

Brain—Reward Pathway. Considering the physical, emotional, psychological, familial, and community toll of drug use, it can be difficult to

Table 6.1
List of Common Drugs Used by Black Women*

	Description & Street Names	Common Forms & Ways Taken	Possible Short-Term (ST) & Long-Term (LT) Health Effects	Withdrawal Symptoms	Treatment Options
Alcohol	Ethyl alcohol, or ethanol, is an intoxicating ingredient found in beer, wine, and liquor. It is produced by the fermentation of yeast, sugars, and starches. Booze, Juice, Sauce, Brew.	Beer, wine, liquor/spirits/malt beverages. Ingested by drinking.	ST: Injuries and risky behavior, including drunk driving and inappropriate sexual behavior; impaired judgment, coordination, and reflexes; slurred speech, memory problems. LT: Irregular heartbeat, stroke, high blood pressure; cirrhosis and fibrosis of the liver; mouth, throat, liver, breast cancer.	Trouble sleeping, shakiness, irritability, depression, anxiety, nausea, sweating.	Naltrexone, acamprosate, disulfiram. CBT, 12-step facilitation therapy, mobile medical application: reset.
Cocaine	A powerfully addictive stimulant drug made from the leaves of the coca plant native to South America. Blow, Bump, C, Candy, Charlie, Coke, Crack, Flake, Rock, Snow, Toot.	White powder, whitish rock crystal. Snorted, smoked, injected.	ST: Narrowed blood vessels; enlarged pupils; increased body temperature, heart rate, and blood pressure; headache; abdominal pain and nausea; euphoria; increased energy, alertness; insomnia, restlessness; anxiety; erratic and violent behavior, panic attacks, paranoia, psychosis; heart rhythm problems, heart attack; stroke, seizure, coma. LT: Loss of sense of smell, nosebleeds, nasal damage and trouble swallowing from snorting; infection and death of bowel tissue from decreased blood flow; poor nutrition and weight loss; lung damage from smoking.	Depression, tiredness, increased appetite, insomnia, vivid unpleasant dreams, slowed movement, restlessness.	No FDA-approved treatment medications. CBT, contingency management, or motivational incentives, including vouchers, the matrix model, community-based recovery groups such as 12-step programs, mobile medical application: reset.

Drug	Description	Short-Term (ST) / Long-Term (LT) Effects	Withdrawal Symptoms	Treatment
Heroin	An opioid drug made from morphine; a natural substance extracted from the seed pod of the various opium poppy plants. Brown sugar, China White, Dope, H, Horse, Junk, Skag, Skunk, Smack, White Horse with OTC cold medicine and antihistamine: Cheese. White or brownish powder, or black sticky substance known as "black tar heroin." Injected, smoked, snorted.	ST: Euphoria, dry mouth, itching, nausea, vomiting, analgesia, slowed breathing and heart rate. LT: Collapsed veins, abscesses (swollen tissue with pus), infection of the lining and valves in the heart, constipation and stomach cramps liver or kidney disease.	Restlessness, muscle and bone pain, insomnia, diarrhea, vomiting, cold flashes with goose bumps ("cold turkey")	Methadone, buprenorphine, naltrexone (short- and long-acting forms), contingency management or motivational incentives, 12-step facilitation therapy.
Marijuana	Marijuana is made from the hemp plant, Cannabis sativa. The main psychoactive (mind-altering) chemical in marijuana is delta-9-tetrahydrocannabinol, or THC. Blunt, Bud, Dope, Ganja, Grass, Green, Herb, Joint, Mary Jane, Pot, Reefer, Sinsemilla, Skunk, Smoke, Trees, Weed Hashish: Boom, Gangster, Hash, Hemp. Greenish-gray mixture of dried, shredded leaves, stems, seeds, and/or flowers; resin (hashish) or sticky, black liquid (hash oil). Smoked, eaten (mixed in food or brewed as tea).	ST: Enhanced sensory perception and euphoria followed by drowsiness/relaxation; slowed reaction time; problems with balance and coordination; increased heart rate and appetite; problems with learning and memory; anxiety. LT: Mental health problems, chronic cough, frequent respiratory infections. In rare cases, risk of recurrent episodes of severe nausea and vomiting.	Irritability, trouble sleeping, decreased appetite, anxiety.	No FDA-approved treatment medications. CBT, contingency management or motivational incentives, motivational enhancement therapy (MET), behavioral treatments geared to adolescents, mobile medical application: reset.

(Continued)

Table 6.1
(Continued)

	Description & Street Names	Common Forms & Ways Taken	Possible Short-Term (ST) & Long-Term (LT) Health Effects	Withdrawal Symptoms	Treatment Options
MDMA	A synthetic, psychoactive drug that has similarities to both the stimulant amphetamine and the hallucinogen mescaline. MDMA is an abbreviation of the scientific name 3,4-methylenedioxymethamphetamine. Adam, Clarity, Eve, Lover's Speed, Peace, Uppers.	Colorful tablets with imprinted logos, capsules, powder, liquid. Swallowed, snorted.	ST: Lowered inhibition, enhanced sensory perception, increased heart rate and blood pressure, muscle tension, nausea, faintness, chills or sweating, sharp rise in body temperature leading to kidney failure or death. LT: Long-lasting confusion, depression, problems with attention, memory, and sleep; increased anxiety, impulsiveness; less interest in sex.	Fatigue, loss of appetite, depression, aggression, trouble concentrating.	There is conflicting evidence about whether MDMA is addictive. No FDA-approved treatment medications. More research is needed to find out if behavioral therapies can be used to treat MDMA addiction.
Methamphetamine	An extremely addictive stimulant amphetamine drug. Crank, Chalk, Crystal, Fire, Glass, Go Fast, Ice, Meth, Speed.	White powder or pill; crystal meth looks like pieces of glass or shiny blue-white "rocks" of different size. Swallowed, snorted, smoked, injected	ST: Increased wakefulness and physical activity; decreased appetite; increased breathing, heart rate, blood pressure, temperature; irregular heartbeat. LT: Anxiety, confusion, insomnia, mood problems, violent behavior, paranoia, hallucinations, delusions, weight loss, severe dental problems ("meth mouth"), intense itching leading to skin sores from scratching.	Depression, anxiety, tiredness.	No FDA-approved treatment medications. CBT, contingency management or motivational incentives, the matrix model, 12-step facilitation therapy, mobile medical application: reset.

Tobacco	Plant grown for its leaves, which are dried and fermented before use.	Smoked, snorted, chewed, vaporized. Cigarettes, cigars, bidis, hookahs, smokeless tobacco (snuff, spit tobacco, chew).	ST: Increased blood pressure, breathing, and heart rate. LT: Greatly increased risk of cancer, especially lung cancer when smoked and oral cancers when chewed; chronic bronchitis; emphysema; heart disease; leukemia; cataracts; pneumonia.	Irritability, attention and sleep problems, depression, increased appetite.	Bupropion (Zyban), varenicline (Chantix), nicotine replacement (gum, patch, lozenge). CBT; self-help materials; mail, phone, and Internet quit resources.

Source: Adapted from: National Institute on Drug Abuse (n.d.). *Commonly abused drugs.* https://www.drugabuse.gov/sites/default/files/nida_commonlyuseddrugs_final_printready.pdf.

*Note: Not included: Inhalants, LSD, PCP, synthetic cannabinoids, synthetic cathinones ("bath salts").

understand how someone continues use in the face of great negative consequence. Understanding of the reward pathway in the brain can help to explain substance use, dependence and addiction. An individual's motivation for using a substance can be viewed through the capacity of positive and negative reinforcement to activate internal sensory or affective processes within certain systems in the body (Lowinson, Ruiz, & Millman, 2004). When an individual experiences pleasant sensations from drug or alcohol use, such as euphoria or relaxation, the "reward pathway" becomes activated. The reward pathway is called the mesolimbic dopamine pathway because it refers to the dopamine neurotransmitter signaling in specific areas of the brain (Koob & Le Moal, 2008). Both positive and negative reinforcement contribute to problematic substance use. Activating the reward pathway is a positive reinforcement as the user is motivated to reengage in use to activate the pathway again. Conversely, individuals are motivated to continue or increase substance use to remove a negative stimulus. For example, using more substances to stop symptoms of withdrawal.

Dopamine is naturally produced in the body and is responsible for the desire to repeat pleasurable activities. To appreciate the surge of dopamine released through substance use, we compare dopamine rates to common activities. Dr. Richard Rawson, retired co-director of UCLA Integrated Substance Abuse Programs, summarized an animal study finding that showed eating food may increase dopamine levels 100 units and sex by 200 units, while alcohol can release dopamine to 100–200 units, cocaine can raise dopamine levels 350 units and methamphetamines to levels of 1,250 units (Frontline, 2006). Drugs produce a much larger surge of dopamine, in comparison to satisfying hunger or sex/orgasm. NIDA (2020b) states that this large surge powerfully reinforces the connection between "consumption of the drug, resulting pleasure, and all the external cues linked to the experience" (17). The brain learns to seek drugs at the expense of other nondrug use activities, including necessary activities like eating (NIDA, 2020b). As individuals are unlikely to experience the same pleasure from nondrug use activities, they will continue to "chase the high" provided only through substance use.

The transition from drug use to dependence is complex. Simply stated, drug use begins as a solitary episode or instance, which can create a "liking" for the drug, and the release of dopamine influences people to want to use again. Humans have a relatively small supply of dopamine, in which prolonged release depletes it. Drug use shifts to drug abuse when liking the drug becomes "wanting" the drug, and a habit is created. Patterned use is a marker of drug abuse when the amount or methods of use are not approved or supervised. This leads to compulsive use, which shifts the "wanting" of the drug to the body "needing" and craving it. With increased drug use, the body develops a tolerance for the drug in which the body will need more of it for the same effect to occur. As related to addiction, when the body begins to crave a drug, the individual becomes preoccupied with obtaining it. The person who has become addicted to the drug(s) experiences a psychological dependence, where they are using to maintain the pleasure and avoid discomfort (Koob & Le Moal, 2008). Thus, social value, decision making, control and inhibition, motivation, drive, and values are all disrupted.

Families and Community. Substance use by Black women impacts not only the individual, but also their families and communities. In many families, Black women balance multiple roles of relationships, finances, and socialization; as a result, substance dependence can disrupt the family balance. Related to an individual's use, family members may be experiencing four factors: stress; threat to the family and home; worry; and strain that may appear as personal upset, distress, and poor mental and physical health (Orford et al., 2005). Finding out that a loved one is substance dependent can lead to confusion, sadness, anger, fear, and shock, which could be influenced by the lack of knowledge and experience with substance use. Supporting a loved one with an addiction can be incredibly taxing; it is important for loved ones to remember to prioritize their health as well. Responses to identifying the drug addiction include the impulse to resolve the problem internally, denial and avoidance, minimizing, and seeking help. As Black women are in treatment, it may be helpful to also engage the family in treatment.

TREATMENT CONSIDERATIONS

Theories and Treatment Models

Theories. Several theories exist to explain substance use, dependence, and treatment (see Department of Health, 2004). Five of these models are briefly described. The *disease or medical model* views addiction as a disease and describes the user having an "illness." From this perspective, the disease is irreversible and abstinence is the only treatment option. With African American women, operating from a disease model may normalize substance use and dependence and improve their ability to seek and receive help. Like other diseases, such as cancer or Type I diabetes, viewing substance use as a disease can help to remove the stigma associated with use and open one up to treatment. However, if they view the problem as a preventable disease, such as Type II diabetes or a sexual transmitted infection, African American women may still blame themselves for the choices they made.

The *moral model* views addiction as a weakness or character flaw of the individual. From this view, on the one hand, African American women and those they interact with may blame themselves for their use and dependence. Black women operating from a Strong Black Woman (SBW) archetype may feel especially troubled, as acknowledging their substance use would be akin to acknowledging a fault or weakness. On the other hand, the moral model may provide African American women with motivation and autonomy, as changes to character and willpower can positively influence harm reduction or abstinence.

The *social learning model* extends addiction beyond the physiological and views addiction as something that anyone engaging in high-risk use can develop (i.e., conditioning). Related to this, the *negative reinforcement model* suggests substances are used as a means to gain relief from emotional, physical, psychological, or environmental pain (Baker et al., 2004). From this perspective, African American women can view their substance use on a spectrum, as opposed to all-or-nothing thinking.

The *sociocultural model* purports that drug use must be understood within the context of the overall society. The type of society one lives in can directly impact their use of and dependence on substances, and treatment moves beyond the individual to changes to the overall community and society. Within this model, African American women's use cannot be detached from their sociocultural experiences, including those of gendered racism. This perspective may help to externalize use and dependence, and overarching treatment and legal changes can assist in reducing substance use.

The *attachment model* views addiction as being connected to the attachment process (Flores, 2011). The biological, psychological, and social variables that create unhealthy attachment patterns are the same conditions that produce and maintain the addiction. Issues of attachment may create addiction issues, and addiction issues can also lead to relationship issues. Substances are used as a reparative attempt to cope with and adjust to dysregulated relationships, yet often serves to worsen interpersonal relationships. Regardless of the precipitant, establishing healthy relationships is needed to treat the addiction. This model can be helpful in conceptualizing Black women who place importance on their interpersonal relationships and desire healthier connections in their lives, and whose addiction is connected to relational trauma.

Treatment Models. Based on treatment needs, individuals benefit from abstinence or harm reduction–based models, and psychoeducation about relapses and slips. Abstinence requires a commitment to refrain from substance use. Particularly from the view of the "addicted brain" in which organic changes have occurred in the brain, full abstinence from the dependent substance(s) is warranted (NIDA, 2020b). Any relapse in use can result in full addiction and dependence behaviors and consequences. For example, the individual cannot have one drink; once they start drinking, they feel compelled to drink to intoxication. Harm reduction is focused on reducing the negative consequences related to substance use (Wagener, 2019). This may include strategies to reduce the quantity and frequency of use or interventions focused on making use safer. For example, this could be reducing marijuana use from daily use to use only on the weekend. Additional harm reduction strategies include providing unused needles and disposal sites to those who use intravenously (i.e., reduce HIV/AIDS transmission), providing safe places to use (i.e., reduce overdose and sexual assault), and switching to use of substances with less negative consequences (i.e., methadone maintenance to treat opioid addiction). Harm reduction programs have demonstrated physical health benefits (e.g., reduced alcohol use was associated with improved liver functioning, lower blood pressure, and improved quality of life), and economic and public health benefits (Witkiewitz et al., 2018). Harm reduction may be sufficient in meeting the physical and psychological needs for some individuals, whereas others may engage in harm reduction practices that later lead to abstinence.

Relapse and slips are important subjects to discuss in treatment to prepare clients for the possibility of them. Although not everyone experiences a relapse and/or slip, they are very common during the recovery journey. A relapse is when an individual returns to substances after a sobriety period. A slip (or lapse) refers to a single use or brief revisiting of substances, after which the individual immediately returns to their recovery journey sometimes feeling more motivated for recovery. If a slip or relapse occurs, it is important to process what they think it means and potential triggers. During these times, therapists offer encouragement, express that the client is not a failure, and normalize the relapse/slip.

SUBSTANCE USE TREATMENT

Screening and Assessments

Failure to screen and assess substance use can lead to ineffective treatment, continuance of dependence or problematic use, and treatment dropout. For example, after 10 sessions, a client reports continued motivational problems and increasing feelings of anxiety. Attempts at thought stopping, relaxation training, and mindfulness have been ineffective. At the 10th session, the client shares that they are smoking marijuana twice daily to relax. As a result, therapy strategies have been ineffective because the client is turning to marijuana to regulate her emotions instead of allowing herself the opportunity to experience emotional discomfort and practice self-regulation.

Even if a clinician believes that substance use treatment is beyond their scope of competence, awareness of substances and strong assessment skills are required to provide an appropriate referral. This begins with having a working knowledge of commonly used drugs and their effects (see Table 6.1). Holding knowledge of different substances while completing a clinical interview is one strategy for obtaining substance use history and assessing treatment needs. As a part of the intake interview, SAMHSA (2013) advises to complete a thorough psychosocial and cultural history for women. Table 6.2 outlines psychosocial and cultural history and intake specific to Black women.

Table 6.2
Psychosocial and Cultural Assessment Considerations

	Assessment Areas	Cultural Considerations
Medical History and Physical Health	• Review HIV/AIDS and other infectious disease status and risk; • explore history of gynecological problems, use of birth control and hormone replacement therapy; • obtain history of pregnancies, miscarriages, abortions, and history of substance abuse during pregnancy; • and assess need for prenatal care.	• Intravenous drugs and high-risk sex behaviors related to use can increase risk for HIV/AIDS exposure. • Demonstrate empathetic understanding related to gynecological care and pregnancy history. Understanding of cultural mistrust associated with health care, as well as shame that may be connected to pregnancy history, is needed.
Substance Abuse History	• Identify people who initially introduced alcohol and drugs; • explore reasons for initiation of use and continued use; • discuss family of origin history of substance abuse; • history of use in previous and present significant relationships; • and history of use with family members or significant others.	• Some Black women are raised to believe secrecy is attached to familial protection. As such, they may feel uncomfortable sharing "family business" to others. This may make it more challenging to disclose family history related to substance use. • Intergenerational trauma could impact self-reporting. High risk and dependency within family could be seen as a norm; thus, use history could be underreported.
Mental Health and Treatment History	• Explore prior treatment history and relationships with prior treatment providers and consequences, if any, for engaging in prior treatment; • review history of prior traumatic events, mood or anxiety disorders (including PTSD), as well as eating disorders; • evaluate safety issues including parasuicidal behaviors, previous or current threats, history of interpersonal violence or sexual abuse, and overall feeling of safety; • review family history of mental illness; • and discuss evidence and history of personal strengths and coping strategies and styles.	• Gendered racism, racial trauma, and minority stress are linked to numerous psychological and health-related complications. Given this, assessment of comorbidity with mental and physical health issues is warranted. • Black women have high comorbidity with mood issues, PTSD, anxiety, and other substances. • Co-occurring substance use disorder (SUD) is associated with greater suicidality for African American adults (SAMHSA, 2019).

Interpersonal and Family History	• Obtain history of substance abuse in current relationship; • explore acceptance of client's substance abuse problem among family and significant relationships; • discuss concerns regarding childcare needs; • and discuss the types of support that she has received from her family and/or significant other for entering treatment and abstaining from substances.	• When assessing substance use and treatment concerns, considerations for childcare may need to be explored (i.e., a single mother entering rehab treatment for 30 days). • The SBW archetype could present as an obstacle in acknowledging substance use and seeking treatment. • Black women may take on many different roles. Their treatment and recovery may have positive and negative impacts on many of the roles in their life.
Sociocultural History	• Evaluate client's social support system, including the level of acceptance of her recovery; • discuss level of social isolation prior to treatment; • discuss the role of her cultural beliefs pertaining to her substance use and recovery process; • explore the specific cultural attitudes toward women and substance abuse; • review current spiritual practices (if any); • and discuss current acculturation conflicts and stressors.	• Fear and shame may make it difficult for some Black women to share their substance use with others, which can limit opportunities for support. • Stereotype threat may delay treatment and extend use history. • In general, religion and spirituality are well ingrained within the Black community. On one hand, spirituality can serve as a strength in recovery. On the other hand, how substance use is perceived in the church may increase feelings of shame, preventing Black women from exploring treatment options.
Vocational, Educational, and Military History	• If employed, discuss the level of support that the client is receiving from her employer; • review military history, then expand questions to include history of traumatic events and violence during employment and history of substance abuse in the military; • and assess financial self-reliance.	• Many Black women may be the main financial provider for her family. Considerations related to treatment needs and income are warranted. • Related to the SBW archetype, Black women may feel their employment or career will be negatively impacted by disclosure of use to employer or the need to take leave from work for treatment.

Table 6.2
(Continued)

	Assessment Areas	Cultural Considerations
Legal History	• Discuss history of custody and current involvement with child protective services, if any; • obtain a history of restraining orders, arrests, or periods of incarceration, if any; • and determine the history of child placement with women who acknowledge past or current incarceration.	• If a legal history is present, consider that detention and incarceration rates are higher for Black women. • Validate concerns related to childcare and custody, and systemic biases within child protective services.
Barriers to Treatment and Related Services	• Explore financial, housing, health insurance, childcare, case management, and transportation needs; • and discuss other potential obstacles the client foresees.	• Financial, health, and housing disparities continue to exist and negatively impact treatment access to Black women.
Strengths and Coping Strategies	• Discuss the challenges that the client has faced throughout her life and how she has managed them; • review prior attempts to quit substance use and identify strategies that did work at the time; • and identify other successes in making changes in other areas of her life.	• Strengths and coping strategies may come in the form of ethnic and gender pride, role as a caregiver (mother, wife, daughter), career success, and/or spirituality. • Explore concepts of self-defined and culturally sanctioned healing and recovery processes.

Source: Adapted from SAMHSA, 2013.

In addition to the interview, there are numerous assessments available to help ascertain substance use needs and potential interventions. Substance use screening identifies the presence of a particular problem and triggers more extensive evaluation, the goal being to identify women who have or are at risk for substance dependence; whereas assessment is used to define the problem, determine the diagnosis, and develop treatment plans and recommendations (SAMHSA, 2013). Among other variables, factors of influence to consider in competent screening and assessment include comorbidity, ethnicity and culture, acculturation and language skills, socioeconomic status, and pregnancy.

SAMHSA (2013) provides an extensive list of screenings and assessments appropriate for use with women; ideally, selected assessment instruments are normed and validated with Black women. If normed assessments are not available, interpretations are made with caution and are considerate of culture, language, and acculturation needs. Self-administered tools (vs. face-to-face interview only) may better detect substance use; this is particularly true for practitioners with limited confidence in substance use assessment. As part of establishing an informed and egalitarian relationship, Black women are informed of what they are being screened or assessed for and why. Triangulation can also be an asset by gaining information from multiple sources including behavioral examples, direct observations, and information provided by others (family, other agencies, and retrospective data from previous treatment). With Black women in which SBW and cultural mistrust of health care may be at play, extending the assessment process over time may help as the therapeutic relationship has additional time to build.

Types of Treatment

In 2017, Black individuals made up 17 percent of substance use treatment admissions, 12 percent being Black men and 5 percent being Black women (White individuals made up 61 percent of treatment admissions) (SAMHSA, 2019). Black Americans' admissions were primarily for smoked cocaine, marijuana/hashish, heroin, and alcohol treatment. With the exception of cocaine/crack admissions, non-Hispanic White individuals were the most likely to enter into treatment for all other substances. When African American women present for treatment, they are typically entering on their own accord (self-referral) (SAMHSA, 2013; 2019) and more likely to engage in outpatient services.

Substance use treatment may come in the form of outpatient, detoxification (detox), inpatient, and rehabilitation treatment. Outpatient care includes non-intensive care such as individual, family or group counseling; intensive outpatient care (IOP), and partial hospitalization (PHP), which includes at least two hours of therapy per day for three to four days per week (then returning home). The individual, family, or group therapist would be responsible for continued assessment of substance treatment needs to determine if a higher level of care is warranted. When providing a referral to more intensive treatment and/or hospitalization, working with African American women, the therapist would address any resistance originating from shame and stigma, demystify the treatment process by providing psychoeducation on substance treatment, and ideally have connections with specific treatment referrals to provide detailed information about the assessment and treatment process.

Detox, a medical intervention providing safe withdrawal, can occur in ambulatory (outpatient pharmacological or non-pharmacological) or inpatient (either hospital or residential program with 24-hour medical care) settings. Medically assisted detox may be necessary for severe alcohol addiction or benzodiazepines use, as withdrawal can lead to life-threatening consequences (Sharp, 2020). Although not life-threatening, detox can also be used to ease the symptoms for opiate, cocaine, and amphetamines withdrawal.

During rehab, residential, and hospital care, individuals receive 24-hour medical care in conjunction with substance and dependency treatment. Short-term rehab is typically 30 days or less, whereas long-term rehab is treatment of 30 days or more, often with the option to transfer to transitional living arrangements (i.e., halfway houses) (SAMHSA, 2019). Considerations for referral to and continuance in inpatient treatment include childcare arrangements, costs of treatment, and location of treatment. Furthermore, inpatient treatment facilities would be culturally sensitive to the needs of Black women with inclusion of culturally informed therapy interventions and nontherapeutic needs (e.g., haircare, spirituality).

Theories and Interventions

Overall, those in substance use treatment tend to do better than those who have no treatment or receive a placebo treatment; however, individuals must participate in treatment for it to be effective. With lower retention rates, treatment with Black women would include increasing retention in treatment. A component of this may be focused on the therapy relationship. In the first study exploring specific therapeutic factors that predicted the working alliance with African American women abusing substances, Davis, Ancis, and Ashby (2015) found that in addition to common therapeutic alliance skills (empathy, unconditional positive regard, and genuineness), African American women benefitted from working with therapists who demonstrated Population Sensitive Therapist Characteristics (PSTCs) of cultural competence, egalitarianism, and empowerment. Stronger working alliances were formed with therapists who operated from an intersectional approach, including the impact of gendered racism, stigma associated with gender and substance use, and internalized feelings of shame and powerlessness into treatment.

A number of evidence-based and clinically informed treatment options exist for treating alcohol and other drug (AOD) use. Some of the more well studied interventions include motivational interviewing (MI), motivational enhancement therapy (MET), contingency management (CM), and CBT; as well as support groups such as Alcoholics Anonymous (AA) and Narcotics Anonymous (NA). The following section will explore MI, CBT, AA/NA, and Afrocentric treatment.

MI, as well as other culturally tailored interventions, has been found to be superior in treatment over methods such as behavioral counseling or health education (Montgomery et al., 2017). MI is a brief intervention targeted at increasing motivation and commitment to change/reduce addictive and problematic behaviors (Rollinick, Miller, & Butler, 2007). It includes basic strategies of empathy expression, building discrepancy between maladaptive behaviors and future goals, avoiding arguing with clients, "rolling with resistance," and supporting self-efficacy. The approach is collaborative, egalitarian, respectful of client autonomy, and evocative (client-driven wisdom vs. therapist-led insights) (Burlew et al., 2013). Burlew and colleagues (2013) suggest use of the transtheoretical model of change to explore African American clients' readiness for change. With African American women, understanding their readiness to change can help in building discrepancies related to continued use and views of parenting, family, spirituality, and career; viewing resistance as an active protective strategy and working to develop alternative protections; and empowering and building on the small changes of self-efficacy.

CBT focuses on identifying and changing problematic thought patterns to alter emotions and behaviors. This may be done through interventions such as psychoeducation, cognitive restructuring, systematic desensitization, role-plays, journaling, and assigning homework. With ethnic minority groups, culturally adapted forms of CBT (ACBT) have been more effective than traditional CBT (Windsor, Jemal, & Alessi, 2015). This may be because nonadaptive CBT relies heavily on cognitive factors to create change in self and external environment, which may be dismissive of the social and cultural factors that impact one's mental health and substance use.

AA and NA are peer-led support groups for individuals with alcohol and/or drug dependency. They are 12-step programs, in which members move through the different steps/principles to support and sustain sobriety. In addition, there are 12-step family and friend support programs— Adult Children of Alcoholics (ACOA), Nar-Anon, and Narateen family groups. AA/NA attendance may have many benefits for Black women. One, they are free and frequent. There are AA/NA meetings all over the world, at different times of the day, and some meetings can be attended virtually; making them very accessible. Two, AA/NA principles are spiritual in nature. The spiritual components to AA/NA may connect well with religious Black women. Black women who feel less connected to the spiritual component of AA/NA may feel better served in alternative groups, such as Secular Organizations for Sobriety (SOS) or Atheistic in

Recovery. Further, a primary tenet of AA/NA is anonymity, which may make it easier for Black women to share vulnerabilities.

AA/NA are not without their challenges to Black women. Principles focus heavily on "self" and do not account for systemic issues that support the development and maintenance of addiction. For Black women, who are already disenfranchised, this focus on self-responsibility and minimization of social action may not account for all variables connected to addiction. Although meetings are plentiful, AA/NA meetings tend to be dominated by White individuals (Tonigan et al., 1998). Some Black women may feel less connected in groups that are absent of ethnic and gender representation. Although these limitations exist, African American women who attended women-only groups and made efforts to creatively include social precipitants to addiction (e.g., SES, discrimination) acknowledged feeling empowered in their recovery and reported greater success than did African American men in similar treatment (Kornfield, 2014).

Afrocentric and Black feminist approaches to therapy may specifically address many of the race and gender needs of Black women. Clinicians must keep in mind that not all Black women will identify with Afrocentric perspectives and cannot assume group homogeneity. One particular program, the Iwo San Program (Jackson, 1995), was developed specifically for African American women. The program integrated Afrocentric and CBT components into the existing 12-step framework by exploring ethnic identity and self-pride, and encouraging Black women to embrace their history and culture. The program was founded on the seven Swahili principles of Nguzo Saba—Umoja (Unity), Kujichagulia (Self-Determination), Ujima (Collective Work and Responsibility), Ujamaa (Cooperative Economics), Nia (Purpose), Kuumba (Creativity), and Imani (Faith).

Recent Developments

Although this chapter is focused on substance dependency and treatment, authors want to point readers to the growing research of psychedelic-assisted therapies. Psychedelics have historically been used as medicine. Dating back to Indigenous people in the Americas, psychedelics were experienced as part of holistic care including spiritual practices, plant-based medicines, and community involvement (George et al., 2019). More recently, psychedelic substances are finally being embraced by modern medicine for treatment of psychological disorders, including addiction, depression, anxiety, posttraumatic stress disorder, "treatment resistant" conditions, and others (George et al., 2019). Plant-based psychedelics and synthetic substances such as LSD, psilocybin, MDMA, ayahuasca, ibogaine, and ketamine have been administered in conjunction with psychotherapy to facilitate the therapeutic process. A general overview of the therapeutic process includes a drug-free preparatory session(s), safe administration of the substance (the amount of sessions vary depending on the drug and client), and drug-free integrative sessions. There are several theories on the healing properties of psychedelic-assisted therapy. However, regardless of the model, clients that experienced psychedelic-assisted therapy reported that hallucinogens appear to have the capacity to accelerate emotional processes, which in turn aids in a corrective emotional experience (George et al., 2019).

CASE STUDY

Abstinence-Based Treatment—Melinda

Melinda, a 45-year-old Black woman, entered therapy as her marriage and family were "falling apart." Melinda explained that her husband of 10 years demanded she get treatment; otherwise, they would divorce and he would pursue full custody of their 9-year-old daughter. Melinda felt especially concerned as she had a 22-year-old son that she currently had no relationship with. At present, Melinda reported drinking daily and occasional use of cocaine. She stated that she began drinking alcohol at age 10. She was introduced to alcohol by an older female cousin, who molested her. She was frequently in her cousin's care, as she explained that her father was not a part of her life and that her mother was a "drug addict." Melinda explained that by age 15, she had tried "every drug" and began having sex with boys and men who would give her drugs and alcohol.

Somehow, Melinda explained, she made it through high school, and at age 18 moved in with her 30-year-old boyfriend, who used cocaine. She reported physical and emotional abuse by her boyfriend. By age 18, Melinda reported heavy drinking and use of crack. She stated that her boyfriend would bring men home for her to have sex with to support their crack habit. When she was 20 years old, her boyfriend was arrested for drug trafficking and was sentenced to 15 years in prison due to prior felonies. Melinda then had nowhere to live and began her life "on the streets." While homeless, Melinda reported going deeper into her addiction, repeated sexual and physical assault, and multiple arrests. At age 23, Melinda found out she was pregnant, and was referred to a treatment facility by her physician. Melinda reported living in a women's shelter during her pregnancy and for approximately six months after giving birth. She denied use of cocaine while pregnant, but reported that she did occasionally drink while pregnant. Post pregnancy, Melinda reported getting high with another shelter resident. They were discovered by a shelter worker, which resulted in her son being removed from her custody and placed in foster care.

For the next 10 years, Melinda reported periods of sobriety or moderated use in which she would work and take a class or two, mixed with periods of binge alcohol and cocaine use. During a period of sobriety, Melinda met her now husband at a shared job. She described her husband as supportive and caring and in recovery himself. Although her husband did not drink, Melinda reported that she continued to drink alcohol during their courtship and marriage, which has always been a problem in the relationship. She was unsure of the reason, but explained that she began smoking crack six months ago and has found herself unable to stop. In the last six months, she has been fired from her job, her husband has come looking for her after she has stayed away for days at a time, and she has stolen from their home and bank account. When she is unable to use crack, she reported having to drink, having cravings, and getting "the shakes" if she wasn't drinking. She stated she wasn't sure if she could stop drinking and using drugs, but feared that her husband would leave her and she would be estranged from her second child.

Melinda's therapist immediately suggested she enter into drug treatment. Her therapist explained that given her history and current level of use, coupled with comorbid trauma history, weekly outpatient therapy was unlikely to be an effective treatment route. Furthermore, with Melinda's physiological dependence on alcohol, medically assisted detox was warranted. Melinda and her therapist contacted Melinda's husband, discussed the treatment plan, and identified childcare assistance for their daughter. Melinda immediately entered a combined detox/rehabilitation treatment center, where she remained for 60 days. During that time, she received individual and group therapy and began working with a psychiatrist who prescribed an antidepressant. During her time in treatment, she reported regularly listening to gospel music and joining a prayer group with other women. While at the rehab center, Melinda learned about ketamine-assisted psychotherapy for trauma, but expressed hesitancy in trying this route at this point in her recovery.

Post rehab, Melinda returned to individual counseling, focusing heavily on her trauma history. Through therapy, she realized that her daughter had been close to turning 10, which is when Melinda's sexual abuse and substance use began. She also explained that she had never dealt with her feelings of worthlessness and felt triggered by seeing herself in her daughter. In therapy, Melinda processed intergenerational trauma, explored her identity development, and integrated cultural strengths associated with healing. She participated in EMDR treatment, her daughter entered individual counseling, and she and her husband began marriage counseling. Her therapist suggested Melinda join a healing circle for Black women in recovery; yet Melinda denied interest in attending this group, as she felt she still carried great shame and would feel embarrassed opening up to Black women. However, she began attending AA and NA meetings, expressing feeling most comfortable at women-only meetings.

Harm Reduction—Nubay

Nubay is a 19-year-old African American college student. She identified as cisgender, heterosexual, and single, majoring in sports medicine and kinesiology with the hope to become a sports trainer or rehabilitation therapist. Nubay presented to the college counseling center with feelings of depression and existential angst. She stated that she is "trying to find herself" and has made poor decisions in this process. She explained that in high school, she "followed all the rules," meaning she was successful academically, but had very little social life. Since beginning college, Nubay reported being more social, attending parties, and binge drinking. With follow-up and prompting questions from her therapist, Nubay explained that she has been drinking every weekend, with some weekends starting on Thursday. She would have between four and six mixed drinks per sitting, and once a month, she smoked "weed." Nubay acknowledged that she initially has more fun when she is drinking and that it is easier for her to be social; however, she explained that there have been times when she has been in "compromising" situations that she feels she would not have been in if she had not been drinking. This includes saying things that she later regrets, driving while intoxicated on two occasions, and passing out at places in which others could have sexually harmed her (she denied any sexual assault experiences). She also expressed that there has been a slip in her grades, especially following the weeks she began partying on Thursdays. Nubay's goals were to improve her mood, academic performance, and learn more about herself. Her clinician suggested that Nubay's drinking contributed to her presenting concerns, and that they should integrate harm reduction strategies into their treatment, which Nubay was open to doing.

In therapy, to help reduce her alcohol intake, her therapist provided psychoeducation on standardized drinks and "high-risk drinking." Nubay was surprised to learn that for women, having more than three drinks in a sitting placed her in the high-risk category. Nubay was also surprised to learn that, although she was unaware of a family history of addiction, continued high-risk drinking could lead to alcohol dependence. Particularly salient to her future career and her current focus on health, she was motivated to reduce drinking after learning of the caloric count in the number of drinks she consumed (i.e., each week she consumed approximately 2,000–3,000 calories from mixed drinks). As a way to monitor her alcohol use, her therapist suggested Nubay implement the 0-1-2-3 Rule: 0 Blackouts; 1 Drink per hour; Drinking only 2 days per week; No more than 3 drinks per sitting. They discussed that this would still allow Nubay to drink socially but would reduce the likelihood of becoming intoxicated.

In therapy, Nubay explored how drinking impacted her in social situations. She connected to how pressures to be a Strong Black Woman and perfectionism contributed to her stress level and her need to unwind. She felt more outgoing, fun, and relaxed when drinking. She and her therapist identified times when Nubay felt similarly without drinking and explored ways to bring those parts of her personality to social environments when sober. They also explored other social situations in which she could feel connected without the use of alcohol. Nubay expressed interest in joining a business sorority and also began attending events sponsored by the Black

Student Association. She noted that some of the events involved alcohol, but overall, she was able to develop friendships with other women who did not engage in high-risk drinking. She also expressed a stronger sense of community in doing self-care activities with other Black women who felt similar pressures as she felt.

Within a month, Nubay expressed that it was easier for her to focus in class and complete her assignments. She felt that her mood was more stable, as she did not have to recover after a night or weekend of partying. She liked the new friendships she was developing and realized that she was okay spending less time with friends who encouraged her drinking, explaining, "I don't judge them, but I don't feel like they have my best interest at mind." She also reported working out more, which, coupled with studying, gave her an excuse not to go out since she was tired. After 10 therapy sessions, Nubay was ready to terminate. She was drinking approximately two to three days a month and having one to three drinks per sitting. She noted no blackouts, hangovers, or compromising experiences. She continued to smoke marijuana one time monthly with no noted problematic side effects. She identified warning signs that would alert her that her alcohol use was becoming problematic again and was invited to return to therapy if so needed.

REFERENCES

American Addictions Centers. (2020, July). *Addiction among African Americans.* https://sunrisehouse.com/addiction-demographics/african-americans/

American Civil Liberties Union (ACLU). (2020). *A tale of two countries: Racially targeted arrests in the era of marijuana reform.* ACLU Research Report. https://www.aclu.org/report/tale-two-countries-racially-targeted-arrests-era-marijuana-reform

American Psychiatric Association (APA). (2013). *Diagnostic and statistical manual of mental disorders, (DSM-5),* 5th ed. Arlington, VA: American Psychiatric Association

Baker, T. B., Piper, M. E., McCarthy, D. E., Majeskie, M. R., & Fiore, M. C. (2004). Addiction motivation reformulated: An affective processing model of negative reinforcement. *Psychological Review, 111*(1), 33–5.

Burlew, A. K., Montgomery, L., Kosinski, A. S., & Forcehimes, A. A. (2013). Does treatment readiness enhance the response of African American substance users to motivational enhancement therapy? *Psychology of Addictive Behaviors, 27*(3), 744–753. https://doi.org/10.1037/a0031274

Curtis-Boles, H., & Jenkins-Monroe, V. (2000). Substance abuse in African American women. *Journal of Black Psychology, 26*(4), 450–469.

Davis, T. A., Ancis, J. R., & Ashby, J. S. (2015). Therapist effects, working alliance, and African American women substance users. *Cultural Diversity and Ethnic Minority Psychology, 21*(1), 126–135. https://doi.org/10.1037/a0036944

Department of Health, Australia. (2004). *Models that help us understand AOD use in society.* https://www1.health.gov.au/internet/publications/publishing.nsf/Content/drugtreat-pubs-front5-wk-toc~drugtreat-pubs-front5-wk-secb~drugtreat-pubs-front5-wk-secb-3~drugtreat-pubs-front5-wk-secb-3-4

Desalu, J. M., Goodhines, P. A., & Park, A. (2019). Racial discrimination and alcohol use and negative drinking consequences among Black Americans: A meta-analytical review. *Addiction, 114*(6), 957–967. https://doi.org/10.1111/add.14578

Flores, P. J. (2011). *Addiction as an attachment disorder.* New York, NY: Jason Aronson.

Frontline. (2006). *Meth and the brain.* https://www.pbs.org/wgbh/pages/frontline/meth/body/methbrainnoflash.html

George, J. R., Michaels, T. I., Sevelius, J., & Williams, M. T. (2019). The psychedelic renaissance and the limitations of a White-dominant medical framework: A call for Indigenous and ethnic minority inclusion. *Journal of Psychedelic Studies, 4*(1), 4–15. https://doi.org/10.1556/2054.2019.015

Jackson, M. (1995). Afrocentric treatment of African American women and their children in a residential chemical dependency program. *Journal of Black Studies, 26*(1), 17–30.

Kaliszewski, M. (2020, February 19). *Alcohol and drug abuse among African Americans.* https://americanaddictioncenters.org/rehab-guide/addiction-statistics/african-americans

Koob, G. F., & Le Moal, M. (2008). Addiction and the brain antireward system. *Annual review of psychology, 59,* 29–53. https://doi.org/10.1146/annurev.psych.59.103006.093548

Kornfield, R. (2014). (Re)working the program: Gender and openness in Alcoholics Anonymous. *ETHOS: Journal of the Society of Psychological Anthropology, 42*(4), 415–439.

Lowinson, J. H., Ruiz, P., & Millman, R. B. (Eds.). (2004). *Substance abuse: A comprehensive textbook.* https://ebookcentral.proquest.com/lib/tcsesl/detail.action?docID=2032589

Montgomery, L., Robinson, C., Seaman, E. L., & Haeny, A. M. (2017). A scoping review and meta-analysis of psychosocial and pharmacological treatments for cannabis and tobacco use among African Americans. *Psychology of Addictive Behaviors, 31*(8), 922–943. https://doi.org/10.1037/adb0000326

National Institute on Drug Abuse (NIDA). (2020a). *The science of drug use: Talking points.* https://www.drugabuse.gov/drug-topics/criminal-justice/science-drug-use-discussion-points

National Institute on Drug Abuse (NIDA). (2020b). *Drugs, brains, and behavior: The science of addiction.* https://www.drugabuse.gov/sites/default/files/soa.pdf

Orford, J., Natera, G., Copello, A., Atkinson, C., Mora, J., Velleman, R., Crundall, I., Tiburcio, M., Templeton, L., & Walley, G. (2005). *Coping with alcohol and drug problems: The experiences of family members in three contrasting cultures.* New York, NY: Routledge.

Rollinick, S., Miller, W. R., & Butler, C. C. (2007). *Motivational interviewing in health care: Helping patients change behavior.* New York, NY: Guilford Press.

The Sentencing Project. (n.d.). *Federal crack cocaine sentencing.* https://www.sentencingproject.org/publications/federal-crack-cocaine-sentencing/

Sharp, A. (2020). *Drug withdrawal symptoms, timelines, and treatment.* American Addiction Centers. https://americanaddictioncenters.org/withdrawal-timelines-treatments

Stevens-Watkins, D., Perry, B., Harp, K. L., & Oser, C. B. (2012). Racism and illicit drug use among African American women: The protective effects of ethnic identity, affirmation, and behavior. *Journal of Black Psychology, 38*(4), 471–496. https://doi.org/10.1177/0095798412438395

Substance Abuse and Mental Health Services Administration (SAMHSA). (2013). *Substance abuse treatment: Addressing the specific needs of women. Treatment improvement protocol (tip) series, no. 51.* HHS Publication No. (SMA) 13-4426. Rockville, MD: Substance Abuse and Mental Health Services Administration.

Substance Abuse and Mental Health Services Administration (SAMHSA). (2020a, April). *The opioid crisis and the Black/African American population: An urgent issue*(Rep.).https://store.samhsa.gov/sites/default/files/SAMHSA_Digital _Download/PEP20-05-02-001_508 Final.pdf

Substance Abuse and Mental Health Services Administration (SAMHSA). (2020b). *2018 National Survey on Drug Use and Health (NSDUH): African Americans.* https://www.samhsa.gov/data/report/2018-nsduh-african-americans

Substance Abuse and Mental Health Services Administration (SAMHSA), Center for Behavioral Health Statistics and Quality. (2019). *Treatment Episode Data Set (TEDS): 2017. Admissions to and discharges from publicly-funded substance use treatment.* Rockville, MD: Substance Abuse and Mental Health Services Administration.

Tonigan, J. S., Connors, G. J., & Miller, W. R. (1998). Special populations in Alcoholics Anonymous. *Alcohol Health & Research World, 22*(4), 281–285.

Turner, W. L., & Wallace, B. (2003). African American substance use: Epidemiology, prevention, and treatment. *Violence Against Women, 9*(5), 576–589.

U.S. Sentencing Commission (USSC). (2007, May). *Report to congress: Cocaine and federal sentencing policy.*

U.S. Sentencing Commission (USSC). (2018). *2019 race of drug trafficking offenders: Fiscal Year 2018.* U.S. Sentencing Commission, 2018 Datafile, USSCFY18. https://www.ussc.gov/sites/default/files/pdf/research-and -publications/annual-reports-and-sourcebooks/2018/TableD2.pdf?_ga =2.143275509.153537049.1599965609-1189796722.1598630202)

Wagener, D. (2019). *Harm reduction.* American Addiction Centers. https:// drugabuse.com/harm-reduction/

Windsor, L. C., Jemal, A., & Alessi, E. J. (2015). Cognitive behavioral therapy: A meta-analysis of race and substance use outcomes. *Cultural Diversity and Ethnic Minority Psychology, 21*(2), 300–313.

Witkiewitz, K., Kranzler, H. R., Hallgren, K. A., O'Malley, S. S., Falk, D. E., Litten, R. Z., Hasin, D. S., Mann, K. F., & Anton, R. F. (2018). Drinking risk level reductions associated with improvements in physical health and quality of life among individuals with alcohol use disorder. *Alcoholism: Clinical and Experimental Research, 42*(12), 2453–2465.

World Health Organization (WHO). (2010). *Lexicon of alcohol and drug terms published by the World Health Organization.* https://www.who.int/substance_abuse /terminology/who_lexicon/en/

CHAPTER 7

Eating Disorders

Judi-Lee Webb
Kimber Shelton

When people think of eating disorder (ED) diagnoses and disordered eating (DE) attitudes and behaviors, they typically think of White women in Western societies. We may be more inclined to imagine emaciated bodies, and less inclined to picture women in average, athletic, larger, or Black bodies. Furthermore, as noted by Claire Mysko, CEO of the National Eating Disorders Association (NEDA), ED research primarily focuses on young, White, affluent, heterosexual females (Beebe, 2018); thus, treatment and interventions are developed with this population in mind. Beyond systemic issues associated with ED research, diagnosis and treatment, and the myth that EDs are primarily created by body image issues, Black women contend with the added layer of cultural stigma associated with mental health issues and the misperception that women of color do not experience EDs.

Some research studies support Black women being less susceptible to EDs. The assumptions are that Black cultures tend to embrace a broader, more flexible definition of beauty; larger, curvier bodies; and strength in ethnic identity, therefore providing protection from EDs (Talleyrand, 2012). However, EDs and DE do not discriminate. They can affect anyone regardless of race, ethnicity, age, gender, culture, sexual orientation, religion, size, and socioeconomic status. Recent studies show that EDs have become a major health issue for Black women (Ross, 2019; Shuttlesworth & Zotter, 2011). There is increasing evidence that the prevalence rates of EDs among women of color, including Black women, are similar to those found among White Americans (Gilbert et al, 2009; Talleyrand, 2012). In a study researching the prevalence of EDs among Black individuals, Taylor et al. (2007) report that African Americans may be more at risk for anorexia nervosa than Black people of Caribbean descent. Researchers further noted that, although anorexia nervosa is uncommon among African Americans, the age of onset (14.89 years) for this particular ED in African Americans was lower than the age of onset for the general U.S. population (18.9 years). Furthermore, Black women who experience anorexia have a longer battle with the disorder (Taylor et al., 2007).

Although some studies indicate that anorexia nervosa and bulimia nervosa are less common among Black women in comparison to other ethnic groups, binge eating occurs at higher rates (Ross, 2019; Shuttlesworth & Zotter, 2011; Talleyrand, 2012; Taylor et al., 2007). In fact, the National Survey of American Life report indicates binge eating was the most prevalent ED among Black Americans (Taylor et al., 2007). Shuttlesworth and Zotter (2011) add that some research suggests Black women with strong ethnic identities may engage in DE to obtain the fuller-figured ideal of feminine beauty that is supported in Black cultures. However, binge eating has been linked to obesity, which may play a role in the high levels of excess weight or obesity among African American women (Talleyrand, 2012).

EATING DISORDER DIAGNOSES AND DISORDERED EATING

Eating Disorder Diagnoses

As per the *Diagnostic and Statistical Manual of Mental Disorders*, 5 (DSM-5, 2013), eating and feeding disorders include eight diagnoses. They are characterized by persistent disturbance of eating or eating-related behavior that significantly impairs physical health or psychosocial functioning and must meet certain criteria such as frequency and duration. The following are brief descriptions of each diagnosis. Please refer to the DSM-5 for specific diagnostic criteria.

Anorexia Nervosa

- Significantly low body weight
- An intense fear of gaining weight or becoming fat
- Restriction of food intake
- Behaviors that interfere with weight gain
- Disturbance in self-perceived weight or shape

Binge-Eating Disorder

- Recurrent episodes of eating that includes eating in a discrete period of time (e.g., within any two-hour period) an amount of food that is larger than what most people would eat in a similar period of time under similar circumstances
- Eating large amounts of food when not feeling physically hungry

- Eating much more rapidly than normal
- Eating until feeling uncomfortably full
- A sense of lack of control over eating during the binge episode
- Feeling disgusted with oneself, depressed, or very guilty afterward
- Eating alone due to embarrassment of how much one is eating

Bulimia Nervosa

- Recurrent binge eating episodes
- Use of inappropriate compensatory behaviors to prevent weight gain such as vomiting; misuse of laxatives, diuretics, or other medications; fasting; or excessive exercise
- A sense of lack of control over eating during the binge episode

Avoidant/Restrictive Food Intake Disorder (ARFID)

- A lack of interest in eating or food
- The avoidance of food is based on the sensory characteristic of food or concern about an aversive consequence of eating, such as choking, vomiting, or an allergic reaction.
- The individual fails to meet appropriate nutritional and/or energy needs that may result in weight loss, failure to gain the appropriate amount of weight, or faltering growth in children.

Rumination Disorder

- Repeated regurgitation of food over the period of at least one month
- The regurgitation behavior is not attributable to an associated gastrointestinal or other medical condition.

Pica

- Persistent and compulsive eating of nonnutritive, nonfood substances over a period of at least one month (e.g., paper, soap, cloth, hair, paint, ice)
- The behavior is inappropriate to the developmental level of the individual; not a part of a culturally supported or socially normative practice.

Other Specified Feeding or Eating Disorder (OSFED)

- Applies to symptoms of feeding and EDs that do not meet the full criteria of any specific feeding or ED
- The diagnosis of OSFED is also used to diagnose night eating syndrome that involves recurrent episodes of eating after awakening from sleep or by excessive food consumption after the evening meal.

Unspecified Feeding or Eating Disorder

- Used when the full criteria have not been met or the clinician chooses not to specify the reason that the criteria are not met (e.g., insufficient information).

Disordered Eating

According to NEDA (2018b), DE behaviors may include similar behaviors and symptoms of diagnosable EDs, but at a lesser frequency or lower level of severity. However, DE can be problematic and may develop into an ED. Like EDs, DE patterns can affect an individual's level of functioning including their social and family lives and is used to cope with aversive emotions such as stress, anxiety, and depression.

There are several common DE behaviors and negative body image behaviors that are not clinical diagnoses, but can lead to significant psychological, emotional, physical, and medical problems if not appropriately addressed. According to NEDA (2018b), common terms include:

- Emotional eating—using food in response to emotions, including positive and negative emotions.
- Compulsive overeating—involves eating behaviors that feel out of control such as eating past satiety, impulsive eating, and night eating, and/or compulsive behaviors such as hiding food or eating food out of the garbage.
- Dieting—rigid eating practices that restrict one to small amounts of food or specific foods in order to lose weight.
- Food restriction—eating fewer calories than the body needs to maintain weight and/or adequate growth, or eliminating/minimizing certain types of food (e.g., meat, sugar, or dairy) for the purpose of altering one's weight, body, or size.
- Diabulimia—insulin-dependent diabetics may restrict or omit insulin in order to lose weight or purge calories.
- Drunkorexia—modifying eating behaviors to either offset the calories consumed from alcohol or to increase/speed the effects of alcohol.
- Pregorexia—pregnant women who are obsessed with and fearful of weight gain and engage in unhealthy behaviors such as restrictive eating, dieting, binge eating, and/or purging behaviors.
- Orthorexia—an obsession with proper, "healthy," or "clean" eating that involves a preoccupation with the quality and purity of the food one consumes.
- Food rituals—obsessive, rigid, compulsive ways in which a person interacts with food that produces anxiety when not followed.
- Body checking—obsessive, intrusive thoughts, and behaviors about body shape and size that can involve repeatedly checking one's

appearance in the mirror, checking the size and appearance of certain body parts, and/or asking others how you look.

- Fear foods—foods a person believes will lead to weight gain, even in small amounts.
- Safe foods—foods that are generally low calorie and less anxiety-provoking.

RISK FACTORS ASSOCIATED WITH BLACK WOMEN

Approximately 13 percent of women experience an ED (Dakanalis et al., 2017), of which 80 percent never receive treatment (Swanson et al., 2011). According to the NEDA (2021), risk factors for all eating disorders involve various biological, psychological, and sociocultural issues. Biological issues may include having a close relative with an eating disorder or mental health condition, a history of dieting behaviors, and Type 1 (insulin-dependent) diabetes. Psychological factors may include personality traits such as perfectionism, body image dissatisfaction, a history of an anxiety disorder, and behavioral inflexibility. Lastly, sociocultural factors may include weight stigma, bullying, internalization of the "ideal" image, acculturation, isolation and loneliness, and historical trauma (NEDA, 2021).

Furthermore, theories purport that girls and women coming from domineering families, feeling as though they have little control over their lives, and/or those with body shame and body self-objectification (internalized socially conditioned sexualizing and objectifying of thin bodies) (Fredrickson & Roberts, 1997), are the most susceptible to developing problematic eating issues. However, these markers may not fully capture the unique experiences of Black women with EDs. These models do not assess or account for the impact of gendered racism and other societal oppression on eating patterns of Black women.

Stress and Strong Black Woman Ideology

EDs and DE patterns are not about food; they are about the underlying emotional or psychological distress one is experiencing (Ross, 2019). Therefore, one's ability to manage stress can have a significant impact on their relationship with food, their bodies, as well as their eating patterns (i.e., unhealthy coping through emotional eating). Stress associated with traditional risk factors of EDs, such as the drive for thinness, body dissatisfaction, and dietary restraint, may not be applicable when understanding, assessing, treating, and preventing EDs among Black women.

Stress comes from a variety of sources including, but not limited to, one's personal life, family, work life, health issues, financial concerns, community, and society. In addition to the stressful life events and daily hassles that people face on a regular basis, for decades the Black community, particularly women, have been plagued with negative body image issues related to skin tone, hair texture and style, facial features, eye color, and body shape (see Chapters 10 and 15). Additional factors creating feelings of inferiority and damaging self-esteem include discrimination (including racial, gender, and wage), heterosexism, trauma, acculturative stress, segregation, forced assimilation, microaggressions, sexual harassment, poverty, and systemic oppression (Holder, Jackson, & Potteronto, 2015; see Chapters 4 and 11). These issues can factor into engaging in maladaptive eating behaviors and EDs to manage negative emotions.

Internalizing the Strong Black Woman (SBW) archetype can also impact the stress experience of Black women. On the one hand, the SBW ideal encompasses attributes such as pride, determination, self-efficacy in the face of challenges, resilience, self-reliance, and self-containment. Harrington, Crowther, and Harrington (2010) explain that the symbol of an SBW originated as a rationalization/justification for slavery because Black women were touted as physically and psychologically stronger and more resilient than White women. Over time, this image was adopted within Black communities in response to derogatory images of Black womanhood (Harrington et al., 2010). As a result of the SBW ideal, Black women have defined themselves in a positive light.

On the other hand, as a component of the SBW schema, Black women experience pressure to perform multiple roles at the same time including mother, wife, career woman, homemaker, nurturer, and caretaker without relying on help from others. Ross (2019) states that the SBW may feel responsible for the larger Black community, and may take on a dominant role in intimate relationships, be a single mother, and feel a responsibility to meet everyone else's needs before her own. There is an expectation to be perfect without showing signs of weakness or vulnerability.

Due to the SBW schema, some women may not feel they have permission to feel stress or show they are struggling. This can lead to experiencing negative physical and psychological symptoms. If these symptoms are not managed appropriately and the individual does not have healthy coping skills, significant medical and emotional issues can arise, including EDs. Harrington, Crowther, and Harrington (2010) emphasize that the ideal/excessive form of the SBW image may be especially problematic for women prone to using food as self-medication or a coping mechanism. Therefore, it is important that Black women are given permission to express negative emotions and vulnerabilities and develop healthy coping mechanisms to manage distress.

Gendered Racism

Another risk factor for the development of EDs in women of color is feeling marginalized and powerless in society, which is created by simultaneous membership in two oppressed demographic identity groups—race and gender (Harrington et al., 2006; Talleyrand, 2012). Harrington et al. (2006) explain that EDs in women of color are viewed as a form of internalized oppression and note a significant relationship between discriminatory stress and binge eating in Black women. Feeling powerless and a lack of control could drive women of color to use food (e.g., restrictive eating, binge eating, purging) to cope with feelings of internalized racism or to reject the Westernized White culture's standard of beauty (Kempa & Thomas, 2000; Talleyrand, 2012).

Gendered racism undoubtedly impacts the socioeconomic position of Black women. Gendered racism resulting in classism provides Black women with less access to resources and positions of power and authority than White men and women and their Black male counterparts. Although educational attainment of Black women has surged in the last two decades (U.S. Census Bureau, 2018), Black women remain disproportionately impacted by poverty and are at greater risk of experiencing health concerns related to not having access to economic resources (Talleyrand, 2006).

Some findings have suggested middle-class Black women who adopt White middle-class values have a higher risk of developing anorexia nervosa and bulimia nervosa (Talleyrand, 2006). There has also been evidence that some Black women who experience poverty-related stress use emotional overeating or binge-eating behaviors to cope, whereas others may suffer from malnutrition or food intake high in fat and sugars. Thus, it is important to explore how one identifies their socioeconomic status and how it may affect their eating habits (Talleyrand, 2006).

Acculturative Stress and Ethnic Identity

As numerical and sociocultural minorities, Black women's experience of acculturative stress may be more aligned with traditional motivating factors of EDs that are connected to body dissatisfaction. Ross, Gipson-Jones, and Davis (2018) describe acculturative stress as "the pressure to adapt or adopt the dominant culture's values and beliefs along with difficulties that manifest while adjusting to a different culture" (69). In this process of acculturation, Black women may adopt Westernized (and White) cultural norms values, behaviors, and beliefs related to beauty, health, and lifestyle practices (Talleyrand, 2012). For example, studies have found African American women who internalize the Western standards of beauty and are less affirming of their own ethnicity endorse more ED symptoms (Talleyrand, 2012; Watson et al., 2013).

Acculturative stress presents significant psychological and physical challenges (Talleyrand, 2006). It has been found to cause psychological illnesses such as depression, substance abuse, and EDs, which can also lead to physical disturbances such as cardiovascular disease, obesity, and other stress-related illness (Ross, Gipson-Jones, & Davis, 2018). Kroon Van Diest et al. (2014) add that acculturative stress is also associated with anxiety, substance abuse, and suicide.

Black women with an affirming and accepting view of their ethnic identity and who ascribe to norms within Black cultures (i.e., enculturation) tend to be more satisfied with their body image and report fewer eating disturbances (Watson et al. 2013); typically reporting less acculturative-related stress. Some research suggests positive and affirming racial and ethnic identities buffer against body image and DE issues (Watson et al., 2013; Zhang, Dixon, & Conrad, 2009). Ross et al. (2018) explain the "buffering hypothesis" proposes Black women have decreased weight consciousness, increased body acceptance, and suppressed weight loss goals as a protective mechanism against the White culture's standard of beauty. Shuttlesworth and Zotter (2011) found that, compared to White women, African American women who were more accepting, affirming, and strongly identified with their ethnic identity had lower rates of anorexic behaviors, binge eating, and bulimia.

Of note, research on the correlation between acculturation and the prevalence of EDs and ethnic identity buffering has yielded inconsistent results. Despite differing cultural values with White Americans, particularly those who ascribe high value to Afrocentrism (Kroon Van Diest et al., 2014), Black Americans are not regularly included in acculturation/ED research as they are not considered immigrants. Furthermore, the buffering effect has not been shown to be protective of binge-eating behaviors. On the contrary, Black women acculturated to Black American cultures may experience higher levels of binge-eating behaviors since this way of coping with emotions is somewhat acceptable within the Black community and does not typically violate the cultural standards of beauty (i.e., curvaceous body type).

Trauma

Trauma is defined as a deeply distressing or disturbing experience such as abuse, bodily injury or threat, or exposure to a traumatic event (American Psychiatric Association, 2020). Trauma is typically accompanied by negative emotions such as fear, helplessness, and horror, in addition to symptoms of post-traumatic stress disorder (PTSD), depression, anxiety, substance abuse, and eating problems. Therefore, trauma survivors may have difficulty managing and regulating their emotions (Harrington, Crowther, & Shipherd, 2010). Exposure to trauma or experiencing a traumatic event has been implicated in the development of EDs (Harrington et al., 2006). Ross (2019) explains that the hypervigilance traumatized people experience causes continual feelings of tension and discomfort. This often leads to self-soothing behaviors such as binge eating and emotional eating, particularly among Black women. Binge eating in trauma survivors has been conceptualized as a maladaptive behavior for regulating negative emotions through distraction, avoiding emotional distress, or escaping trauma reminders (Harrington et al., 2010).

Ross (2019) explains that stress and trauma can cause neurological changes in the brain that increase the risk of binge eating and compulsive overeating. Specifically, cortisol and adrenaline released as part of the stress response interferes with the development of certain parts of the brain, especially areas associated with judgment and impulse control (Ross, 2019). In addition, prenatal stress and early life stress can increase the risk of developing an ED, obesity, addiction issues, mood disorders, impulsivity, and compulsivity, as this can result in difficulty managing distress and regulating emotions later in life (Ross, 2019). Women embodying the SBW image may hold more rigidly to these ideals following trauma and use binge eating to regulate emotions, particularly since this form of self-soothing behavior is socially sanctioned (or, at least, not culturally prohibited) in Black cultures (Harrington et al., 2010).

MEDICAL COMPLICATIONS AND COMORBIDITY

EDs are serious conditions that can have profound mental and medical impacts, including death. In fact, anorexia nervosa has the highest mortality rate of any psychiatric disorder due to the medical complications that typically develop and the prevalence of death by suicide (Arcelus et al., 2011). In addition, individuals with EDs can also suffer from a life-threatening condition called refeeding syndrome. Refeeding syndrome occurs in significantly malnourished individuals during the early phase of the nutritional replenishment. As a result of the significant weight loss, the heart can be adversely affected; therefore, heart failure can result during the refeeding process. In addition, changes in serum levels of phosphorus, magnesium, and potassium can also complicate this process. Therefore, it is imperative that individuals at risk for refeeding syndrome be admitted to a hospital and treated by medical professionals trained in ED treatment (Mehler & Anderson, 2010).

Medical complications are primarily due to the behaviors associated with particular EDs such as food restriction, malnutrition, and purging behaviors (i.e., vomiting, laxative and diuretic abuse, and excessive exercise). These complications include, but are not limited to: electrolyte abnormalities, gastrointestinal symptoms, gynecological and obstetric changes such as infertility and complications during pregnancy, neurological problems, cardiac symptoms, endocrine abnormalities, hematological indicators, renal complications, opportunistic infections, dental/oral problems, dermatological issues, problems with bone mass, and refeeding syndrome (APA, 2011).

In addition to medical complications, EDs and DE behaviors can also involve psychological, emotional, social, behavioral, and spiritual problems. They can affect multiple facets of one's life including family relationships, friendships, and work relationships. Other psychiatric disorders typically accompanying EDs include depression, bipolar disorder, dysthymia, anxiety disorders, obsessive-compulsive disorder, PTSD, alcohol and other substance abuse, and personality disorders. According to NEDA (2018a), these co-occurring mental health diagnoses can begin around the same time as an ED, precede it, or emerge after the ED has begun. In addition, some mental health issues, including genetic predispositions, can be risk factors for EDs, indicating a person may be more likely to develop an ED (NEDA, 2018a). Harrington et al. (2006) also found a significant relationship between discriminatory stress and binge eating among African American women, which is consistent with the growing body of research connecting racism to a host of adverse physical and mental health outcomes such as hypertension, depression, anxiety, feelings of inadequacy, and low self-esteem.

TREATMENT CONSIDERATIONS AND RECOMMENDATIONS

Clinician Competence

Despite the risks of EDs, the great news is that EDs are treatable. Reviews of evidence-based clinical treatment guidelines for EDs validate treatment of EDs (Hilbert, Hoek, & Schmidt, 2017). The American Psychiatric Association (APA) Practice Guideline for the Treatment of Patients with Eating Disorders (2006; 2011) suggests:

(a) Psychiatric Management—Coordinating care and collaboration with other clinicians, Assessing and monitoring ED symptoms and behaviors, Assessing and monitoring the patient's general medical condition, Assessing and monitoring the patient's safety and psychiatric status, and Providing family assessment and treatment.
(b) Choosing a Treatment Site—Outpatient, Intensive Outpatient, Partial Hospitalization, Residential care or Inpatient Hospitalization.
(c) Choice of Specific Treatments for Anorexia, Bulimia, Binge Eating, and other eating disorders—Nutritional rehabilitation, Psychosocial interventions, and Medications and other somatic treatments.

Given these guidelines, proficient practice with EDs would include an understanding of EDs and DE diagnosis and symptoms, clinical assessment skills, assessment and treatment of comorbid disorders, and skill in evidence-based practices such as cognitive behavioral therapy (CBT).

Despite existing guidelines, clinicians remain ill prepared in treating Black women with EDs. According to NEDA (2018c), when presented with identical case studies, treatment professionals were less likely to identify if an African American woman's eating behavior was problematic. In general, there is little information on the inclusion of cultural diversity within ED guidelines, with APA treatment guidelines being no exception. These guidelines provide no specific details on the treatment of Black women; however, they note the importance of building a therapeutic rapport with the client and broadly suggest that clinicians lead informed and sensitive discussions on struggles, experiences, and perceptions of attractiveness and body satisfaction; weight and shape concerns; and assimilation experiences when working with cultural minorities. Clinicians must be trained and prepared to recognize and treat populations that are often considered to be least likely to develop EDs (Taylor et al., 2007). As such, integration of multicultural counseling competences (MCC) (Sue, Arredondo, & McDavis, 1992) can be utilized as a starting point in culturally competent practice with Black women.

Multicultural Counseling Competence Principles—Eating Disorders & Disorder Eating:

1. Clinician Self-Awareness
   - Awareness into one's own view of healthy and problematic eating behaviors.
   - Address own expectations about eating and thinness (Henrickson, Crowder, & Harrington, 2010).
   - Insight and challenging biases related to Black women bodies.
2. Knowledge
   - Knowledge of treatment and recovery barriers and exploring strategies for reducing or removing said barriers.
   - Intersectional understanding of the impact race, ethnicity, gender, and sex (as well as additional variables such as economic status and sexual orientation) have on the development, presentation, maintenance, treatment, and recovery experience.
   - Recognition of issues of stress-related factors, family and culture of origin issues, emotion regulation, distress tolerance, appropriate expression of aversive emotions, and healthy coping among Black women.
3. Skill
   - Identifying and combating treatment barriers (i.e., internalized stigma and external advocacy efforts).
   - Utilization assessment procedures that capture the ED experiences of Black women.
   - Using or developing culturally adaptive assessment and treatment interventions inclusive of nuanced experiences of Black women.

Assessment

EDs are not about the food; they are about emotions and the strategies people use to manage negative emotions. As previously discussed, the traditional risk factors and symptoms associated with assessing and diagnosing EDs may not be appropriate for African American women. Furthermore, inadequate assessment can result in misdiagnoses such as weight management issues or metabolic conditions (diabetes). According to Dr. Charlynn Small, a member of the International Association of Eating Disorder Professionals Board of Directors, misdiagnosis of EDs occurs as a result of practitioner fear of having difficult conversations related to the correlation of systemic oppression on Black women's overall health (Veritas Collaborative, 2020). Having honest conversations about the lived experiences of Black women can shine light on problematic eating behaviors connected to social oppression.

These difficult and honest conversations would incorporate the unique sociocultural experiences of Black women, and an understanding of how each woman's level of acculturation to her culture of origin or the dominant culture influences her beliefs regarding food and physical appearance is also necessary (Talleyrand, 2006). The worldview, values, belief systems, and assimilation of the client needs to be understood as well as the effects of oppression, racial identity, and ethnic identity on the client (Kempa & Thomas, 2000). Additionally, clinicians should also explore and address stress from identity-based discrimination and trauma. Ross (2019) encourages clinicians to conceptualize EDs as a strategy for coping with stress, anxiety, depression, and trauma, rather than as a preoccupation with appearance. Therefore, in addition to obtaining a thorough individual, family, and cultural history, it is imperative to explore all forms of stressful and traumatic events the individual has faced in their past, present, and daily lives. Assessing Adverse Childhood Experiences (ACEs) is also highly recommended since these experiences have been linked to risky health behaviors and chronic health conditions. Lastly, assessing the degrees of racial and gender oppression and the unhealthy coping mechanisms used will help the clinician develop an appropriate treatment plan.

Commonly used ED assessment measures may not capture the full presentation of DE of Black women as they are not normed on this population. Cultural genograms may be more effective in identifying and processing individual and family-related coping strategies and competing cultural demands. A cultural genogram could potentially help clients uncover the messages related to the role of food and eating behaviors and attitudes, body image, and overall appearance that have been passed down from family members. Racial identity assessment measures may also provide insight into acculturation level and perception of food and body. The use of the Minority Identity Development model is encouraged for use in the assessment phase of ED treatment for Black women (Kempa & Thomas, 2000; Talleyrand, 2012). This allows clinicians to have the necessary understanding of a client's stage of ethnocultural identity using vetted models (Harris & Kuba, 1997). It may also be helpful if clinicians ask questions related to the client's culture, spirituality, and religious practices and how these factors impact their relationship with food and their bodies. Post hospitalization, Harris and Kuba (1997) explain that understanding food and food patterns in the client's family, community, and culture is important and should be incorporated into treatment modalities as it will prepare the client for her return home. Questions surrounding family roles, expectations, and messages about beauty and physical features could also be helpful in assessing ethnic identity (Kempa & Thomas, 2000). A combination of commonly used assessment measures, a cultural genogram, racial and ethnic identity measures, an understanding of food patterns, and questions related to culture, spirituality, and religious practices will yield a more comprehensive assessment.

Levels of Care and Treatment Considerations

Levels of Care. APA Guidelines (2011) and directives specific to Black women (Ross, 2019) support use of integrative medicine and multidisciplinary treatment teams in EDs recovery work. Given the complexity and interconnection of factors, the treatment team can include a therapist, physician, registered dietitian, and a psychiatrist as well as other professionals if needed. As a member of the treatment team, providing psychological and psychoeducational resources to family members can help support Black women's recovery. Harris and Kuba (1997) emphasize the importance of role models in the recovery process. They explain that having women and men of color as part of the treatment team may help in creating cultural acceptance and sensitivity. This also includes addressing ethnocultural differences among staff members and an understanding of the roles staff carry in the lives of the women in treatment.

EDs are complex illnesses that vary in the level of intervention needed. As per the Guidelines (APA, 2011), non-physician providers are significant in the management and treatment of EDs; however, certain conditions and symptoms would require specific medical interventions provided by medical health professionals. The level of care recommended to those struggling with DE and EDs is determined by the degree of their psychological and medical state based on a comprehensive evaluation. Levels of care include outpatient treatment, intensive outpatient programs (IOP), partial hospitalization programs (PHP), residential programs, and inpatient hospitalization treatment. Outpatient care may include individual, couples, family, and/or group counseling, with mental health professionals and services provided by a registered dietitian, physician(s), and a psychiatrist. IOP and PHP provide treatment two or more times a week for multiple hours each day (frequency and length of treatment is more intensive for PHP). IOP and PHP treatment may involve individual, couples, family, and group counseling; nutrition counseling (i.e., weight restoration, normalize eating patterns, behavioral weight management options); and medical support including a psychiatrist, physician, and/or nurse.

Residential treatment includes support 24 hours a day and seven days a week. Treatment may include individual, family, couples and group therapy along with nutrition, medical, and psychiatric support. Hospitalization, the most intensive treatment, is utilized to treat individuals at risk for serious health consequences and death related to their EDs. As well as treatment options provided at lower levels of care, hospitalization includes many medical-based interventions such as monitoring of vital, electrolytes, and cardiac conditions; addressing gastrointestinal issues; restrictions on compulsory behaviors such as purging through vomiting and exercise; restoration of bone mineral density; and addressing any suicidality. In addition to medical and nutritional stability in a hospital setting, individual, family, couples, and group counseling may be utilized along with psychiatric care. In conjunction with the aforementioned treatment team members and therapies, adjunctive therapies such as exercise physiology, physical therapy, experiential therapies, occupational and activities therapies, educational activities, and support groups may be utilized to support the client during various phases of the recovery process (Mehler & Anderson, 2010).

In demystifying the treatment process, Black women need to be included in conversations regarding treatment options. People of color, including Black women operating from the SBW archetype, are significantly less likely to receive help for their eating issues (Becker et al., 2003; Marques et al., 2011). Psychoeducation regarding treatment levels and what to expect in treatment can increase buy-in in assessing care. Given the prevalence of cultural incompetence that continues in ED care, conversations and preparation for treatment can help Black women to advocate for their needs within differing treatment levels.

The costs associated with treatment may also impact the level of care and can serve as a barrier or stressor for individuals and families. Fortunately, many ED treatment centers and clinicians accept various insurance plans. Those without insurance or the financial ability to pay for treatment may qualify for reduced-fee services. Some treatment centers even collaborate with nonprofit organizations to help sponsor treatment services. Some programs and professionals are also able to advocate on behalf of the client in an effort to request extended treatment from insurance companies as well as a "single case agreement" where the insurance company agrees to consider the treatment services as in-network rather than out-of-network. If outpatient services are appropriate, group therapy as well as support groups also provide low-cost or free services for those in need.

Therapy Models. There are several treatment modalities and therapies used to treat EDs. These include nontraditional approaches such as yoga, meditation, and dance to increase awareness of mind-body connections and emotional states (Watson et al., 2013) as well as traditional therapy approaches, including acceptance and commitment therapy (ACT), CBT, dialectical behavioral therapy (DBT), interpersonal therapy (IPT), and family-based treatment (FBT). CBT and IPT are discussed in further detail below.

CBT, an evidence-based approach, has been found to be effective in treating DE (APA, 2011). It may be particularly effective when working with women of color because of its emphasis on a solution-focused, time-limited approach; educational and practical focus; and use of homework. This approach may need to be adapted to include an exploration of the relevant contextual factors and cultural values in understanding how a client perceives her problem (e.g., body satisfaction for African American women may include facial features, skin color, and hair in addition to other body parts) (Talleyrand, 2012).

IPT is an evidence-based therapy that is time-limited and semi-structured. IPT focuses on assisting the client to identify and cope with interpersonal difficulties they face in their lives, rather than focusing specifically on their DE thoughts and behaviors (Choate, 2010). As previously discussed, African American women face multiple life stressors due to the intersecting marginalized identities they hold. This could impact their interpersonal relationships. The use of IPT can provide the contextual framework necessary in understanding DE attitudes and behaviors (Talleyrand, 2012). IPT can be used to help women who have been focusing on trying to control their weight and shape recognize that interpersonal difficulties may be the root of their DE thoughts and behaviors. By taking the emphasis off the ED symptoms and behaviors, clients can explore the underlying problems that are driving their ED. Best practices also indicate that IPT for bulimia nervosa is beneficial for those who are reluctant to engage in CBT (Choate, 2010).

Clinicians are advised to collaboratively discuss the benefits of acceptance and positive identification with one's cultural group(s) as well as discussing the role of internalized oppression, challenging their clients to consider how they may have internalized the dominant culture's values and beauty standards. This might involve clinicians educating their clients on how these objectifying experiences may negatively alter their relationship with their bodies and teaching them empowering coping skills to use when faced with these experiences and the ability to discern identity-based oppressive acts for what they are without internalizing these experiences (Watson et al., 2013). These culturally adaptive strategies fit well in the purview of either CBT or IPT.

Williams, Frame, and Green (1999) explain that group counseling may be another effective model when working with women of color because of the nature of the experience, since group counseling can create close relationships among group members and a sense of community. The emphasis on close relationships and community is consistent with the collectivistic values embedded in African American cultures, and it may feel less threatening than individual therapy (Talleyrand, 2012). Reducing isolation and providing connections with other women who can help each other confront conflicting cultural standards that contribute to internalized oppression can be rewarding for women of color. Kroon Van Diest et al. (2014) add that treatments that are designed to reduce acculturative stress and increase social support may increase overall treatment effects, producing greater reduction in ED symptoms. In addition, the empowering and egalitarian nature of the group counseling process may be appealing to women of color, who tend to face several forms of oppression (Talleyrand, 2012).

Honoring and respecting the client's community and culture are vital to effective therapeutic treatment. Harris and Kuba (1997) emphasize the involvement of the individual, family, and community in the treatment process. Family therapy is typically utilized in treating EDs because it oftentimes involves family relational problems that may contribute to the development of an ED (Talleyrand 2012). In addition, participation in family therapy can provide education for the family members as well as provide a supportive family unit to assist the client throughout the recovery process. Family therapy can extend beyond the immediate family, particularly if the immediate family is not emotionally available or is dysfunctional. This can also include clergy and other members of the client's community. Based on the strong value placed on family in African American culture, family therapy may be an effective and culturally relevant form of therapy, and it may also create a sense of unity among family members and the mental health provider and allow the provider to learn more about specific cultural values in the family that could potentially contribute to the development of EDs (Talleyrand, 2012).

In addition to aforementioned counseling theories and approaches, Ross (2019) suggests five levels of change to help African American women heal from DE:

Level 1: Let go of superficial behaviors such as dieting, restrictive eating, and obsessing about food as these behaviors distract from the underlying emotional issues.

Level 2: Building new ways of coping with stress that better acknowledge and address the painful emotions sustaining the ED.

Level 3: Develop body awareness of one's body, reconnect with sensations, and view the body as a source of wisdom.

Level 4: Eliminate destructive core beliefs and cultivating new beliefs that are functional and rational.

Level 5: Discover healthy ways to satisfy the profound human need for authenticity and meaning as these experiences are essential to a good life and serve as natural, positive reinforcers to help heal the brain's reward system. This involves satisfying the soul rather than the scale (paragraph 18).

CASE STUDY

Zoe* is a Caribbean Black woman in her fifties. Her parents are Jamaican, and she was born in the United Kingdom (UK). Zoe migrated to the United States with her parents when she was an adolescent. She described this transition as "abrupt and traumatic," given the significant cultural differences and because her mother made the decision to move without input from Zoe, her father, and siblings. Zoe described her mother as an authoritarian person and therefore typically did not seek feedback from others. Since her siblings were older, Zoe was the only child who migrated with her parents. Soon after settling in the United States, her mother returned to the United Kingdom, leaving Zoe and her father with a relative. She shared that this relative was emotionally and verbally abusive, making her new life in the United States very daunting and depressing. Her mother's departure led to feelings of abandonment and the need to be a "responsible adult at an early age." Zoe added that her mother's decision to return to the United Kingdom and leave her with an abusive relative was re-traumatizing.

Zoe earned her undergraduate degree at a historically Black college in the South. This experience was another culture shock given that she was raised in predominately White communities and experienced European colonial racial issues, which were different from racial issues prevalent in the South. This was also when Zoe became more aware of her racial and ethnic identities. She shared that at times, she was teased for having an accent, and some people continue to make negative statements about her accent, including current colleagues.

After graduation, Zoe moved to Atlanta and started her career. Soon thereafter, her mother returned to the United States and settled in Atlanta as well. Sadly, her father passed away while Zoe was in college. She described her relationship with her mother at that time as "volatile," which led to feelings of anger. However, today she reports having a better relationship with her mother, attributing this to being more assertive with her mom and feeling more comfortable with using her voice.

During the initial evaluation, Zoe shared that she has been experiencing distress due to racial and gender biases in her industry and work setting. She explained she is oftentimes the only Black female in the room, which is usually dominated by White males. She shared several microaggressions made by colleagues and supervisors over the years. Zoe described herself as having a very strong work ethic due to her family of origin and her Jamaican heritage. She also admitted to struggling with the "Strong Black Woman" ideology. Although she feels accomplished and successful, she began to question her career path and sought counseling to address these issues and to explore how she can feel more fulfilled and happier within her career and personal life.

---

* Identifying information has been altered to protect this client's confidentiality.

Zoe also revealed her unhealthy relationship with food and her body. She reported that throughout her childhood she was given the message by her mother that she "must eat." She explained that her mother displayed love and affection through food rather than physical and verbal affection, and her family viewed having access to a large amount of food as a symbol of wealth and abundance. Interestingly, when Zoe began to gain weight, her mother made negative comments, suggesting she should lose weight. She reported receiving many mixed messages about food and her body for years, including while she was an athlete.

Zoe shared that she engaged in binge-eating episodes throughout her adult life. She acknowledged she rapidly ate large amounts of food until she was uncomfortably full. At times, she would eat in response to an aversive emotion even though she wasn't hungry. This then led to feelings of guilt and shame. Her poor body image resulted in excessive exercising and frequent dieting. She shared that these behaviors intensified when she felt she needed to look a certain way for an important life event. This created a cycle of unhealthy eating and exercise patterns mixed with negative emotions.

Zoe has responded well to outpatient individual therapy. Therapy began with building rapport, safety, trust, and collaboration. Utilizing mainly CBT and IPT, she has been able to challenge her dysfunctional/ unhealthy thoughts and recognize interpersonal difficulties in the workplace and her personal life, addressing them with healthier coping and communication skills. By restructuring her cognitions, Zoe developed rational/healthy thoughts that help her externalize the chaos of gendered racism in her workplace and manage her negative emotions in a healthy way without dishonoring herself and her body.

Through discussions on the impact colonization has on the bodies of Black women, Zoe works to deconstruct narratives that do not support her health. She has embraced a healthier perspective of nutrition and exercise and is now able to listen to her body and treat it with the respect she and her body deserve. She now appreciates a variety of exercise activities including those that are not excessive. Additionally, Zoe joined a support group with other women of color from the United Kingdom as well as a professional group with women within her industry. She has normalized her eating by listening to her body's internal cues, which has allowed her body to stabilize at its natural weight. She has worked hard to accept her body in its natural state; the state it is when she is truly honoring herself, nourishing her body, and engaging in a variety of physical movements and exercises, including gentle movements.

Zoe has also learned how to tolerate distress and manage her emotions with healthier coping skills. In fact, she reported she has been allowing herself to relax more and engage in activities she had previously neglected, such as reading and spending time outdoors. As a result, Zoe has also been able to confront the Strong Black Woman ideology by no longer prioritizing achievement and career success; instead, she prioritizes her emotional and physical well-being and allows herself to be vulnerable.

Zoe has cultivated environments of acceptance for herself in the workplace, with her mother, as well as within her body. She has developed more compassion and grace for herself and her body and as a result improved her relationship with food and exercise and enhanced interpersonal skills and coping mechanisms. She has freed herself from the diet mentality and expectations set by others and society. The skills Zoe is learning in therapy can be used throughout her life and in various areas of her life.

REFERENCES

American Psychiatric Association (APA). (2011). *Treating eating disorders: A quick reference guide.* https://psychiatryonline.org/pb/assets/raw/sitewide/practice_guidelines/guidelines/eatingdisorders-guide.pdf

American Psychiatric Association (APA). (2013). *Diagnostic and statistical manual of mental disorders*, 5th ed. Washington, DC: Author.

American Psychiatric Association. (2020). *Trauma.* https://www.apa.org/topics/trauma

Arcelus, J., Mitchell, A. J., Wales, J., & Nielsen, S. (2011). Mortality rates in patients with anorexia nervosa and other eating disorders. *Archives of General Psychiatry, 68*(7), 724–731.

Becker, A. E., Franko, D. L., Speck, A., & Herzog, D. B. (2003). Ethnicity and differential access to care for eating disorder symptoms. *International Journal of Eating Disorders, 33*(2), 205–212.

Beebe, J. (2018). Black women suffer from eating disorders too. Daily Beast. https://www.thedailybeast.com/black-women-suffer-from-eating-disorders-too

Choate, L. (2010). Interpersonal group therapy for women experiencing bulimia. *Journal for Specialists in Group Work, 35*(4), 349–364. https://doi.org/10.1080/01933922.2010.514977

Dakanalis, A., Clerici, M., Bartoli, F., Caslini, M., Crocamo, C., Riva, G., & Carrà, G. (2017). Risk and maintenance factors for young women's DSM–5 eating disorders. *Archives of Women's Mental Health, 20*(6), 721–731.

Fredrickson, B. L., & Roberts, T. A. (1997). Objectification theory: Toward understanding women's lived experiences and mental health risks. *Psychology of Women Quarterly, 21*(2), 173–206.

Gilbert, S. C., Crump, S., Madhere, S., & Schutz, W. (2009). Internalization of the thin ideal as a predictor of body dissatisfaction and disordered eating in African, African-American, and Afro-Caribbean female college students. *Journal of College Student Psychotherapy, 23*(3), 196–211. https://doi.org/10.1080/87568220902794093

Harrington, E. F., Crowther, J. H., Payne Henrickson, H. C., & Mickelson, K. D. (2006). The relationships among trauma, stress, ethnicity, and binge eating. *Cultural Diversity and Ethnic Minority Psychology, 12*(2), 212–229. https://doi.org/10.1037/1099-9809.12.2.212

Harrington, E. F., Crowther, J. H., & Shipherd, J. C. (2010). Trauma, binge eating, and the "Strong Black Woman." *Journal of Counseling and Clinical Psychology, 78*(4), 469–479. https://doi.org/10.1037/a0019174

Harris, D. J., & Kuba, S. A. (1997). Ethnocultural identity and eating disorders in women of color. *Professional Psychology: Research and Practice, 28*(4), 341–347.

Henrickson, H. C., Crowther, J. H., & Harrington, E. F. (2010). Ethnic identity and maladaptive eating: Expectations about eating and thinness in African American women. *Cultural Diversity and Ethnic Minority Psychology, 16*(1), 87–93. https://doi.org/10.1037/a0013455

Hilbert, A., Hoek, H. W., & Schmidt, R. (2017). Evidence-based clinical guidelines for eating disorders: International comparison. *Current Opinion in Psychiatry, 30*(6), 423–437.

Holder, A, M. B., Jackson, M. A., & Ponterotto, J. G. (2015). Racial microaggression experiences and coping strategies of Black women in corporate leadership. *Qualitative Psychology, 2*(2), 164 –180.

Kempa, M. L., & Thomas, A. J. (2000). Culturally sensitive assessment and treatment of eating disorders. *Eating Disorders, 8*(1), 17–30.

Kroon Van Diest, A. M., Tartakovsky, M., Stachon, C., Pettit, J. W., & Perez, M. (2014). The relationship between acculturative stress and eating disorder symptoms: Is it unique from general life stress? *Journal of Behavioral Medicine, 37*, 445–457. https://doi.org/10.1007/s10865-013-9498-5

Marques, L., Alegria, M., Becker, A. E., Chen, C., Fang, A., & Diniz, J. B. (2011). Comparative prevalence, correlates of impairment, and service utilization for eating disorders across U.S. Ethnic Groups: Implications for reducing ethnic disparities in health care access for eating disorders. *International Journal of Eating Disorders, 44*(5), 412–420.

Mehler, P. S., & Anderson, A. E. (2010). Nutritional rehabilitation—Practical guidelines for refeeding anorexia nervosa patients. In *Eating disorders—A guide to medical care and complications* (pp. 83–84). Baltimore, MD: Johns Hopkins University Press.

National Eating Disorders Association (NEDA). (2018a). *Co-occurring conditions & special issues.* https://www.nationaleatingdisorders.org/co-occurring-disorders-and-special-issues

National Eating Disorders Association (NEDA). (2018b). *Eating disorders vs. disordered eating: What's the difference?* https://www.nationaleatingdisorders.org/blog/eating-disorders-versus-disordered-eating

National Eating Disorders Association (NEDA). (2018c). *Marginalized voices.* https://www.nationaleatingdisorders.org/marginalized-voices-0

National Eating Disorders Association (NEDA). (2021). *Risk factors.* Retrieved from: https://www.nationaleatingdisorders.org/risk-factors

Ross, C. C. (2019). African-American women and eating disorders: Depression, and the strong Black woman archetype. *Eating Disorders Review, 30*(5). https://eatingdisordersreview.com/wp-content/uploads/2020/05/nl_edr_30_5print.pdf

Ross, S. V., Gipson-Jones, T. L., & Davis, B. L. (2018). Acculturative stress and binge eating in African-American Women: Where do they go from here? *ABNF Journal*, 69–75.

Shuttlesworth, M. E., & Zotter, D. (2011). Disordered eating in African American and Caucasian women: The role of ethnic identity. *Journal of Black Studies, 42*(6), 906–922. https://doi.org/10.1177/0021934710396368

Sue, D. W., Arredondo, P., & McDavis, R. J. (1992). Multicultural counseling competencies and standards: A call to the profession. *Journal of Counseling &*

Development, 70(4), 477–486. https://doi.org/10.1002/j.1556-6676.1992
.tb01642.x

Swanson, S. A., Crow, S. J., Le Grange, D., Swendsen, J., & Merikangas, K. R.
(2011). Prevalence and correlates of eating disorders in adolescents. Results
from the national comorbidity survey replication adolescent supplement.
Archives of General Psychiatry, 68(7), 714–723. http://dx.doi.org/10.1001
/archgenpsychiatry.2011.22

Talleyrand, R. M. (2006). Potential stressors contributing to eating disorder symptoms in African American women: Implications for mental health counselors. *Journal of Mental Health Counseling,* 28(4), 338–352.

Talleyrand, R. M. (2012). Disordered eating in women of color: Some counseling
considerations. *Journal of Counseling and Development,* 90(3), 271–280.

Taylor, J. Y., Caldwell, C. H., Baser, R. E., Faison, N., & Jackson, J. S. (2007). Prevalence of eating disorders among Blacks in the National Survey of American
Life. *International Journal of Eating Disorders,* 40(Suppl), S10–S14.

U.S. Census Bureau. (2018). Educational attainment in the United States: 2018.
Current Population Survey: 2018 Annual Social and Economic Supplement.
https://www.census.gov/data/tables/2018/demo/education-attainment
/cps-detailed-tables.html

Veritas Collaborative. (2020). *Symposium speaker series: Treating Black people with
eating disorders.* https://veritascollaborative.com/veritas-collaborative
/symposium-speaker-series-treating-black-people-with-eating-disorders/

Watson, L. B., Ancis, J. R., White, D. N., & Nazari, N. (2013). Racial identity buffers African American women from body image problems and disordered
eating. *Psychology of Women Quarterly,* 37(3), 337–350. https://doi.org
/10.1177/0361684312474799

Williams, C. B., Frame, M. W., & Green, E. (1999). Counseling groups for African
American women: A focus on spirituality. *Journal for Specialists in Group
Work,* 24(3), 260–273.

Zhang, Y., Dixon, T. L., & Conrad, K. (2009). Rap music videos and African American women's body image: The moderating role of ethnic identity. *Journal of
Communication,* 59, 262–278. https://doi.org/10.1111/j.1460-2466.2009.01415.x

CHAPTER 8

Individual Counseling

Tamara D'Anjou Turner
Mahlet Endale
Michelle King Lyn

Individual counseling is a "personal opportunity to receive support and experience growth during challenging times in life" (American Counseling Association, 2020). It is also known as individual therapy, psychotherapy, or treatment. Psychotherapists use "research-based techniques to help people develop more effective" coping strategies to attend to the concerns bringing them to counseling (American Psychological Association [APA], 2020). Individual counseling is offered by providers with graduate-level training in counseling, psychology, social work, or marriage and family counseling, and who either have a professional license or work under supervision toward these degrees or licensure. Psychotherapists aim to create "a supportive environment that allows [those seeking treatment] to talk openly with someone who is objective, neutral and nonjudgmental" (APA, 2020).

There is limited comprehensive published data on what brings individuals for counseling. University mental health centers collect and release this data in the most systematic way, and year after year report mood disorders and anxiety disorders as the two most common presenting concerns in the population they serve (Glaser, 2008; Pérez-Rojas et al., 2017). Psychiatry departments in university medical centers list mood disorders, substance abuse disorders, and anxiety disorders as the most common treated concerns. As frontline access and a means of last resort, particularly to individuals with limited resources, community mental health centers tend to see the broadest range of presenting concerns (Glaser, 2008). Many individuals also seek counseling services in private practice settings for which comprehensive data on presenting concerns is not typically gathered or published in the same way that agency data is provided.

In the past 50 years, there have been a large number of scientifically sound studies on the efficacy of theoretically based psychotherapy. The cumulative data shows psychotherapy is effective in treating mental health concerns. In fact, psychotherapy has better outcomes than some evidence-based medical practices such as cardiology treatments, the flu vaccine, and cataract surgery (Wampold, 2007). The body of research shows on average 67 percent of those receiving theory-grounded treatment experience improvement of symptoms and functioning, while only 33 percent without treatment show the same gains (Lambert, 2013a). Research shows clients see the benefits of treatment after 12–14 sessions generally, and that the treatment gains are observable even two and three years later (Lambert, 2013b).

Although the majority of psychological research and collected data comes from White participants, research reports the rates of mental health concerns of African Americans are at the same level as that of the general population (U.S. Department of Health and Human Services [HHS], 2001; American Psychiatric Association, 2017). While rates of mental health concerns are comparable to peers, African Americans are less likely to seek out psychotherapy compared to White Americans (HHS, 2001). African Americans face a number of obstacles that interfere with their utilization of mental health treatment, including cultural stigma and norms, financial concerns, and systemic oppression (Shim et al., 2009; HHS, 2001). Despite some evidence of a decrease in stigma associated with seeking mental health care (Shim et al., 2009), for African American women, these barriers are compounded by gendered racism.

This chapter will provide an overview of the mental health needs of African American women and discuss treatment considerations and interventions that can help facilitate culturally competent individual therapy with them. Case examples and vignettes will be used to illustrate concepts and interventions.

OVERVIEW OF AFRICAN AMERICAN WOMEN MENTAL HEALTH

Likely due to a combination of reduced stigma and ongoing stressors, therapy entrance rates of African American women continue rising. For example, compared to White peers, Black women report being less likely to be embarrassed about being in mental health care (Mojtabai, 2007; Shim et al., 2009). African American women share many mental health similarities with their non-Black female counterparts. One in five women experiences a diagnosable mental health condition (American Psychiatric Association, 2017). Women are twice as likely to experience depression, anxiety, and post-traumatic stress disorder (PTSD) as men. However, the symptoms of PTSD manifest differently for women versus men. Women attempt suicide more often than men, but men die by suicide at four times the rate of women. Women generally have a lower income than men, are more likely to live in poverty, be victims of violence, and serve as caregivers for loved ones—all these things are risk factors for experiencing mental health concerns (American Psychiatric Association, 2017). Regarding mental health service utilization, as compared to men, women are: more likely to seek care from a primary care physician and be prescribed psychotropic medication, less likely to report alcohol use concerns, reluctant to report experiencing interpersonal violence (IPV), and more likely to be diagnosed with depression even when reported symptoms are identical to those reported by a man.

Even with improved utilization rates, African American women continue experiencing barriers to compromise their mental health treatment. According to the Substance Abuse and Mental Health Services Administration (SAMHSA) 2018 National Survey on Drug Use and Health, 16 percent of Black or African Americans reported having a mental illness, and of that 16 percent, 22.4 percent reported a serious mental illness over the last year. Dual minority status intensifies the acuity and the rates of mental health concerns for African American women. African American men and women report higher rates of sadness, helplessness, and feeling that everything is an effort (Centers for Disease Control and Prevention [CDC], 2019a). Although suicide rates for African American adults are 60 percent lower than that of White Americans, it must be noted that in 2017, African American girls in grades 9–12 were 70 percent more likely to attempt suicide than White girls of the same age (CDC, 2019b). According to SAMHSA (2015), Black women report higher depression rates and experiences of interpersonal violence (IPV, domestic violence) than women of different ethnicities. African American women experience diagnostic psychological concerns such as mood, anxiety, trauma, psychosis, and substance use disorders (SAMHSA, 2015), as well as a host of nondiagnostic issues such as life transition, professional identity, personal growth, and relationship enrichment.

To understand the mental health needs of African American women, one must understand the roles stress and oppression play in their lives. In general, women as a group struggle to fully participate in therapy due to financial limitations, lack of information about mental health concerns and available support, stigma regarding mental illness, logistical barriers (getting leave from work, care for children, etc.), and limited integrative care based on a woman's unique mental health needs (American Psychiatric Association, 2017). However, the experience of gendered racism further complicates each of these variables.

Between 2008 and 2012, African American women made up 10.3 percent of those utilizing mental health services (American Psychiatric Association, 2017). Utilization rates remain low due to challenges in locating a

Black and/or culturally competent therapists. Some Black clients prefer seeing a Black psychotherapist, yet Black providers are underrepresented, with only 8.0 percent of psychology doctoral degrees being awarded to African American graduates (National Science Foundation, 2015). The most common therapeutic ruptures related to cultural competency include racist attitudes (Constantine, 2007), being misunderstood (Chang & Berk, 2009), lack of cultural knowledge (Chang & Berk, 2009), worrying about being overdiagnosed, and lack of connection (Chang & Berk, 2009). Being misunderstood is a feeling that mimics the isolation that Black women feel in the outside world. Therefore, therapists must employ therapeutic factors that increase feelings of connection and safety in therapy.

THERAPIST CONSIDERATIONS

APA Multicultural Guidelines (2017) on developing cultural competence advises therapists to examine the ways in which bias may affect how they interact professionally with clients. Within the therapy room, biases can affect the therapist's theoretical orientation, treatment recommendations, assessment and diagnosis, expectations, assessment of progress, and communication style. For instance, studies show that nonmedical conversational warm-ups tend to be longer when there is a therapist–client identity match (Ivey, Ivey, & Zalaquett, 2014). Ivey et al. (2014) found that Black counselors tend to communicate more actively and give more direct feedback and interpretations than White counselors. Yet graduate programs continue training counselors to listen and attend. This difference in communication style may lead to less dropout among therapist–client cross-racial pairings.

As a culturally competent therapist, it is vitally important to be aware of Black history and national news that affect women, Black women, Black men, and Black families. Knowledge of both the historical and present-day oppressive experiences of Black Americans can help build a deeper connection with Black clients. Some national news examples include events like the opening of the National Museum of African American History and Culture in 2016, the opening of the National Memorial for Peace and Justice in 2018, and the Inauguration of Barack Obama in 2009. This means being aware of people like Philando Castile, George Floyd, and Tamir Rice. It means understanding the emotional impact of movies like *Antwone Fisher* (Washington, 2002), *Black Panther* (Coogler, 2018), or *When They See Us* (DuVernay, 2019). As a culturally competent counselor treating Black women, it would be important to understand why these significant events and movies resonated within the community. Additionally, understanding that oftentimes Black people feel unheard or silenced from expressing their true feelings. Cultural competence is demonstrated in creating therapeutic relationships in which Black clients are heard and understood in their experience as a Black person (Ward, 2005).

INDIVIDUAL THERAPY TREATMENT MODELS

There are many theoretical orientations guiding conceptualization and intervention in individual therapy with Black women. A review of every theoretical orientation is beyond the scope of this chapter; however, it will focus on exploring several models particularly helpful for work with African American women: cognitive behavioral therapy (CBT), psychodynamic therapy (PT), interpersonal therapy (IPT), and History, Empowerment, Rapport, and Spirituality (HERS). The chapter then explores general themes in culturally adaptive clinical work with Black women. Also note, culturally adaptive evidence-based treatment for group therapy with Black women using relational cultural theory, CBT, and several non-colonized approaches are included in Chapter 10 of this text. Coverage of the use of psychodynamic and cognitive behavioral approaches with African American women in general and inpatient settings is covered in Chapter 11 of this text as well.

Cognitive Behavioral Therapy

CBT, one of the most researched and utilized treatment models, is found to be effective in work with African American women (Carter et al., 2003), particularly when culturally adaptive principles are utilized (Kohn et al., 2002; Ponting et al., 2020). Simply stated, CBT asserts that an individual's automatic thoughts (perception) create an emotional response (feeling), which drives behaviors and actions. These automatic thoughts originate from a schema or set of core beliefs that are well ingrained into the individual's psyche (Fenn & Byrne, 2013). CBT focuses on challenging and refuting maladaptive automatic thoughts to create more realistic and functional feelings and behaviors. Several models fall under the CBT umbrella including trauma focused CBT (TF-CBT), dialectical behavioral therapy, cognitive processing therapy (CPT), cognitive therapy (CT), and rational emotive behavior therapy (REBT).

There are a number of considerations in utilizing CBT with African American women because most CBT research utilizes White participants. In fact, there is evidence that CBT is more effective for White people than Black people. For example, in a substance use treatment meta-analysis, although CBT treatment was effective in reducing substance use among Black participants, Windsor, Jemal, and Alessi (2015) report CBT pre-posttest effect sizes are significantly higher for White participants than for Black participants. Additionally, a CBT approach that focuses primarily on individual responsibility and change, minimizing sociocultural elements that impact mental well-being, may hurt African American women (Windsor & Dunlap, 2010). For example, an African American pregnant woman presents to therapy for anxiety about either she or her baby possibly receiving inferior medical care because of race. A therapist not versed in the role of gendered racism in America's prenatal care system resulting in disproportionate numbers of Black mothers and babies dying may attribute this client's concerns to an internal cognitive process rather than taking into account the validity of this concern in the American health-care system. When utilizing CBT, it is important for clinicians to consider how sociopolitical factors are impacting their client. In this writer's (Endale) 19 years of clinical experience, this is important not just for CBT case conceptualization and clinical intervention, but also for providing psychoeducation and validation for the client's experience. Helping the client differentiate between maladaptive beliefs and accurate helpful instincts around injustices experienced has an empowering effect.

Psychodynamic Therapy

PT, which emerged out of psychoanalytic theory, aims to help clients develop insight on how their subconscious as well as past experiences influence their present-day behavior. This insight is then used to help the client have a better experience in the present by changing components of their identity and/or learning important components of emotional development that were not learned earlier in life (SAMHSA, 1999). PT stands on three assumptions (Bornstein, 2020):

1. Most people's psychological processes take place in the subconscious outside their awareness.
2. Early childhood experiences hold a critical role in personality development, especially if they are out of the norm or traumatic.
3. "Thoughts, motives, emotional responses, and expressed behaviors do not arise randomly, but always stem from some combination of identifiable biological and psychological processes" (Bornstein, 2020).

PT is offered in its original longer form or as a brief model. Traditional PT usually lasts at least two years and takes a global look at all aspects of the person past and present to inform the insight and change (Ackerman, 2020). In brief psychodynamic therapy (BPT), therapy focuses on a specific concern in the client's life and uses traditional psychodynamic interventions to develop insight and change around the agreed-upon focus. Different models of BPT can last anywhere from 12 to 40 sessions (SAMHSA, 1999).

It is important to adapt the application of PT when working with clients of color including Black women because the model was established from a Eurocentric framework. "Communities of color have long been suspicious of psychoanalytic models because of their traditional focus on the individual, as well as their failure to acknowledge racist and sexist assumptions underlying the theory of personality development" (Jackson, 2000, 1).

Researchers have used these models to study the impact of gendered racism on identity development as they attempted to modify PT for African American clients; however, there are still limitations to be aware of in this application (Jackson, 2000). The first step to counter the limitations is to establish a strong lens of cultural competence and humility through which PT is applied. If PT is applied without an intentional consideration of sociopolitical dynamics, the clinician risks "[supporting] and [sustaining] cultural stereotypes and social constructions about" the client while "denying within-group differences and prevents the client from experiencing . . . her individual uniqueness" (Jackson, 2000, 2). Jackson (2000) recommends using the following questions to help circumvent Eurocentric bias in the model:

1. How does the experience of early childhood development (if the nuclear family is not the model) effect the development of healthy or unhealthy personality?
2. When is the development of autonomy or separation an appropriate marker of healthy functioning?
3. How have the effects of slavery, marginalization, and discrimination affected the development of personality?
4. What is the importance of the effects of racial identity development, skin color, and hair (being either idealized or devalued) on the development of African American personality? (p. 3)

Once this critical foundation is established, Jackson (2000) reports it is possible to use the very strengths of PT to enhance the experience of Black women clients. The strengths of PT begin with the strong collaborative therapeutic relationship fostered in PT. Then the traditional effective tools of PT (i.e., utilizing transference, resistance, countertransference, projection, developing defensive functioning) can be used to help the client develop insight and adaptive change strategies for how their personal history set in the sociopolitical context they grew up in came together to lead them to become who they are (Jackson, 2000).

Interpersonal Therapy

Interpersonal therapy is based on attachment theory and presupposes that individuals experience emotional distress when interpersonal relationships are disrupted, similar to painful attachment disruptions in early childhood (Poleshuck et al., 2010). As such, the approach focuses on understanding and strengthening interpersonal relationships for the client as part of symptom reduction and treatment. This includes using the client–therapist relationship as a way of facilitating healing and growth. Some authors have suggested that IPT is especially fitting for female clients because of the focus on relationships (Poleshuck et al., 2010) and appropriate for African American clients given congruence with collectivist values (Brown, Conner, & McMurray, 2012).

Applying the results of a focus group of African American clients as a guide, ITP was adapted to treat African American women with depression in a primary care setting (Brown et al., 2012). The cultural adaptations were also made based on research that showed efficacy of ITP across different racial groups for depression in particular (Poleshuck et al., 2010). The following cultural modifications were made: 1) Addressed stigma related to seeking psychological help, 2) Shortened total number of sessions to eliminate barriers to treatment such as transportation and cost, 3) Facilitated trust in the therapeutic relationship to allow for discussion of cultural differences between therapist and client, and 4) Added a pretreatment session focused on engaging the client to reduce premature termination.

One point to consider in using ITP with African American women is exploration and understanding of relationships that may hinder African American women from seeking out or maximizing therapy based on stigma or role overload (Brown et al., 2012). For example, an African American woman with a close relationship with her mother, or another respected elder who does not see therapy in a positive light, may resist seeking help, fearing judgment from her family or community. Using ITP principles, the therapist would reinforce the client's decision to seek help by identifying other affirming relationships and role-play with the client ways to assert her interpersonal needs. Another consideration is discrimination in relationships, such as teachers, coworkers, and neighbors, and the emotional impact of these relationships. The role of the therapist would be as an advocate to the client navigating these challenging relationships.

HERS Model

Developed by Moore and Madison-Colmore (2005), the HERS model is a four-step holistic approach that integrates cultural history, psychological, emotional, and social needs designed specifically for African American women. The model includes information from traditional approaches to psychological treatment including psychodynamic and feminist therapy, as well as approaches including cultural values of African American women, specifically emergent and Afrocentric therapies. Step one focuses on using a feminist perspective to gather the woman's *herstory*. Therapists integrate their cultural knowledge of Black women in developing assessment questions and/or use interventions such as a cultural–spiritual genogram to explore history. Step two focuses on empowering Black women to participate in therapy in a way that will meet their needs. Acknowledging sociocultural factors that disempower them, Black women may use bibliotherapy, spirituality, community involvement, or other means to empower their positionality within and outside of the therapy space. Step three focuses on creating a therapeutic rapport conducive to meeting Black women's therapy needs. This relationship includes trust, a sense of belonging, and provides opportunity for personal growth. The final step, spirituality is incorporated as consistent with the needs and belief of the African American client. For many African American women, spirituality is a place of support and comfort. Therapists must develop competent inclusion of spiritualty, while not generalizing that this will be a need of all Black women. As a more recently developed multicultural-focused model, HERS is conceptual and research on efficacy is limited.

Cultural Adaptation Interventions

Again, across different theoretical orientations, literature suggest the use of culturally adaptive models to traditional therapy approaches. The American Psychiatric Association developed the Cultural Formulation Interview (CFI) to increase the incorporation of cultural understanding in clinical decision-making (American Psychiatric Association, 2013). The CFI helps the clinician ask questions that allow the client to express the impact of their culture on their worldview and emotional concerns, which can increase the likelihood of developing culturally sensitive interventions and treatment plans. Culturally adapted approaches have been found to be more effective in working with ethnic minorities (Benish, Quintana, & Wampold, 2011) including Black women, (Kohn et al., 2002), and participants are less likely to prematurely terminate (Windsor, Jemal, & Alessi, 2015).

Culturally adapted interventions include:

- Inclusion of cultural values relevant to African American women
- Meeting the African American women's therapist preferences
- Integration of Afrocentric values and beliefs (Banks et al., 1996)
- Name and confront systemic oppression impacting the lived reality of African American women (i.e., sexism, patriarchy, racism, anti-Blackness, harassment, exoticization)
- Inclusion of holistic and nontraditional therapy interventions (i.e., spirituality)

TRANSTHEORETICAL CULTURAL THEMES: STRATEGIES AND INTERVENTIONS

Cutting across theoretical orientation and theory-based research, common themes may emerge in individual therapy with Black women. These themes impact all aspects of life (i.e., thoughts, feelings, beliefs, relationships, motivations, decisions), thus specific clinical intervention strategies and nuanced skills are paramount. This section details the unique lived experiences of Black women and provides culturally grounded interventions appropriate for individual therapy with Black women.

Discrimination

The Black community is aware of biases in treatment and have developed a distrust of the medical field (Marbley, 2011; Sue & Sue, 2016; Terrell & Terrell, 1981). Given this, some Black women may present to counseling with the need to build trust in the clinician and the process. Black women may enter with "healthy cultural paranoia," to which Ward (2005) found participants' skepticism of counselors acted as a form of self-protection. In the therapy room, cultural mistrust may display itself as taking more time for Black clients to disclose the most personal details of their story or doubt in treatment methods. Furthermore, Black women may feel more comfortable after asking questions about the therapist or therapy process (Ward, 2005). It is important not to pathologize these behaviors but to contextualize them within a history of mistreatment. Showing compassion, patience, and understanding will help Black women build trust at a pace that feels comfortable to them.

From an individual standpoint, cognitions and appraisals of discrimination can affect the impact of discrimination on mental health outcomes (Brondolo et al., 2009). Oftentimes, people make the mistake of believing that overt discrimination must be present to affect the health and well-being of people of color. But one only needs to be fearful of or think that discrimination is possible for negative health effects to occur (Cokley, Hall-Clark, & Hicks, 2011; Hall, Everett, & Hamilton Mason, 2012). The intellectual and emotional energy of scanning for threats or deciding if an event was discriminatory depletes emotional resources. Research shows discrimination or perceived discrimination is associated with increased depression, anxiety, substance use, and decreased well-being (Paradies, 2006; Williams & Mohammed, 2009). The cumulative effects of perceived discrimination also affect physical health (Williams et al., 2019).

As a culturally competent therapist treating Black women, it can be helpful to explore both the tangible and intangible effects of discrimination and how they may be affecting the client's clinical concerns. If using cognitive techniques, it is important to adjust them to be sensitive to the reality of discrimination. Even the use of common CBT terms like "distortions" and "maladaptive thoughts" may come across as uninformed if talking about racism, discrimination, or prejudice. Some clients' automatic thoughts may be adaptive, protective, or related to a Black experience worldview. In these cases, typical techniques of challenging the client's automatic thoughts regarding the racist intent of others might come across as dismissive, insensitive, or culturally uninformed. Additionally, there may be previous traumas that are triggered by current sociocultural issues, which would be worth exploring. An effective intervention would be validating the client's concerns and being curious about her fears, environment, and perception of discrimination.

Discrimination can lead to self-doubt, self-hate, defeatist mentality, nihilism, and helplessness. Therefore, it is important to explore if these factors have an influence on beliefs, motivation, and actions. See case vignette below:

> *Tamika was a teacher in a predominantly White town and school. She dreaded going to work, expecting to be discriminated against by her White supervisors, and feared receiving poor ratings from her students. She decided not to buy a house for fear of losing her job one day and systematically sabotaged her dating relationships and friendships. Counseling was used to explore ways in which discrimination and racism tied into her own negative expectations, self-doubt, and self-sabotage. One intervention was noticing when these fears were present with her at work and incorporating deep breathing in those moments to lessen her anxiety. Her therapist validated her concerns, while helping her create self-care practices that reduced stress. Tamika intentionally disengaged from social media and conversations with dismissive individuals at work. She started realizing she was living under constant stereotype threat.*

In a study on stereotype threat, Steele and Aronson (1995) found that when minority group members are exposed to reminders of a common stereotype before engaging in an activity where they could confirm that stereotype, their performance suffers. Similarly, some African American women in counseling have intense shame and fear about confirming negative stereotypes about Black women, which affects how they engage in the counseling process (Williams et al., 1998). It can also affect how Black women operate professionally and personally. In the case of "Ebony," she is concerned about stereotypes of Black mothers.

> *When making a very difficult personal decision about whether to get a divorce, despite being very unhappy in her relationship, Ebony expressed the distress of confirming the stereotype of the Black single mother. Counseling had to go beyond helping her readjust dreams of raising her children in a biological two-parent household. The stereotype concern and her fear of discrimination had to be addressed. It was important to bring her awareness to the stereotype, acknowledge the power it had in her decision-making, help her separate from the narrative, and embrace her unique story.*

Collectivist Values

Collectivist cultures tend to value selflessness, rule following, working together, supporting others, and prioritizing family as the center (Harris,

1992). Individual needs and goals are de-emphasized, and character-istics like generosity, conformity, kindness, harmony, and sacrifice are highly esteemed. Black American culture tends to be collectivistic with an emphasis on respect of elders and family closeness. There is a belief in a shared identity, shared experience, and shared responsibility. Strong family ties usually extend beyond the nuclear family to cousins, aunts, uncles, grandparents, neighbors, church members, and friends (Lincoln, Taylor, & Chatters, 2012).

Due to historical realities, it has been adaptive for Black families to expand their emotional and financial resources by enlarging their social circles (Chatters et al., 2002). As a result, it is not uncommon for some Black children to see their aunts, grandmothers, or neighbors as second mothers; live with family members for periods or their lives; or even lov-ingly call a friend's mother "Mom." Yet the expansion of the idea of fam-ily also increases feelings of responsibility. Some of the expectations of Black women often include being the backbone of the family, caring for siblings, nurturing nieces and nephews, providing financially for the fam-ily members in need, and taking care of parents, even at an early age. These expectations increase when the disenfranchisement of Black men is considered. Due to disproportionately high rates of incarceration, unem-ployment, and death, Black women are left carrying a heavier load. The marginalization of Black men has also contributed to Black women being more likely to pursue higher educational opportunities (U.S. Department of Education, 2019) and become heads of household (Acs et al., 2013) than Black men. Furthermore, studies show Black women who graduate from college are often seen as the most successful in the family and feel com-pelled to help others in the family financially (Rochester, 2018).

> *Growing up as the oldest child, Ruby would take care of her much younger siblings while her single mother worked long hours. In her senior year, Ruby was accepted into several colleges with scholarships to cover tuition—including her dream school out of state. However, Ruby carried a lot of guilt and even anger at wanting to do something for herself at what felt like a cost to her family. She questioned how her mother would take care of the remain-ing kids without her. Childcare would eat up too much of her mom's income. With sadness, and without discussion, Ruby announced she would enroll at the nearby lower-tier college. She explained she would live at home while attending classes. The look of relief on her mother's face was not lost on Ruby, and she felt guilty at the resentment she felt for feeling internal pressure to make this decision.*

Though initially it can feel good to have the ability and resources to help family financially or otherwise, over time those who are regularly put in this role can start feeling resentful, drained, used, and/or taken for granted by family members. If they decide not to give, Black women can feel guilty, avoidant, judged, or uncomfortable with family. It can be challenging for those who are in this role to balance sense of self and familial obligations.

Silence and Secrecy

Many Black clients will feel torn about talking honestly about the negative aspects of their families, even in the safety of the therapy room (Alvidrez, Snowden, & Kaiser, 2008). Often, because of this value, counseling can be the first time that Black women speak honestly about the negative aspects of family. This can feel scary or as if they are betraying their loved ones. This collective value contributes to Black women underreporting perpetrators of violence to authorities. Part of this is based on the history of Black men unfairly being targeted by police for crimes they did not commit (Stone, 2004). The criminalization of Black men has had dire consequences for Black men and their families impacting the father–child bond, financial security, housing security, and educational opportunities (Acs et al., 2013). As a result, women in the Black community often do not want to contribute to the accusation of a Black man (Eligon, 2019; Zellars, 2019) out of fear of retribution, judgment, rejection, or social exclusion (Zellars, 2019).

In the book *No Secrets No Lies*, Robin Stone (2004) describes in detail how the code of silence puts pressure on Black survivors to stay silent and moves the responsibility away from the perpetrator for their abusive behavior. The book details the detrimental impact this silence has on Black survivors of abuse including increasing the duration and severity of PTSD and depressive symptoms. It also discusses the impact of not being believed or supported as a survivor. Black women experience an undue burden of protecting Black men especially in cases of childhood sexual assault, where 82 percent of childhood sexual abuse survivors are girls (Snyder & National Center for Juvenile Justice, 2000). The culture of silence can leave childhood sexual abuse survivors feeling responsible, not only for their own abuse, but for convincing others of the truth, providing their own support, holding the perpetrator responsible, keeping themselves safe, keeping other children safe, and facilitating their own healing.

Kenya was sexually abused by her maternal uncle from age 6 to 14. As an adult she told her mother, who did not believe her initially, but later showed strong support for Kenya. Feeling empowered, Kenya started telling other family members, but was not believed. They continued inviting her uncle to family functions, leaving Kenya feeling unsupported and in need of figuring out ways of protecting herself emotionally. It also made her feel like she lost her family. She reported she did not tell her father fearing he would kill her uncle, and she wanted to protect him from going to jail. During therapy, she reported feeling a need to advocate for childhood abuse survivors and protect other girls from what she experienced. She often spent more time worried about others instead of herself. The therapist helped Kenya explore her beliefs about protection of Black men, Black women, Black children, and Black families and how these values have been fostered throughout her life. She was encouraged to speak her truth to trustworthy and safe individuals and identified that the perpetrator is responsible for what happened.

It is helpful to explore clients' cultural values and how family value is entering the counseling space. Furthermore, explaining that being able to speak freely about the effects of these factors is a necessary component of discovering the unhealthy family patterns that may contribute to the presenting problem will help clients let go of inner conflict in doing so.

The Strong Black Woman Schema

There are some benefits to aspiring to be a Strong Black Woman (SBW). The SBW/Superwoman persona is strong, driven to succeed, emotionless, self-sacrificing, and helpful to others (Watson & Hunter, 2015). She can achieve career aspirations, raise a family, be the head of the household when necessary, care for loved ones, nurture friendships, and look gorgeous while facing gender and racial discrimination. It is protective in that Black women display "higher self-confidence, lower levels of substance abuse, and more positive body images than do White female adolescents" (Sue & Sue, 2008). Yet the SBW schema can take a toll on the mental health of Black women. The SBW schema can lead to perfectionism, pride, and a disconnection from feelings, leaving emotions unrecognizable and unaddressed, thus explaining why Black women are more likely to report physical symptoms when they are in emotional distress (Neal-Barnett et al., 2011) and why Black women are less likely to seek help for mental health concerns (Brown et al., 2010). Furthermore, the SBW archetype negatively impacts African American women who seek mental health care in alternative places. Common places include primary care providers, emergency departments, clergy, and individuals within their own support communities (HHS, 2001; Shim et al., 2009). Sometimes, individuals within these health and spiritual systems miss opportunities to refer someone with need for more specialized mental health care due to their own assumptions that Black women will be resistant to seeing a psychotherapist or psychiatrist (Shim et al., 2009).

The SBW schema is problematic because it is exhausting, unsustainable, and an unrealistic expectation by which Black women and others evaluate and judge themselves. As a result, some Black women judge themselves and feel ashamed of essentially being human, never fully realizing that the initial expectation was unrealistic (Watson & Hunter, 2015). Denial of symptoms and pretending that everything is okay can delay seeking mental health services. When Black women identify with the SBW archetype, therapists might pose questions such as: Where do SBW beliefs originate from? What does being human feel like? How would it change your actions? How would it change your relationships? How would you see yourself for opening up or asking for help? By addressing these questions, clients may gain a more balanced perspective and approach to their concerns.

CONCLUSION

Pursuing culturally competency is an endeavor which can feel daunting. This chapter is just a beginning to growing awareness around the unique needs of Black women in counseling. Hopefully, the chapter will help increase clinicians' knowledge of the cultural beliefs and values that may enter the therapy room, and clients will feel more understood and connected. The interventions included illustrate how common therapeutic techniques can be adapted for Black women experiencing some of these cultural factors. Yet each technique can be tailored to a client's clinical concerns, diagnosis, and background, and interventions will ultimately be determined collaboratively between the client and the therapist.

REFERENCES

Ackerman, C. (2020). *What is psychodynamic therapy? 5 tools & techniques.* https://positivepsychology.com/psychodynamic-therapy/

Acs, G., Braswell, K., Sorensen, E., & Turner, M. A. (2013). *The Moynihan Report revisited.* The Urban Institute. https://www.urban.org/sites/default/files/publication/23696/412839-The-Moynihan-Report-Revisited.PDF

Alvidrez, J., Snowden, L. R., & Kaiser, D. M. (2008). The experience of stigma among Black mental health consumers. *Journal of Health Care for the Poor and Underserved, 19*(3), 874–893. https://doi.org/10.1353/hpu.0.0058

American Counseling Association. (2020). *What is professional counseling?* https://www.counseling.org/aca-community/learn-about-counseling/what-is-counseling

American Psychiatric Association (APA). (2013). *Diagnostic and statistical manual of mental disorders,* 5th ed. Washington, DC: American Psychiatric Association.

American Psychiatric Association (APA). (2017). *Mental health disparities: African Americans.* https://www.psychiatry.org/psychiatrists/cultural-competency/education/african-american-patients

American Psychological Association (APA). (2017). *Multicultural guidelines: An ecological approach to context, identity, and intersectionality, 2017.* https://www.apa.org/about/policy/multicultural-guidelines

American Psychological Association (APA). (2020). *Therapy.* https://www.apa.org/topics/therapy/

Banks, R., Hogue, A., Timberlake, T., & Liddle, H. (1996). An Afrocentric approach to group social skills training with inner-city African American adolescents. *Journal of Negro Education, 65*(4), 414–423.

Benish, S. G., Quintana, S., & Wampold, B. E. (2011). Culturally adapted psychotherapy and the legitimacy of myth: A direct-comparison meta-analysis. *Journal of Counseling Psychology, 58*(3), 279–289.

Bornstein, R. (2020). The psychodynamic perspective. In R. Biswas-Diener & E. Diener (Eds.), *Noba textbook series: Psychology*. Champaign, IL: DEF publishers. http://noba.to/zdemy2cv

Boyd-Franklin, N. (1987). Group therapy for Black women: A therapeutic support model. *American Journal of Orthopsychiatry, 57*(3), 394–401. https://doi.org/10.1111/j.1939-0025.1987.tb03548.x

Brondolo, E., Brady ver Halen, N., Pencille, M., Beatty, D., & Contrada, R. J. (2009). Coping with racism: A selective review of the literature and a theoretical and methodological critique. *Journal of Behavioral Medicine, 32*(1), 64–88. https://doi.org/10.1007/s10865-008-9193-0

Brown, C., Conner, K. O., Copeland, V. C., Grote, N., Beach, S., Battista, D., & Reynolds, C. F. (2010). Depression stigma, race, and treatment seeking behavior and attitudes. *Journal of Community Psychology, 38*(3), 350–368. https://doi.org/10.1002/jcop.20368

Brown, C., Conner, K. O., & McMurray, M. (2012). *Toward cultural adaptation of interpersonal psychotherapy for depressed African American primary care patients*. In G. Bernal & M. M. Domenech Rodríguez (Eds.), *Cultural adaptations: Tools for evidence-based practice with diverse populations* (pp. 223–238). Washington, DC: American Psychological Association. https://doi.org/10.1037/13752-011

Carter, M. M., Sbrocco, T., Gore, K. L., Marin, N. W., & Lewis, E. L. (2003). Cognitive–behavioral group therapy versus a wait-list control in the treatment of African American women with panic disorder. *Cognitive Therapy and Research, 27*(5), 505–518.

Centers for Disease Control and Prevention (CDC). (2019a). *Summary health statistics: National health interview survey: 2017. Table A-7*. https://www.cdc.gov/nchs/nhis/shs/tables.htm

Centers for Disease Control and Prevention (CDC). (2019b). *High school youth risk behavior survey data*. https://nccd.cdc.gov/youthonline

Chang, D. F. & Berk, A. (2009). Making cross-racial therapy work: A phenomenological study of clients' experiences of cross-racial therapy. *Journal of Counseling Psychology, 56*(4), 521–536. https://doi.org/10.1037/a0016905

Chatters, L. M., Taylor, R. J., Lincoln, K. D., & Schroepfer, T. (2002). Patterns of informal support from family and church members among African Americans. *Journal of Black Studies, 33*(1), 66–85.

Cokley, K., Hall-Clark, B., & Hicks, D. (2011). Ethnic minority–majority status and mental health: The mediating role of perceived discrimination. *Journal of Mental Health Counseling, 33*(3), 243–263. https://doi.org/10.17744/mehc.33.3.u1n011t020783086

Constantine, M. G. (2007). Racial microaggressions against African American clients in cross-racial counseling relationships. *Journal of Counseling Psychology, 54*(1), 1–16. https://doi.org/10.1037/0022-0167.54.1.1

Coogler, R. (Director). (2018). *Black Panther* [Film]. Marvel Studios.

DuVernay, A. (Director). (2019). *When They See Us* [Film]. Harpo Films, Tribeca Productions, ARRAY, Participant Media.

Eligon, J. (2019, March 22). "You're not supposed to betray your race": The challenge faced by Black women accusing Black men. *New York Times*. https://www.nytimes.com/2019/03/22/us/meredith-watson-duke-justin-fairfax.html

Fenn, K. & Byrne, M. (2013). The key principles of cognitive behavioural therapy. *Sage Journals, 6*(9), 579–585. https://doi.org/10.1177/1755738012471029

Glaser, B. (2008). Clinical presenting issues. In F. T. L. Leong, E. M. Altmaier, & B. D. Johnson (Eds.), *Encyclopedia of counseling: Changes and challenges for counseling in the 21st century* (Vol. 2, pp. 491–493). Sage.

Hall, J. C., Everett, J. E., & Hamilton Mason, J. (2012). Black women talk about workplace stress and how they cope. *Journal of Black Studies, 43*(2), 207.

Harris, N. (1992). Afrocentrism—Concept and method: A philosophical basis for an Afrocentric orientation. *Western Journal of Black Studies, 16*(3), 154–159.

Ivey, A. E., Ivey, M. B., & Zalaquett, C. P. (2014). *Intentional interviewing and counseling: Facilitating client development in a multicultural society* (8th ed.). Belmont, CA: Brooks/Cole.

Jackson, L. (2000). The new multiculturalism and psychodynamic theory: Psychodynamic psychotherapy and African American women. In L. Jackson & B. Greene (Eds.), *Psychotherapy with African American women.* New York, NY: Guilford Press.

Kohn, L. P., Oden, T., Muñoz, R. F., Robinson, A., & Leavitt, D. (2002). Adapted cognitive behavioral group therapy for depressed low-income African American women. *Community Mental Health Journal, 38,* 497–504. http://dx.doi.org/10.1023/A:1020884202677

Lambert, M. J. (2013a). Outcome in psychotherapy: The past and important advances. *Psychotherapy, 50*(1), 42–51.

Lambert, M. J. (2013b). The efficacy and effectiveness of psychotherapy. In M. J. Lambert (Ed.), *Bergin & Garfield's handbook of psychotherapy and behavior change* (6th ed.). New York, NY: Wiley.

Lincoln, K. D., Taylor, R. J., & Chatters, L. M. (2012). Correlates of emotional support and negative interaction among African Americans and Caribbean Blacks. *Journal of Family Issues, 34*(9), 1262–1290.

Marbley, A. F. (2011). *Multicultural counseling: Perspectives from counselors as clients of color.* New York, NY: Routledge/Taylor & Francis Group.

Mojtabai, R. (2007). Americans' attitudes toward mental health treatment seeking. *Psychiatric Services, 58*(5), 642–651.

Moore, J. L., III, & Madison-Colmore, O. (2005). Using the H.E.R.S. model in counseling African-American women. *Journal of African American Studies, 9*(2), 39–50.

National Science Foundation (2015). Doctorate recipients from U.S. universities. Summary Report, 2014. Survey of earned doctorates. Special report. *National Science Foundation.*

Neal-Barnett, A., Stadulis, R., Murray, M., Payne, M. R., Thomas, A., & Salley, B. B. (2011). Sister circles as a culturally relevant intervention for anxious Black women. *Clinical Psychology: Science and Practice, 18*(3), 266–273. https://doi.org/10.1111/j.1468-2850.2011.01258.x

Neighbors, H. W. (1985). Seeking professional help for personal problems: Black Americans' use of health and mental health services. *Community Mental Health Journal, 21*(3), 156–166.

Neighbors, H. W. (1988). The help-seeking behavior of Black Americans. *Journal of the National Medical Association, 80*(9), 1009–1012.

Paradies, Y. C. (2006). Defining, conceptualizing and characterizing racism in health research. *Critical Public Health, 16*(2), 143–157. https://doi.org/10.1080/09581590600828881

Pérez-Rojas, A. E., Lockard, A. J., Bartholomew, T. T., Janis, R. A., Carney, D. M., Xiao, H., Youn, S. J., Scofield, B. E., Locke, B. D., Castonguay, L. G., & Hayes, J. A. (2017). Presenting concerns in counseling centers: The view from clinicians on the ground. *Psychological Services, 14*(4), 416–427. https://doi.org/10.1037/ser0000122

Poleshuck, E. L., Gamble, S. A., Cort, N., Hoffman-King, D., Cerrito, B., Rosario-McCabe, L. A., & Giles, D. E. (2010). Interpersonal psychotherapy for co-occurring depression and chronic pain. *Professional Psychology: Research and Practice, 41*(4), 312–318. https://doi.org/10.1037/a0019924

Ponting, C., Mahrer, N. E., Zelcer, H., Dunkel Schetter, C., & Chavira, D. A. (2020). Psychological interventions for depression and anxiety in pregnant Latina and Black women in the United States: A systematic review. *Clinical Psychology and Psychotherapy, 27*(2), 249–265. https://doi.org/10.1002/cpp.2424

Rochester, S. (2018). *The Black tax: The cost of being Black in America.* Southbury, CT: Good Steward Publishing.

Shim, R. S., Compton, M. T., Rust, G., Druss, B. G., & Kaslow, N. J. (2009). Race-Ethnicity as a predictor of attitudes toward mental health treatment seeking. *Psychiatry Services, 60*(10), 1336–1341.

Snyder, H. N., & National Center for Juvenile Justice. (2000). *Sexual assault of young children as reported to law enforcement: Victim, incident, and offender characteristics. A NIBRS Statistical Report.*

Steele, C. M., & Aronson, J. (1995). Stereotype threat and the intellectual test performance of African Americans. *Journal of Personality and Social Psychology, 69*(5), 797–811. https://doi.org/10.1037/0022-3514.69.5.797

Stone, R. D. (2004). *No secrets no lies: How Black families can heal from sexual abuse.* New York, NY: Broadway.

Substance Abuse and Mental Health Services Administration (SAMHSA). (1999). Brief interventions and brief therapies for substance abuse. Treatment Improvement Protocol (TIP) Series, No. 34. *HHS Publication No. (SMA) 12-3952.* Rockville, MD: Substance Abuse and Mental Health Services Administration. https://www.ncbi.nlm.nih.gov/books/NBK64947/pdf/Bookshelf_NBK64947.pdf

Substance Abuse and Mental Health Services Administration (SAMHSA). (2015). Racial/Ethnic differences in mental health service use among adults. *HHS Publication No. SMA-15-4906.* Rockville, MD: Author.

Substance Abuse and Mental Health Services Administration (SAMHSA). (2018). *National survey on drug use and health: African Americans.* https://www.samhsa.gov/data/sites/default/files/reports/rpt23247/2_AfricanAmerican_2020_01_14.pdf

Sue, D. W., & Sue, D. (2008). *Counseling the culturally diverse: Theory and practice* (5th ed.). John Wiley & Sons.

Sue, D. W., & Sue, D. (2016). *Counseling the culturally diverse: Theory and practice* (7th ed.). John Wiley & Sons.

Terrell, F., & Terrell, S. L. (1981). An inventory to measure cultural mistrust among Blacks. *Western Journal of Black Studies, 5*(3), 180–184.

U.S. Department of Education's National Center for Education Statistics (NCES). (2019). *Status and trends in the education of racial and ethnic groups 2018* (NCES 2019–038). https://nces.ed.gov/pubs2019/2019038.pdf

U.S. Department of Health and Human Services (HHS). (2001). *Mental health: Culture, race, and ethnicity—A supplement to mental health: A report of the Surgeon General.* Rockville, MD: U.S. Department of Health and Human Services, Substance Abuse and Mental Health Services Administration, Center for Mental Health Services.

Wampold, B. E. (2007). Psychotherapy: The humanistic (and effective) treatment. *American Psychologist, 62*(8), 857–873.

Ward, E. C. (2005). Keeping it real: A grounded theory study of African American clients engaging in counseling at a community mental health agency. *Journal of Counseling Psychology, 52*(4), 471–481. https://doi.org/10.1037/0022-0167.52.4.471

Washington, D. (Director). (2002). *Antwone Fisher* [Film]. Fox Searchlight Pictures, Antwone Fisher Productions.

Watson, N. N., & Hunter, C. D. (2015). Anxiety and depression among African American women: The costs of strength and negative attitudes toward psychological help-seeking. *Cultural Diversity and Ethnic Minority Psychology, 21*(4), 604–612.

Whaley, A. L. (2001). Cultural mistrust: An important psychological construct for diagnosis and treatment of African Americans. *Professional Psychology: Research and Practice, 32*(6), 555–562. https://doi.org/10.1037/0735-7028.32.6.555

Williams, D. R., Lawrence, J. A., Davis, B. A., & Vu, C. (2019). Understanding how discrimination can affect health. *Health Services Research, 54*(S2), 1374–1388. https://doi.org/10.1111/1475-6773.13222

Williams, D. R., & Mohammed, S. A. (2009). Discrimination and racial disparities in health: Evidence and needed research. *Journal of Behavioral Medicine, 32*(1), 20–47. https://doi.org/10.1007/s10865-008-9185-0

Williams, K. E., Chambless, D. L., & Steketee, G. (1998). Behavioral treatment of obsessive-compulsive disorder in African Americans: Clinical issues. *Journal of Behavior Therapy and Experimental Psychiatry, 29*(2), 163–170.

Windsor, L., & Dunlap, E. (2010). What is substance use all about? Assumptions in New York's drug policies and the perceptions of drug using low-income African-Americans. *Journal of Ethnicity in Substance Abuse, 9*(1), 64–87.

Windsor, L. C., Jemal, A., & Alessi, E. J. (2015). Cognitive behavioral therapy: A meta-analysis of race and substance use outcomes. *Cultural Diversity and Ethnic Minority Psychology, 21*(2), 300–313. https://doi.org/10.1037/a0037929

Zellars, R. B. (2019). "As if we were all struggling together": Black intellectual traditions and legacies of gendered violence. *Women's Studies International Forum, 77.* https://doi.org/10.1016/j.wsif.2019.04.008

CHAPTER 9

Couple and Family Therapy with African American Women

Ayanna Abrams
Ticily Medley

Couple and family treatment has seen an increase in utilization by African American women as negative stigma surrounding seeking support has decreased; however, there are still several treatment factors related to African American women's experience and outcomes that have been insufficiently researched (Kelly & Boyd-Franklin, in Rastogi & Thomas, 2009). Most of the existing research comes from studying White clinical and research populations and is rooted in theories created by White scholars and clinicians. In order to address how African American women utilize couple and family therapy, it is important to understand the social, historical, and political lenses through which African American women have been viewed, recognizing that this impacts how, why, and when they choose to seek professional help. Therapeutic interventions that validate experiences of racism and how couples and families are negatively impacted not only can create a safer therapeutic environment and stronger alliance, but also can help African American families better understand what may be exacerbating their presenting concerns (Kelly & Boyd-Franklin, in Rastogi & Thomas, 2009).

While the information in this chapter is an overview, it can be used to contextualize experiences that African American clients may have and create an opportunity for learning and growth in cultural humility for clinicians. First, it is important to understand that African Americans and their experiences are not a monolith. Lincoln, Taylor, and Jackson (2008) found that immigration by individuals of African descent, gender norms, ratios of men and women, and socioeconomic statuses largely influenced how African Americans trended toward or away from marital unions. It is also important to highlight the lasting impact that racism, segregation, and the prison industrial complex has had on African American family cohesion and stability across generations. While these factors are often used to point to deficits in African American kinship, romance, and parenting, this chapter seeks to support the resilience of African American couples and families without pathologizing generational traumas (Lyles & Carter, 1982).

AFRICAN AMERICAN COUPLES AND FAMILIES

The history of African Americans in the United States and current dating and marriage constellations present great diversity in the ethnic and cultural composition of African American couples and families. As noted in other chapters (see Chapters 4 and 14), a history of enslavement and rape impacted the dynamics of African American families. As descendants of mothers who were enslaved and raped by enslavers, there is variety in the phenotypical appearance and genetic makeup of African Americans. Post-enslavement, interracial marriage and children with multiracial identities continue to infuse diversity within the African American family composition. Legally and anecdotally relevant today, the "one-drop rule," meaning that if a person had "one drop of African blood" they were considered Black, persists (Livingston & Brown, 2017). Therefore, a wide range of individuals may identify themselves as African American. As such, African American couples and families may be comprised of two (or more) Black individuals, a Black partner and a partner(s) of a different ethnicity, or Black individuals with multiracial identities.

Fortunately, it is not for therapists to identify who is an African American couple or family. Therapists, entering with a knowledge of and respect for African Americans, allow these couples and families the space to self-identify and honor their race and ethnic identity in ways that are most meaningful to them as an individual, partner, and family member.

Marriage and Divorce Rate Statistics

As of 2018, 6.5 out of every 1,000 people in the United States were married and 2.9 per thousand were divorced (excluding five states). A 2019 Pew Research Center study showed that rates of marriage and unmarried cohabitation have broadly changed over the past few years; notably, marriage rates have declined by 5 percent since 1995, and adults living with an unmarried partner increased from 3 to 7 percent (Horowitz, Graf, & Livingston, 2019). Among other trends noted, African American rates of marriage stabilized at 33 percent, in comparison to White counterparts at 57 percent, Asian Americans at 63 percent, and Hispanics at 48 percent. Compared to other racial groups, African Americans marry later, and

Couple and Family Therapy with African American Women   169

African American women exhibit less marital stability (Raley, Sweeney, & Wondra, 2016). Cohabitation rates are generally more consistent across racial categories.

The ability to marry for same-sex couples became nationally legalized with a June 2015 Supreme Court ruling, following the important precedent of a provision within the federal Defense of Marriage Act that restricted the federal recognition of marriages to heterosexual couples being declared unconstitutional in 2013 (Gates, 2015). Since then, according to national social surveys, the number of adults who are accepting of same-sex marriage has consistently increased. It is estimated that almost 40 percent of same-sex couples were married as of 2015. As the social dynamics impacting same-sex couples begin to parallel those that affect heterosexual couples, the significant differences in behavior between the groups has begun to diminish (e.g., cohabiting rates). Based on census estimates, it is believed that same-sex married couples make up about 0.5 percent of U.S. households and 1 percent of cohabiting couples. These couples also display similar divorce rates to that of heterosexual couples (Kim & Stein, 2018), though same-sex relationships, overall, have higher rates of separation compared to heterosexual couples (Joyner, Manning, & Bogle, 2017). In heterosexual and same-sex couples, women are more likely to file for divorce than men (Kim & Stein, 2018).

Healthy Couples and Families

There are many ideas about what is considered a healthy and functional couple or family. For example, the National Center on African American Marriages and Parenting (NCAAMP, n.d.) lists the following 10 elements of healthy marriage: relationship satisfaction, commitment, friendship, intimacy, trust and honesty, fidelity, supportiveness, effective communication, effective conflict management, and nonviolent interactions. There is some overlap in healthy relationship components supported by Gottman's Sound Relationship House Theory, which also includes understanding a partner's inner world (i.e., stress, fears, goals, etc.), as well as fondness and admiration for one another. Some attributes of healthy African American couples and families include the ability to provide support and comfort regarding issues of racial discrimination and injustice, which promotes resilience (Smith et al., 2019). Positive couple and family interactions show benefits across time such as increased self-esteem, sharing in caregiving roles across generations, and mitigating the negative impacts of disability (Pienta, Hayward, & Jenkins, 2000; Thomas, Liu, & Umberson, 2017).

In this author's (Abrams) experience with couples and families who report overall relationship satisfaction, factors that are consistent are emotional and physical safety, playfulness/ability to have fun with one another, feeling physically attracted to and attractive to their partner, and an ability to display vulnerability with one another. Though the reasons that bring them to therapy may not always reflect the above, therapy is utilized to illuminate how these factors can significantly mitigate conflict and emotional disconnection.

AFRICAN AMERICAN WOMEN IN COUPLE AND FAMILY THERAPY

Presenting Concerns

Relationship Distress. Clients commonly present for therapy reporting "communication issues," "not feeling connected anymore," an expression of role strain, or emotional/sexual infidelity that has eroded trust and resulted in increased anxiety and hypervigilance. When dysfunction is present within couple and parenting roles, this can also be related to the paradox of rigid Westernized gender roles for men and women that do not account for the long-standing impact that enslavement has had on African American family stability, or the physical presence of African American men in families and their economic contributions (Nightingale, Awosan, & Stavrianopoulos, 2019). The overwhelming feeling that comes with mitigating the complexities of these roles in a partnership can contribute to conflict, unmet expectations of partners, and overall marital dissatisfaction.

Financial decisions, along with household and parenting roles, are often rooted in learned gender roles and must be explored in depth for partners and families to assess fit with each other. Considering disparities in African American women and men's educational patterns, economic earnings and earning potential, and socialization, traditional gender roles can sometimes create distress and instability in relationships (Cutrona et al., 2011). Conflicting norms around self-sufficiency and dependence can make it harder for African American women to determine when it is safe to challenge those norms or when their personal value is being undermined, which can create feelings of overwhelm and maintenance of unrealistic relationship and parenting expectations (Nightingale, Awosan, & Stavrianopoulos, 2019).

Educational and Behavioral Issues. Compared to White peers, African American boys and girls are overrepresented in special education classes and juvenile detention facilities (Serwatka, Deering, & Grant, 1995), receive educational and behavioral discipline (i.e., suspension vs. detention) with greater penalty (Civil Rights Project, 2000), and are more likely to be diagnosed with oppositional and conduct disorders, behavioral problems, and attention deficit hyperactivity disorder (ADHD) (Fadus et al., 2020). It is not unusual that schools and the juvenile justice system refer children and families for therapy when the above concerns are encountered.

For some families, issues with children may serve as a precursor to relationship and personal concerns later explored in therapy. Whether it be limited insight, shame, or limited rapport with the therapist, children's issues may be common clinical presenting concerns that mask underlying relational or familial problems (Boyd-Franklin, Nelly, & Durham, 2015).

Trauma

Trauma is defined as a response to a distressing event that overwhelms a person's emotional ability to cope with its effects. Whether directly or vicariously, trauma can lead to psychological, relational, and occupational disruptions including anxiety, depression, mistrust, and sleep and appetite dysregulation. The 5th edition of the *Diagnostic and Statistical Manual of Mental Disorders* (*DSM-5*) describes post-traumatic stress disorder as involving exposure to a stressor with the consequent presence of one intrusive symptom, avoidance of reminders of said stressor, a negative change in thoughts and mood, and physiological arousal that persists for at least one month (American Psychiatric Association, 2013).

Using this criterion and applying it broadly to the African American experience in the United States, Dr. Joy DeGruy developed a theory called post-traumatic slave syndrome, defined as "multigenerational trauma together with continued oppression and absence of opportunity to access the benefits available in the society" (DeGruy & Robinson, 2005/2017, 105). This trauma is often passed down through epigenetics (i.e., scientific research with evidence that the environment can influence people at the genetic level and across generations) (DeGruy & Robinson, 2005/2017). DeGruy further explains that trauma is reflected in behaviors and beliefs, which impacts how African Americans operate in all relationships, including how they parent their children, understand romantic and familial love and connection to others, and learn to cope with stressors. Trauma through generations can present as secrecy in families; physical, emotional, or sexual abuse between partners or directed toward children; dysregulated anger; and psychological symptoms like anxiety, depression, and addiction.

Intimate partner violence (IPV) is described by the World Health Organization (WHO) as "one of the most common forms of violence against women and includes physical, sexual, and emotional abuse and controlling behaviours by an intimate partner" (WHO, 2012, 1). In the United States, as many as 6 million Black women are believed to have survived IPV, and Black women typically experience severe violence at higher rates than White women (Smith et al., 2017). Though most of the people experiencing IPV are women and the majority of perpetrators are men, IPV does sometimes occur in same-sex relationships (WHO, 2015). Regardless of the makeup of the couple, the WHO identifies the following significant consequences for women who experience intimate partner violence: physical injury, negative physical health, mental health disorders and suicide, sexual health diagnoses, reproductive health concerns, violence during pregnancy and related birth complications, homicide risk, and physical and psychological effects for children who are exposed to the violence. Therapists may find that women who have been victimized by IPV will present to counseling for the physical and psychological health consequences of their abuse or for assistance with keeping them or their children safe (Nnawulezi & West, 2018).

COMMON COUPLE AND FAMILY THERAPY TREATMENT METHODS

Numerous therapy models and theoretical orientations exist for treating couples and families. These modalities may differ in treatment length, therapist training requirements and certification, and evidence of success, depending on the presenting concerns. Regardless of the treatment modality, some basic premises exist when working with couples and families. First, when couples and families present for treatment, they have typically been dealing with the presenting concern for some time. Doss, Atkins, & Christensen (2003) noted that distressed couples presented to counseling six years after the issue began. Competent couple and family therapists should be prepared to handle high levels of conflict and chronic discord (Sullivan & Davila, 2014). Second, couples and families who present in crisis may prematurely leave therapy in continued distress. Overall, couples and families benefit from treatment (Christensen et al., 2004; Shadish et al., 1995); however, given the prominence of discord, many couples and families may find their problems persisting even after therapy has ended (Prince & Jacobson, 1995). Third, couple and family therapists working with African Americans may find themselves underprepared for using or adapting existing couple and family therapy models with their clients because traditional models were not designed with African American couples and families as a focus. Therefore, practitioners working with African American couples and families must be adaptive in how they approach adherence to existing therapy models. Furthermore, beyond adaptability, competent therapists working with African American couples and families should be prepared to approach clients from a place of cultural respect, dignity, and humility. This chapter is not able to comprehensively explore all couple and family models. However, this section highlights the following models: emotionally focused therapy (EFT), brief strategic family therapy (BSFT), the Gottman Method, and parent management training (PMT).

Emotionally Focused Therapy

EFT is an empirically supported intervention with a 70–75 percent effectiveness rate for reducing relationship distress. It is based on adult attachment theory, which stipulates that *all* people, regardless of their culture of origin, have innate needs for safety, comfort, and emotional closeness (Greenman, Young, & Johnson, in Rastogi and Thomas, 2009). This model uses the impact of negative emotion, how couples exchange emotions in a cycle of interactions, and positive and vulnerable emotion to predict relationship stability and security (Johnson, 2019). Though impressive in its level of effectiveness and like other clinical models, EFT does not thoroughly address racial, ethnic, and cultural dynamics that influence relationship cohesion, safety, and unmet needs.

Brief Strategic Family Therapy

BSFT is a short-term evidence-based practice originally developed for Hispanic families that focuses on changing the structure of family interactions to create stability. This model was expanded to facilitate cross-cultural implementation to families navigating conflict that can result from acculturation after emigration and possible separation. This model asserts that families are more likely to seek therapy when parts of the family system become dysfunctional and negative symptoms are displayed (Hervis, Shea, & Kaminsky, 2009). According to BSFT, children's functioning within the family is the result of how their parents are functioning because all parts of the family system are interdependent. BSFT aims to change the emotional affect of family members to help them reframe how they understand and interpret family interactions and, consequently, change the behavioral responses in the family unit.

The Gottman Method

Another popular approach to couple therapy, the Gottman Method, is a robust theoretical model based on decades of research that uses a thorough assessment process, including individual interviews with partners, questionnaires, and feedback sessions to help couples create or recreate their "Sound Relationship House" (Gottman & Gottman, 2015, 140). This figurative structure helps couples learn ways to minimize conflict, create shared meaning, and emotionally connect as friends (Gottman & Gottman, 2015). This model's interventions work to increase intimacy using specific steps to help couples understand one another, repair conflict, and act in ways that consider each other's value within the relationship.

Parent Management Training

As mentioned above, children's behavioral issues are a common presenting concern for family therapy. PMT is a research-based intervention primarily used for families with a child or adolescent presenting with social, emotional, and/or behavioral concerns. Based on views of human functioning, parents are taught specific skills and strategies to improve their child's functioning through techniques like role-playing and modeling. Kazdin (2005) notes that this theory is heavily rooted in *operant conditioning*, a type of learning that suggests that the environment has an influence on one's behavior.

CONSIDERATIONS FOR COUPLE AND FAMILY THERAPY WITH AFRICAN AMERICAN WOMEN

Help-Seeking Behaviors

Given the history of mistreatment of African American individuals and families, pathologizing of Black culture, and systemic oppression serving to rupture Black families, it is a wonder that African American couples and families present for therapy. Although African Americans are more open to attending couple and family counseling (compared to individual counseling), their entrance is often complicated by cultural and social factors. Cultural narratives such as "You don't tell family business," combined with therapist misinformation and a lack of cultural competence, can impact entrance into treatment and relationship building with African American couples and families. Coined "healthy cultural suspicion," African Americans may not trust the investment in therapy, the intent of therapists, or the mental health system as a whole (Boyd-Franklin, 2003). Unfortunately, African American consumers of mental health care are often seen as "resistant" to treatment or "noncompliant with recommendations," without due diligence to understand their culturally healthy suspicions and fears of mis- or overdiagnosis by treatment providers.

Because they are often the matriarch of the family, therapy and theoretical orientations aimed at challenging family and relationship dynamics can negatively impact help-seeking in African American women. With seeking therapy potentially being perceived as a sign of weakness, African American women contend with overcoming fears of being perceived as an inadequate partner or parent. Although therapist transparency is often beneficial and necessary for deep healing, offering therapeutic challenges or criticisms about family structure and hierarchy without cultural sensitivity and rapport can negatively impact engagement in the therapeutic process. African American women who do connect with culturally sensitive care can receive benefits from consistent therapy, including a greater understanding of their strengths, resilience, and struggles through consciousness raising, gender-role analysis. and social activism (Jones & Guy-Sheftall, 2017).

For African American women who identify as members of the LGBT community, their triple minority status (black, female, lesbian) or quadruple status (for those who identify as transgender or gender nonconforming) exposes them to multiple types of prejudice and systemic oppression (Bridges, Selvidge, & Matthews, 2003; Greene, 1994a). The effects of various social pressures, such as family loyalty and racism, are what sometimes lead Black women who identify as LGBT into therapy (Bridges et al., 2003). Therefore, in working with lesbian or bisexual women of color, counselors should attempt to assess the salience of each part of the client's identity (race/ethnicity, sexual orientation, and gender) and each's impact on the clinical presenting concerns. For transgender or gender nonconforming women of color, also addressing gender identity is a recommendation. Counselors who work with LGBT African American women should work to assess their own awareness of cultural identity factors, while informing themselves of ways to affirm the complex identities of this population (Bridges et al., 2003).

Religion

Although not generalizable to all African American families, religion and spirituality are well cemented with the Black community. African American families may identify faith community members as part of their family unit and as a means of emotional, economic, social, and parenting support. They are more likely to seek support and refuge within these communities compared to other resources that are outside the home (e.g., non-African American contacts, people outside of their faith, or medical/health professionals).

Religion has both direct and indirect associations with marital quality for heterosexual couples. Directly, participation in religion equates to increased social support of norms and values of marriage and relationship-enhancing behaviors (e.g., partner forgiveness), while indirect effects include fostering increased psychological well-being, temperance, and sexual fidelity (Wolfinger & Wilcox, 2008). Indirectly, religion has provided a foundation of traditional norms that can buffer distress and reground couples when they feel disconnected from each other. "The implication is that faith-based organizations (including churches and synagogues) may have a particularly strong role to play in nurturing the spiritual lives and enhancing the quality of the intimate marital relationships of their flocks" (Lichter & Carmalt, 2009, 168).

The role of religion with nonheterosexual and non-cisgender populations is a bit more complex. Members of the LGBTQ+ community may find it challenging to reconcile aspects of their sexual or gender identity with their religious values (Rostosky et al., 2008). Though it seems that adopting a sense of spirituality can offer protective mechanisms, strong connections to organized religion may create a greater experience of identity conflict for people who identify as LGBTQ+.

Same-Sex Couples and Gender Diversity

Historically, research with the LGBTQ+ community was created on a foundation of assumptions oft rooted in heterosexist and cisgender ideas of normalcy (Greene, 1994b). These and other assumptions have created not only barriers to understanding more about LGBTQ+ experiences, but also ways to support and care for their unique needs. With the legalization of same-sex marriage in 2015 and increases in positive social perceptions regarding same-sex relationships, there is greater access to research centering on LGBTQ+ populations (Gates, 2015). However, gaps still remain in areas that address the intersectional identities of women of color who identify as LGBTQ+ (Bridges, Selvidge, & Matthews, 2003). What we do know is that the triple minority status of African American women who are lesbian contributes to an additive effect when it comes to experiences of oppression (Greene, 1994a). Addressing these threats to mental wellness in counseling requires that therapists work to inform themselves, explore and address their personal biases, and become intentional about implementing therapeutic strategies that do not replicate racist, heterosexist, or cissexist norms (Bridges et al., 2003).

The professional codes for therapists in various fields each address work with LGBTQ+ populations in different ways. The American Psychological Association (APA) published guidelines for working with LGB, transgender, and gender nonconforming clients. The guidelines are aspirational principles that clinicians should strive toward; however, they do not override state or federal laws that govern the practice of clinicians (APA, 2015). The *Guidelines for Psychological Practice with Lesbian, Gay, and Bisexual Clients* (APA, 2012) encourage therapists to educate themselves on the social stigmas faced by the LGB community, to understand that nonheterosexual orientations do not constitute mental illness, and to accept that reparative/conversion therapies are detrimental to the health of LGB clients. Other guidelines encourage practitioners to increase their self-awareness regarding social biases, understand differences between sexual orientation and gender identity, and engage in affirmation of the various ways that LGB clients may present in identity, family patterns, and cultural practices. The *Guidelines for Psychological Practice with Transgender and Gender Nonconforming People* (APA, 2015) are similar to those for LGB clients in recommending that practitioners increase their knowledge base regarding gender and explore personal biases, as well as inform themselves about the range of identities and cultural experiences that may impact the lives of their clients. Also, these guidelines encourage practitioners to embrace foundational knowledge about the nonbinary construct of gender. Practitioners who implement these guidelines may be less likely to enact microaggressions against their LGBTQ+ clients, who may already be experiencing negative impacts on their mental health due to homophobic and transphobic stigma (McCullough et al., 2017).

Similar guidelines can be found in a set of competencies published by the American Counseling Association (ACA) that address the needs of LGBTQ+ clients in therapy (ALGBTIC, 2009a; ALGBTIC, 2009b). The core competencies published by the American Association for Marriage and

Family Therapy (AAMFT, 2004) and the National Association of Social Workers (NASW, 2001) generally address clinical work with diverse populations, but neither includes specific guidelines for work with LGBTQ+ populations.

Though LGBTQ+ African Americans have been central forces in changing the landscape and acceptance of sexual orientation and gender identity minorities, they have often been relegated to the margins of societal and familial acceptance (Pew Research Center, 2013). Increased visibility and acceptance of LGBTQ+ individuals have brought greater attention to the relationship and family needs of same-sex couples, gender identity diversity, and LGBTQ+ youth. It is estimated that 3.6 percent of adult women in the United States identify as LGBTQ+ and that anywhere from 2 million to 3.7 million minor children have a parent who identifies as LGBTQ+ (Gates, 2015). Approximately 200,000 children in the United States are being raised by married or cohabiting same-sex couples. Though the acceptance of same-sex relationships continues to rise, the number of same-sex couples who report raising children has declined since 2000 (Gates, 2015). This trend is likely due, at least in part, to the fact that a greater proportion of children who were previously raised by same-sex couples were the product of heterosexual relationships, whereas now, there are more same-sex couples who are seeking parenthood through the use of reproductive technologies and adoption (Gates, 2015; Meezan & Rauch, 2005). Overall, African Americans who identify as LGB or who are a member of a same-sex couple report a higher likelihood of raising or having children, compared to their White counterparts (Gates, 2015).

It is believed that the stigma of being LGBTQ+ contributes to a higher likelihood that LGBTQ+ individuals and same-sex couples with children will live in poverty (Gates, 2015). This finding is surprising because same-sex couples typically obtain greater levels of education compared to different-sex couples. However, the educational attainment of those same-sex couples who have children is not as high as those couples who are childless. Despite the greater likelihood of living in poverty mentioned above, overall, research has shown that children raised by LGB parents do not experience any significant disadvantages compared to the children of heterosexual parents (Gates, 2015; Meezan & Rauch, 2005). In fact, children of same-sex parents who are married are likely to experience multiple benefits, such as financial well-being, life stability, and reduced social stigma (Meezan & Rauch, 2005).

In those families where the person with the LGBTQ+ identity is a child, there are different dynamics and needs. For example, one study found that African American LGBTQ+ youth underscored the need for safe schools and communities, comprehensive feelings of safety across multiple contexts or environments, consistent support from people with whom they felt close, and resources to help their family members adjust to the minor's LGBTQ+ identity (Craig, McInroy, & Austin, 2018). Family acceptance was found to play a significant protective role against depression, suicidality, and social isolation, and in improving the self-esteem and overall health identity of LGBTQ+ youth (Ryan et al., 2010). AAMFT notes that while there are similarities in couple and family functioning between hetero-sexual and same-sex couples, negative social conditions (like alienation), stage discrepancies in awareness of same-sex attraction, and gender role confusion or strain impact LGBTQ+ relationships in distinct ways.

Greene and Boyd-Franklin (1996) found that African American lesbian women, due to historically strong cultural ties to family, may be less likely to face ostracism from their families in response to their sexual orienta-tion. This family support can help to allay the negative effects of racism. However, the absence of ostracism should not be interpreted as full inclu-sion; particularly within religious contexts, the intimate relationships of African American lesbian women may be ignored, denied, or recatego-rized as platonic friendships.

Due to stigma also associated with the LGBTQ+ community, LGBTQ+ African Americans find it harder to seek professional help, McGeorge and Carlson (2011) posit: "It is important for heterosexual therapists to engage in this critical self-exploration on an ongoing basis as it is not possible for heterosexual therapists to arrive at a place where they are completely free from their heteronormative assumptions and heterosexual privileges" (3). This can also be said for cisgender clinicians providing treatment to gen-der nonconforming clients.

Furthermore, "in contrast to the (White, middle-class) hetero-normative arrangement of two biological parents who preside over their children within close proximity, parenting by lesbians and gays oftentimes does not follow this model" (Cahill, Battle, & Meyer, 2004, 86). These supports are viewed as just as integral to the family structure as blood relatives. While this creates an in-group safety net that has widely been a means of survival and protection against racist and discriminatory violence from other races and ethnicities, it can limit African American couples and fam-ilies to only have as much access to resources as their network has, which may not be enough to meet their full needs.

Please refer to Chapter 12 of this text for additional information on work-ing with African American sexual and gender minority clients, includ-ing dynamics of providing family and couple counseling with LGBTQ+ populations.

Attachment

Like many couples seeking couple therapy, African American women may present with struggles identifying healthy attachment role models. Healthy attachment is defined as "an emotional connection with a sig-nificant other that offers comfort, reassurance and protection in the face of adversities in life" (Johnson, as cited in Atkinson & Goldberg, 2004,

209) and is often modeled by affect regulation (co-regulation), knowledge of expectations and beliefs of one another, and an interest in what the other is thinking and feeling (Bowlby, 1982). Lack of adequate modeling can make it difficult to practice healthier patterns of engagement in families they create with partners and if they choose to begin raising children. Additionally, if poor relationship models continue to persist in their lives, this impacts how women operate in these relationships and what they understand to be healthy, based on familiarity and pattern.

With strong and persistent messages of independence and self-sufficiency, ideas of attachment and reliance on another person can feel threatening to African American women, even when romantic relationships and parenting with a love partner are desirable. There are "unique challenges this population faces in terms of mate availability, gender, power and vulnerability," that impact openness to relationships, and once engaging, can make them more difficult to sustain (Chambers, 2009). African American women across age, sexual orientation, able-bodiedness, spirituality, and cohabitation arrangement can struggle with ideas of how to be themselves and simultaneously feel emotionally connected to and safe with others. Establishing long-lasting healthy relationships amidst messaging of relational and love deficiency can prove difficult because relationships require the very aspects that feel risky: trust and acceptance. Without these, romantic partnership and familial dynamics become eroded and sometimes irreparable.

Cultural Considerations

African American women often look for treatment providers of similar race or culture to feel emotionally safer and "seen." Cabral and Smith (2011) found African Americans preferred to be matched with African American therapists for treatment and evaluated African American therapists more positively than other therapists. Even with providers who may meet this racial and/or cultural criteria, African American women have learned vulnerability can be more risky than beneficial. Appearing "strong"—meaning capable, resilient, independent, and intelligent—has served as an armor for African American women against a world that has not seen or treated them as valuable.

Additional contributors to distress and impairment in African American women, though more subtle, are microaggressions, micro-assaults and micro-invalidations (Sue et al., 2007). As a result of these stressors, African Americans may present to health-care providers as significantly more distressed than White patients, and are then pathologized for the impact of these stressors on their health. It is important to acknowledge the impact of racism, sexism, and classism on how African American women function individually as well as within couple and family roles. Implicit and explicit messages of love worthiness, attachment capacity, and value in partner seeking that are provided through FOO, community, and media narratives heavily impact how African American women relate to others. All these sources are susceptible to infiltration from macro and micro levels of racism.

CLINICAL SKILLS IN COUPLE AND FAMILY THERAPY

As more African American women are open to and economically able to seek mental health treatment, therapists are learning how to provide more culturally appropriate treatment to them as individuals, romantic relationship partners, and family members. Shame, embarrassment, and fear of rejection can make it difficult for African American women to share openly what their struggles are and that they are seeking outside support. Participating in therapy without the social support system knowing can increase anxiety, even if the treatment is working on addressing presenting issues. Additionally, the health-care field, and more specifically the field of mental health, has historically mislabeled, misdiagnosed, and mistreated African American women due to clinician bias, which has understandably created a mistrust of providers (U.S. Department of Health and Human Services, 2001, 67).

Due to the above factors, two specific skills are most helpful in creating emotional safety for African American women in therapy: rapport between client and therapist and the ongoing treatment alliance.

Rapport Building

The unique dilemma presented to African American women in discerning when vulnerability may be helpful or harmful to their well-being, based on mixed messages from media, gendered norms, and the impact of racism, can make it difficult for them to explore these themes with their partners and families. Additionally, women must face the negative stigma that surrounds seeking professional mental health support, leaving them with limited social support and validation. This stigma decreases the likelihood of pursuing treatment and is one of the largest barriers to seeking care (Awosan et al., 2011).

When African American women enter therapy, it can be difficult to quickly embrace vulnerability with the therapist or their partner/children in front of a therapist. Sharing details of what they are struggling with, with someone they do not know, can feel threatening to their sense of capability and self-efficacy, even if they have reached the point of recognizing they need help. In order to build rapport and maintain emotional safety within the therapeutic alliance, it is imperative to understand this dilemma and offer strengths-based models of care that account for the impact of racism on the client's functioning as well as the clinician's own treatment biases

(Kelly & Boyd-Franklin, 2009; Nightingale, Awosan, & Stavrianopoulos, 2019). See the section on the Strong Black Woman Schema in Chapter 7 for more information.

Therapeutic Alliance

Building a therapeutic alliance with African American women may require ongoing assessment and rapport building across multiple sessions, not disclosing much personal information so as to not disrupt their narrative, not challenging cultural views or norms without rapport, and not presenting immediate solutions to problems without listening to their narrative fully. An understanding of potential racial, ethnic, social, and political differences present between client and therapist is imperative to building a safe and empathic treatment model for therapy. Addressing how these factors affect the client's ideas of partnership and parenting will help in collaborating on treatment goals that are tailored to specific clients.

Self of the Therapist and Implicit Bias

There is no expectation that non-Black therapists should be void of bias to successfully treat couples and families. However, it is important to develop awareness and humility and understand how systemic constructs reinforce racist systems. Examining one's own racial identity and biases and how they may impact the treatment relationship is required for transformative cross-racial couple and family therapy. Bias informs how we view others and subconsciously make assumption about motives, abilities, and possibility for change. Acknowledgment of strengths and affirmations in the initial assessment and initial sessions with African American women and families can create openness to feedback about areas of change, and lead to less defensiveness.

Culturally Responsive Therapeutic Intervention

Culturally responsive therapeutic intervention for couple and family therapy with African American women requires humility, curiosity, and active listening skills. Research, statistics and treatment modalities must be viewed from a culturally sensitive lens; this comes with recognizing and accepting that implicit bias exists and is inherent in clinical training. Indicators for culturally competent care based on race, sexual orientation and gender identification, and age, from APA, AAMFT and NASW provide the most up-to-date and ethical frameworks for clinicians to use best practices. Additionally, required and peer-supportive supervision and consultation offer ongoing support in providing adequate services to African American women through discussions of race, learning appropriate interventions, and exploring biases.

From a relational perspective, curiosity about African American women's experiences and expectations can be addressed directly by asking clients about their choice in therapist and if they share any ideas about how this may impact the therapeutic alliance. When assessing childhood and family histories, valuable information can be gathered by asking clients about implicit or explicit messages received across their life span about race, ethnicity, and gender, and if they have experienced discrimination or racism in the past. Some African American clients may minimize, or not even recognize, some of their experiences, and it could be helpful for a therapist to provide psychoeducation about this norm and collaborate with curiosity.

Further, Boyd-Franklin, Kelly, & Durham (2015) point out that therapists often err on one of two extremes in terms of the question of raising cultural or racial differences or similarities in treatment. Some therapists have been taught not to raise these issues in treatment until they are mentioned by their client(s); therefore, they are uncomfortable initiating this discussion. At the other extreme are therapists who, through their training in multicultural approaches, are aware these issues need to be raised; therefore, they raise them prematurely, before a therapeutic relationship has been established.

Greater emphasis should be placed on the quality of relationships than on structures that are not inclusive of African American culture, acknowledging African American families possess a variety of power structures and family systems and that some are perhaps matriarchal or do not fit traditional White norms. While helping clients build insight into family structures and roles, it is imperative African American women feel emotionally supported by other family members, who may only learn to offer appropriate support through therapeutic intervention. Considering couples and families with non-Black members, helping these family members understand the impact of the sociopolitical climate and how this can create distress for African American women in the family, would prove helpful.

Some options to improve assessment and treatment with African American women include use of the Inventory of Microaggressions Against Black Individuals (IMABI), mindfulness-based interventions to promote stress management and self-efficacy, incorporating Afrocentric theoretical approaches like NTU psychotherapy and a willingness to modify currently available interventions to adequately meet the needs of African American women.

CASE STUDY

The clinical case presented below offers a look into the intersections of how childhood and past relationship experiences, cultural expectations, and relationship role modeling can impact how couples and families present in therapy. This case provides an example of clinical intervention with a couple who exhibit a severed attachment and a pursuer–distancer cycle of interaction. This writer uses EFT theory to present a fuller scope of the couple's functioning. Beneficial techniques included slowly building the therapeutic alliance to look at relational themes that predated their marriage, and using interventions tailored to their racial/ethnic identities. Names have been changed to protect confidentiality.

Jerry and Faye identified as cisgender, heterosexual African American individuals in their mid-30s who were married for seven years and shared one child together. Faye, who held a leadership position at the corporate level, initiated counseling after a series of conflicts with Jerry, reporting that they were feeling "stuck in a bad rut," and wanted to "improve communication, understanding, and affection in the marriage because divorce was not an option." Faye was prompted to seek help because she did not want their daughter to be raised in a "broken home," but found Jerry's stoic communication patterns, hostility, and dependence on her unsustainable. Jerry, who worked full-time developing a company of his own, agreed to begin therapy if it would "help Faye feel better" about their marriage and "stop the fighting." Faye and Jerry dated for three years prior to marriage but broke up briefly when Jerry was unsure about taking a more serious step toward engagement.

The assessment consisted of four sessions: one joint session to gather the history of their relationship, conflict patterns, what *is* working in their marriage, as well as parenting values; two individual sessions to assess individual attachment patterns, medical and mental health histories, and relationship histories. Also included were questions about racial, gender, ethnic, and religious identity rooted within messages received from caregivers, media, and other sources, and how these messages impact their views of themselves and others. The couple was then brought back together for a fourth session to cover any additional information that would be helpful for the assessment, provide feedback on presenting issues, psychoeducation about EFT, and treatment planning. The presenting concern at the time of intake was each other's experience of emotional hostility.

Therapeutic intervention included addressing roles that each partner played in their partnership regarding parenting, household norms, financial decisions, and physical intimacy. Faye identified role strain that created resentment and disappointment toward Jerry. Dissension between the two began when Jerry felt pressured to propose to Faye, which led to a breakup after a series of arguments and impasses. After time apart and consulting with family, Jerry agreed to propose, and the couple married one year later. The couple expanded their family 1.5 years later with a child. They both shared values in child-rearing, however, several parenting conflicts arose, with Faye feeling isolated and resentful at what was expected of her in motherhood. Jerry admitted that he did not know much about children, and the ways that he provided support "never seemed like enough." He compared Faye to his mother, stating that Faye needed more than his mother ever needed from his father. Faye reported that she felt more supported by other parents, research, and blogs than by Jerry, which was "not what [she] signed up for."

It was important to use the assessment sessions, as well as the few sessions following, to build rapport with this couple. Neither had participated in therapy before, so psychoeducation about how early childhood experiences could impact adult functioning was helpful to them.

This therapist was intentional about building rapport individually with both partners. Two main rapport-building techniques, empathy and validation, were used to disrupt the negative cycle of communication between Jerry and Faye. Central to EFT's stage model, both interventions allowed the spouses to be and feel heard by the therapist and slowed down their interactions in order to process primary emotional states. Additionally, assessing racial and ethnic relationship models was important diagnostic information, as this impacted how they initially viewed each other and the implicit expectations they had. When Jerry was able to place Faye's fear of divorce in the context of her own childhood experiences, he expressed empathy and exhibited an emotional softening that she had not felt before. Faye also built insight into her patterns of taking control and how this served as an understandable adaptive function of her adolescence, though not useful as a strategy in her adult relationships. Both shared their respective experiences with racism in the workplace, the unspoken trauma this caused, as well as the support they had been implicitly needing from one another that went unmet. The couple was allowed time to practice displaying active listening and empathy, and building insight toward vulnerability, which helped to de-escalate hostility across the first few months of treatment. Then underlying narratives that motivated their behaviors were directly addressed. Once emotional safety was reestablished, therapy offered a space for depth, emotional risk-taking, and reframing their beliefs about their marriage. Treatment was terminated after a maintenance period of 18 months, when the couple was able to sustain a positive shift in how they understood one another's behaviors, they engaged in and repaired conflict, and they envisioned a stable future for their family.

REFERENCES

American Association for Marriage and Family Therapy (AAMFT). *Therapeutic issues for same-sex couples.* Retrieved September 29, 2020, from https://www.aamft.org/Consumer_Updates/Therapeutic_Issues_for_Same-sex_Couples.aspx

American Association for Marriage and Family Therapy (AAMFT). (2004). *Marriage and family therapy core competencies.* Alexandria, VA: Author.

American Psychiatric Association (APA). (2013). *Diagnostic and statistical manual of mental disorders* (5th ed.). Arlington, VA: Author.

American Psychological Association (APA). (2012). Guidelines for psychological practice with lesbian, gay, and bisexual clients. *American Psychologist, 67*(1), 10–42. https://doi.org/10.1037/a0024659

American Psychological Association (APA). (2015). Guidelines for psychological practice with transgender and gender nonconforming people. *American Psychologist, 70*(9), 832–864. https://doi.org/10.1037/a0039906

American Psychological Association (APA). (2019). *Race and ethnicity guidelines in psychology: Promoting responsiveness and equity.* https://www.apa.org/about/policy/summary-guidelines-race-ethnicity

Association of Lesbian, Gay, Bisexual and Transgender Issues in Counseling (ALGBTIC). (2009a). *ALGBTIC competencies for counseling LGBQQIA.* Alexandria, VA: Author.

Association of Lesbian, Gay, Bisexual and Transgender Issues in Counseling (ALGBTIC). (2009b). Competencies for counseling transgender clients. Alexandria, VA: Author. https://www.counseling.org/docs/default-source/competencies/algbtic_competencies.pdf?sfvrsn=d8d3732f_12

Atkinson, L., & Goldberg, S. (Eds.). (2004). *Attachment issues in psychopathology and intervention.* New York, NY: Routledge.

Awosan, C. I., Sandberg, J. G., & Hall, C. A. (2011). Understanding the experience of Black clients in marriage and family therapy. *Journal of Marital and Family Therapy, 37*(2), 153–168. https://doi.org/10.1111/j.1752-0606.2009.00166.x

Bowlby, J. (1982). Attachment and loss: Retrospect and prospect. *American Journal of Orthopsychiatry, 52*(4), 664–678. https://doi.org/10.1111/j.1939-0025.1982.tb01456.x

Boyd-Franklin, N. (2003). *Black families in therapy: Understanding the African American experience.* New York, NY: Guilford Press.

Boyd-Franklin, N., Kelly, S., & Durham, J. (2015). African American couples in therapy. In A. Gurman, *Clinical handbook of couple therapy* (4th ed). (pp. 681–697). New York, NY: Guilford Press.

Bridges, S. K., Selvidge, M. M. D., & Matthews, C. R. (2003). Lesbian women of color: Therapeutic issues and challenges. *Journal of Multicultural Counseling and Development, 31*(2), 113–130.

Cabral, R. R., & Smith, T. B. (2011). Racial/ethnic matching of clients and therapists in mental health services: A meta-analytic review of preferences, perceptions, and outcomes. *Journal of Counseling Psychology, 58*(4), 537–554. https://doi.org/10.1037/a0025266

Cahill, S., Battle, J., & Meyer, D. (2004). Partnering, parenting, and policy: Family issues affecting Black lesbian, gay, bisexual, and transgender (LGBT) people. *Race and Society, 6,* 85–98.

Chambers, A. (2009). Pre-marital counseling with middle-class African Americans: The forgotten group. In M. Rastogi & V. Thomas (Eds.), *Multicultural couple therapy* (pp. 217–234). Newbury Park, CA: Sage.

Christensen, A., Atkins, D. C., Berns, S., Wheeler, J., Baucom, D. H., & Simpson, L. E. (2004). Traditional versus integrative behavioral couple therapy for significantly and chronically distressed married couples. *Journal of Consulting and Clinical Psychology, 72*(2), 176–191. https://doi.org/10.1037/0022-006X.72.2.176

Civil Rights Project (Harvard University), Advancement Project., & National Summit on Zero Tolerance. (2000). *Opportunities suspended: The devastating consequences of zero tolerance and school discipline policies: Report from a National Summit on Zero Tolerance, June 15–16, 2000, Washington D.C.* Cambridge, MA.: Civil Rights Project, Harvard University, Advancement Project, A project of Community Partners.

Craig, S. L., McInroy, L. B., & Austin, A. (2018). "Someone to have my back": Exploring the needs of racially and ethnically diverse lesbian, gay, bisexual, and transgender high school students. *Children & Schools*, 40(4), 231–239. https://doi.org/10.1093/cs/cdy016

Cutrona, C. E., Russell, D. W., Burzette, R. G., Wesner, K. A., & Bryant, C. M. (2011). Predicting relationship stability among midlife African American couples. *Journal of Consulting and Clinical Psychology*, 79(6), 814–825. https://doi.org/10.1037/a0025874

DeGruy, J., & Robinson, R. (2017). *Post traumatic slave syndrome: America's legacy of enduring injury and healing*. Milwaukie, Oregon: Uptone Press. (Original work published 2005)

Doss, B., Atkins, D., & Christensen, A. (2003). Who's dragging their feet? Husbands and wives seeking marital therapy. *Journal of Marital and Family Therapy*, 29(2), 165–177. https://doi.org/10.1111/j.1752-0606.2003.tb01198.x

Fadus, M. C., Ginsburg, K. R., Sobowale, K., Halliday-Boykins, C. A., Bryant, B. E., Gray, K. M., & Squeglia, L. M. (2020). Unconscious bias and the diagnosis of disruptive behavior disorders and ADHD in African American and Hispanic youth. *Academic Psychiatry*, 44, 95–102. https://doi.org/10.1007/s40596-019-01127-6

Gates, G. J. (2015). Marriage and Family: LGBT individuals and same-sex couples. *The Future of Children*, 25(2), 67–87.

Gottman, J. M., & Gottman, J. S. (2015). Gottman Method couple therapy. In A. Gurman (Ed.), *Clinical handbook of couple therapy* (4th ed). (pp. 138–166). New York, NY: Guilford Press.

Greene, B. (1994a). Lesbian women of color: Triple jeopardy. In L. Comas-Diaz & B. Greene, (Eds)., *Women of color: Integrating ethnic and gender identities in psychotherapy* (pp. 389–427). New York, NY: Guilford Press.

Greene, B. (1994b). Ethnic-minority lesbians and gay men: Mental health and treatment issues. *Journal of Consulting and Clinical Psychology*, 62(2), 243–251. https://doi.org/10.1037/0022-006X.62.2.243

Greene, B., & Boyd-Franklin, N. (1996). African American lesbian couples: Ethnocultural considerations in psychotherapy. In M. Hill & E. D. Rothblum (Eds.), *Couples therapy: Feminist perspectives* (pp. 49–60). Philadelphia, PA: Harrington Park Press/Haworth Press.

Greenman, P. S., Young, M. Y., & Johnson, S. M. (2009). Emotionally focused couple therapy with intercultural couples. In M. Rastogi & V. Thomas (Eds.), *Multicultural couple therapy* (pp. 143–166). Thousand Oaks, CA: Sage.

Hervis, O. E., Shea, K. A., & Kaminsky, S. M. (2009). Brief strategic family therapy. In M. Rastogi & V. Thomas (Eds.), *Multicultural couple therapy* (pp. 167–186). Thousand Oaks, CA: Sage.

Horowitz, J. M., Graf, N., & Livingston, G. (2019, Nov 6). Marriage and cohabitation in the U.S. https://www.pewsocialtrends.org/wp-content/uploads/sites/3/2019/11/PSDT_11.06.19_marriage_cohabitation_FULL.final_.pdf

Johnson, S. M. (2004). An antidote to posttraumatic stress disorder: The creation of secure attachment in couples therapy. In L. Atkinson & S. Goldberg (Eds.), *Attachment issues in psychopathology and intervention* (pp. 207–228). Mahwah, NJ: Lawrence Erlbaum Associates.

Johnson, S. M. (2019). *Attachment theory in practice: Emotionally focused therapy (EFT) with individuals, couples, and families*. Guilford Press.

Jones, L. V., & Guy-Sheftall, B. (2017). *Black feminist therapy as a wellness tool*. In S. Y. Evans, K. Bell, & N. K. Burton (Eds.), *Black women's mental health: Balancing strength and vulnerability* (pp. 201–213). State University of New York Press.

Joyner, K., Manning, W., & Bogle, R. (2017). Gender and the stability of same-sex and different-sex relationships among young adults. *Demography, 54*(6), 2351–2374. https://doi.org/10.1007/s13524-017-0633-8

Kazdin, A. E. (2005). *Parent management training: Treatment for oppositional, aggressive, and antisocial behavior in children and adolescents.* Oxford, England: Oxford University Press.

Kelly, S., & Boyd-Franklin, N. (2009). Joining, understanding, and supporting Black couples in treatment. In M. Rastogi & V. Thomas (Eds.), *Multicultural couple therapy* (pp. 235–254). Thousand Oaks, CA: Sage.

Kim, S. A., & Stein, E. (2018). Gender in the context of same-sex divorce and relationship dissolution. *Family Court Review, 56*(3), 384–398.

Lichter, D. T., & Carmalt, J. H. (2009). Religion and marital quality among low-income couples. *Social Science Research, 38*(1), 168–187.

Lincoln, K. D., Taylor, R. J., & Jackson, J. S. (2008). Romantic relationships among unmarried African Americans and Caribbean Blacks: Findings from the National Survey of American Life. *Family Relationships, 57*(2), 254–266.

Livingston, G., & Brown, A. (2017, May 30). *Intermarriage in the U.S. 50 years after Loving v. Virginia.* https://www.pewsocialtrends.org/2017/05/18/intermarriage-in-the-u-s-50-years-after-loving-v-virginia/

Lyles, M. R., & Carter, J. H. (1982). Myths and strengths of the Black family: A historical and sociological contribution to family therapy. *Journal of the National Medical Association, 74*(11), 1119–1123.

McCullough, R., Dispenza, F., Parker, L. K., Viehl, C. J., Chang, C. Y., & Murphy, T. M. (2017). The counseling experiences of transgender and gender nonconforming clients. *Journal of Counseling & Development, 95*(4), 423–434. https://doi.org/10.1002/jcad.12157

McGeorge, C., & Carlson, T. S. (2011). Deconstructing heterosexism: Becoming an LGB affirmative heterosexual couple and family therapist. *Journal of Marital and Family Therapy, 37*(1), 14–26. https://doi.org/10.1111/j.1752-0606.2009.00149.x

Meezan, W., & Rauch, J. (2005). Gay Marriage, same-sex parenting, and America's children. *The Future of Children, 15*(2), 97–115.

National Association of Social Workers (NASW). (2001). *NASW standards for cultural competence in social work practice.* Washington, DC: Author.

National Center on African American Marriages and Parenting (NCAAMP). (n.d.). *What is a healthy marriage?* http://www.hamptonu.edu/ncaamp/docs/HU_NCAMMP_Healthy_Marriage.pdf

Nightingale, M., Awosan, C. I., & Stavrianopoulos, K. (2019). Emotionally focused therapy: A culturally sensitive approach for African American heterosexual couples. *Journal of Family Psychotherapy, 30*(3), 221–244.

Nnawulezi, N., & West, C. M. (2018). Institutional strategies to promote the health of Black women survivors of intimate partner violence. *Meridians: Feminism, Race, Transnationalism, 16*(2), 276–285. https://doi.org/10.2979/meridians.16.2.08

Pew Research Center. (2013, June 13). *A survey of LGBT Americans.* https://www.pewsocialtrends.org/2013/06/13/a-survey-of-lgbt-americans/#social-acceptance-and-the-publics-perspective

Pienta, A. M., Hayward, M. D., & Jenkins, K. R. (2000). Health consequences of marriage for the retirement years. *Journal of Family Issues, 21*(5), 559–586. https://doi.org/10.1177/019251300021005003

Prince, S. E., & Jacobson, N. S. (1995). *Couple and family therapy for depression*. In E. E. Beckham & W. R. Leber (Eds.), *Handbook of depression* (pp. 404–424). New York, NY: Guilford Press.

Raley, R. K., Sweeney, M. M., & Wondra, D. (2015). The growing racial and ethnic divide in U.S. marriage patterns. *The Future of Children, 25*(2), 89–109. https://doi.org/10.1353/foc.2015.0014

Rastogi, M., & Thomas, V. (Eds.) (2009). *Multicultural couple therapy*. Thousand Oaks, CA: Sage.

Rostosky, S. S., Danner, F., & Riggle, E. D. B. (2008). Religiosity and alcohol use in sexual minority and heterosexual youth and young adults. *Journal of Youth and Adolescence, 37*, 552–563. https://doi.org/10.1007/s10964-007-9251-x

Ryan, C., Russell, S. T., Huebner, D. M., Diaz, R., and Sanchez, J. (2010). Family acceptance in adolescence and the health of LGBT young adults. *Journal of Child and Adolescent Psychiatric Nursing, 23*(4), 205–213.

Serwatka, T. S., Deering, S., & Grant, P. (1995). Disproportionate representation of African Americans in emotionally handicapped classes. *Journal of Black Studies, 25*(4), 492–506. https://doi.org/10.1177/002193479502500406

Shadish, W.R., Ragsdale, K., Glaser, R. R., & Montgomery, L. M. (1995). The Efficacy and effectiveness of marital and family therapy: A perspective from meta-analysis. *Journal of Marital and Family Therapy, 21*: 345-360. https://doi.org/10.1111/j.1752-0606.1995.tb00170.x

Smith, S. G., Chen, J., Basile, K. C., Gilbert, L. K., Merrick, M. T., Patel, N., Walling, M., & Jain, A. (2017). The National Intimate Partner and Sexual Violence Survey (NISVS): 2010–2012 State Report. Atlanta, GA: National Center for Injury Prevention and Control, Centers for Disease Control and Prevention. https://www.cdc.gov/violenceprevention/pdf/NISVS-StateReportBook.pdf

Smith, S. M., Williamson, L. D., Branch, H., & Fincham, F. D. (2019). Racial discrimination, racism-specific support, and self-reported health among African American couples. *Journal of Social and Personal Relationships, 37*(3), 779–799.

Sue, D. W., Capodilupo, C. M., Torino, G. C., Bucceri, J. M., Holder, A. M. B., Nadal, K. L., & Esquilin, M. (2007). Racial microaggressions in everyday life: Implications for clinical practice. *American Psychologist, 62*(4), 271–286. https://doi.org/10.1037/0003-066X.62.4.271

Sullivan, K. T., & Davila, J. (2014). The problem is my partner: Treating couples when one partner wants the other to change. *Journal of Psychotherapy Integration, 24*(1), 1–12. https://doi.org/10.1037/a0035969

Thomas, P. A., Liu, H., & Umberson, D. (2017). Family relationships and well-being. *Innovation in Aging, 1*(3), igx025. https://doi.org/10.1093/geroni/igx025

U.S. Department of Health and Human Services. (2001). *Mental health: Culture, race, and ethnicity—A supplement to mental health: A report of the surgeon general*. Rockville, MD: U.S. Department of Health and Human Services, Substance Abuse and Mental Health Services Administration, Center for Mental Health Services.

Wolfinger, N., & Wilcox, W. (2008). Happily ever after? Religion, marital status, gender, and relationship quality in urban families. *Social Forces, 86*(3), 1311–1337.

World Health Organization. (2012). *Understanding and addressing violence against women*. http://apps.who.int/iris/bitstream/10665/77432/1/WHO_RHR_12.36_eng.pdf

CHAPTER 10

Group Therapy with Black and African American Women

Michelle King Lyn

INTRODUCTION

In contemporary popular media, there are multiple images of beautiful, successful Black and African American women (BAAW) living their best lives as part of a vibrant and close-knit group of sister friends. Feature films such as *Waiting to Exhale* (Whitaker, 1995) and *Girls Trip* (Lee, 2017) and television series such as *Living Single* (Bowser & Shulman, 1993–1998), *Girlfriends* (Grammer, Akil, & Hicks, 2000–2008), and *Insecure* (Rae et al., 2016–present) have reached commercial success within the African American community and among mainstream audiences worldwide. The women in these fictional stories are dealing with ups and downs of their romantic, familial, and professional lives and simultaneously giving and receiving support to one another. Written and/or produced by BAAW, these fictional accounts reflect real-life experiences of BAAW. The women, who are typically highly capable as individuals, are even more effective and victorious in overcoming obstacles as part of a collective group.

Karenga (2008) introduced seven guiding principles for the African American community. The principles are collectively referred to as the Nguzo Saba and include: Umoja—Unity, Kujichagulia—Self Determination, Ujima—Collective Work and Responsibility, Ujaama—Cooperative Economics, Nia—Purpose, Kuumba—Creativity, and Imani—Faith. The Nguzo Saba are at the center of the holiday Kwanzaa, the annual celebration of Afrocentric cultural values and traditions taking place from

December 26 through January 1 (Karenga, 2008). The Nguzo Saba and principles of Kwanzaa are reflective of the Afrocentric worldview based on collectivist values. Similar themes of connection can be found when looking at several of the curative factors of group therapy outlined by Yalom and Leszcz (2005) (e.g., giving of oneself to help others, universality, identification, and group cohesiveness). The similarities between the Afrocentric worldview and the tenets of group therapy are apparent. Furthermore, the interactions between African American sister friends are often portrayed as dynamic and transformative, which can also be said of effective group therapy.

Group therapy is a therapeutic modality that involves one or more trained therapists leading a group of approximately 5 to 15 members and targets a common presenting problem (APA, 2019). For BAAW, group therapy has been proposed to be an optimal treatment modality offering the help of trained behavioral health clinicians and support of others who can relate directly to their unique experience (Pack-Brown, Whittington-Clark, & Parker, 1998; Boyd-Franklin, 1987). The focus of the chapter is to explore the use of group therapy as a means of support and treatment for psychological concerns for BAAW. BAAW may be members of heterogeneous groups with open membership related to diversity, culture, and gender, or may enter groups specifically designed for BAAW. This chapter primarily focuses on the homogeneous group experience of BAAW.

HISTORY AND BACKGROUND

During the 1980s and 1990s, there was an emergence of BAAW clinicians addressing the lack of specific clinical interventions targeting BAAW despite evidence of higher emotional distress and psychological risk factors compared to other groups. An article published in *Essence*, a long-standing popular magazine for BAAW, detailed the rising trend of group therapy for BAAW emphasizing: 1) affordability relative to individual therapy, 2) cultural familiarity as compared to less welcoming professional spaces, and 3) a safe space for mutual support and healing (Pickney, 1994). The article normalized help-seeking behaviors by providing examples of BAAW seeking group therapy to cope with situational stressors such as divorce, and clinical issues like depression and anxiety. Using layperson's terms, the article described the process of group therapy and stands as an example of popular media providing psychoeducation to BAAW promoting group therapy.

Boyd-Franklin (1987) offered pioneering research on the topic. She provided ongoing group therapy in her psychological practice to BAAW based on the theoretical underpinnings of Yalom and Leszcz (2005) and borrowing from psychoanalytic and behavioral theory. The groups were designed to foster support in addition to helping group members meet the therapeutic goal of translating insight into new patterns of behavior.

Boyd-Franklin (1987) noted support remained essential in the groups because Black women reported feeling isolated, especially as professionals in a higher social stratum. They were often geographically and socioeconomically distant from families and sought out sisterhood with other Black women.

Boyd-Franklin (1987) outlined themes and interpersonal observations of the groups including family relationships, the impact of heterosexual romantic relationships, and female friendships. Group members reported feeling weighed down by family responsibilities from their family of origin (FOO). The women often struggled when receiving support due to greater comfort in their typical role as supporter in their outside relationships. Boyd-Franklin (1987) helped group members identify difficult emotions and facilitated the expression of vulnerability. Members being vulnerable with one another often facilitated greater connections in group and greater insight.

The role of the Black church was prominent in the lives of group members. For some members this was expressed by reconciling conflicting feelings about religious upbringings and current values and behaviors, while others expressed the importance of religion in coping with emotional issues. Diversity within the groups allowed the members to process assumptions they had of one another, leading to another important theme, which was fear of rejection by other Black women. The complexities of within-group differences will be explored later in this chapter.

The work of Pack-Brown and colleagues (1998) was also foundational and innovative. In *Images of Me* (1998), Pack Brown et al. illustrated a comprehensive group therapy program for BAAW. The group program incorporates the Nguzo Saba principles (Karenga, 2008). The process of treatment as outlined by Pack Brown et al. (1998) in the Images of Me groups occurs in four stages, with several of the Nguzo Saba principles serving as guides for each stage. The Images of Me group stages also correspond with group stages (e.g., initial stage, working stage, and termination) defined by Yalom and Leszcz (2005) to help members achieve individual and collective goals. Authors emphasize how "symbolism, strength, faith, and creativity" (Pack Brown et al., 1998, 4) are channeled throughout and central to the activities of the group. Images of Me incorporates theories specifically addressing African American mental health concerns as well as theories from broad perspectives. The theoretical orientation for Images of Me groups is eclectic, borrowing from existential and cognitive behavioral approaches in addition to principles of prominent group therapy theories.

One of the traditions from the Afrocentric worldview is to honor elders and ancestors who have paved the way for the community. Authors like Boyd-Franklin (1987) and Pack Brown et al. (1998) pioneered the expansion of group psychological theory and practice to include the experiences of BAAW. This was especially difficult coming out of an era when research and training in the psychological field was dominated by White and male perspectives. Thanks to their efforts, the specific needs of BAAW in group therapy have gained some traction, and many of the foundational concepts and methods are still relevant today; however, psychological literature still has further to go in providing comprehensive understanding and treatment for BAAW in group.

Evidence of the Benefits of Group for BAAW

As mentioned, there is a lag in recent psychological research exploring the therapeutic utility of group therapy with BAAW. Several of the existing studies focus on culturally adapted group interventions that coincide with research on empirically based treatment. The ethical standards of psychological practice require the adaptation of evidence-based interventions to incorporate the cultural values of the intended population (Ward & Brown, 2015). As such, there is a growing body of research focused on culturally adapted evidence-based treatment groups.

Jones and Sam (2018) provided group therapy to BAAW college students using a format they called Cultural Connections, which incorporated tenets of relational cultural theory (RTC). The authors found a lack of studies on culturally adapted groups for BAAW college women with a clear theoretical foundation. They argued that RTC lent itself well to work with BAAW based on the central relationship paradigm that fosters authenticity, vulnerability, and mutuality in relationships. These principles are akin to collectivism and sisterhood encouraged in the Black community. Their case study described group members having a stronger identity as a Black woman, greater self-confidence, and healthier patterns of relating to others post group. The treatment outcomes are based on clinician observations and group members' self-report because assessment measures were deemed by both clients and clinicians to be limited in their ability to accurately measure the benefits of the group intervention.

Another study used formal assessment measures of depression, posttraumatic stress, suicidality, and general psychological functioning to examine the effects of a culturally adapted group intervention for BAAW in an urban, lower SES population. Kaslow et al. (2010) developed a culturally informed 10-week group intervention that was offered as an alternative to standard support groups and psychiatric care in an outpatient setting for BAAW patients. The intervention, referred to as the Grady Nia Project, focused on personal and community empowerment and purpose ("Nia" in Swahili). Characteristics of the culturally informed group included the following: having a least one BAAW coleader, incorporating Afrocentric principles and proverbs, invoking African American female role models, and empowering members regarding self-awareness, connectedness, and racial identity. The women in both the traditional treatment group and the culturally informed group presented with a history of suicide attempts and interpersonal partner violence. The culturally informed group seemed to provide more defined clinical improvement for its members. Data analysis comparing the levels of depression for both groups indicated the culturally informed group members had a faster initial reduction in depressive symptoms than the traditional treatment group. The culturally informed group members also showed lower levels of suicidality, particularly during times of interpersonal partner violence. Given this data, it appears that as well as group therapy being beneficial to BAAW, the use of cultural-specific interventions seems to enhance those benefits (Kaslow et al., 2010).

Manualized group cognitive behavioral therapy (CBT) has been established as effective in treating anxiety disorders and depression (Hofmann et al., 2012). Several researchers have further explored the effectiveness of manualized CBT with diverse groups, including BAAW. Research was designed to examine the effects of CBT in a group format for BAAW with panic disorder. In the intervention, Carter et al. (2003) allowed for discussion of race discrimination as part of the treatment in addition to traditional CBT concepts such as cognitive restructuring. The treatment groups, mostly comprised of professional working women, were led by an African American male counselor who discussed the importance of being vulnerable in group despite messages BAAW may have received about showing emotions being equated with weakness. Other "ethnically-specific changes" (Carter et al., 2003, 514) to the typical treatment protocol included exploration of how being African American influenced *in vivo* treatment exercises, the experience of being a minority at work, and additional pressures resulting in increased anxiety and panic symptoms. The authors found that CBT was particularly effective compared to the control group of BAAW in lowering depression, general anxiety, and symptoms of panic disorder. Carter et al. (2003) supposed the effectiveness of the treatment with BAAW was due to the combination of a culturally competent therapist who identified as African American using cognitive techniques and discussing racial issues in the context of a supportive group therapy. Like Jones and Sam (2018), Carter et al. (2003) suggested that group cohesiveness played a significant role in the group's effectiveness in lowering anxiety and symptoms of panic disorder in BAAW.

Ward and Brown (2015) incorporated their own prior research on the attitudes of African American men and women to culturally adapt a CBT group treatment for depression. The authors learned that the BAAW in their study believed depression was a normal response to life circumstances, and thus found no need to seek help for it. Based on this information, specific psychoeducation about depression was incorporated into the treatment. African American therapists facilitated the group treatment and gave "specific attention to language, persons, metaphors, content, concepts, goals, methods, and context" (Ward & Brown, 2015, 13) according to the ecological validity framework of cultural adaptation of psychological interventions. Principles of Kwanzaa were also discussed in the treatment group. Participant retention was one of the primary benefits of the adaptation of the group compared to a previously high early termination rate with African American patients in this setting. The participants completed the 12-week study with a retention rate of 66 percent of the group's initial 50 participants. Also, the symptoms of depression were significantly less across multiple measures of depression. The sessions included a psychoeducational component each week, as well as assigned weekly topics.

Positive results have been reported for quantitative research on group treatment for BAAW. Similarly, in a qualitative study of older homeless African American women, a quilting workshop served as a helpful group intervention for achieving connectivity and healing among participants (Moxley et al., 2011). In the structured intervention, the women were asked to share personal experiences with homelessness that were ultimately represented on a patch of material. The patches later became part of a larger quilt collectively made by the women. The participants noted they felt heard and understood as they told their personal stories. It was especially meaningful for them to share their stories with women who also experienced homelessness themselves. The qualitative data suggests the process of telling one's story to a group of other BAAW with similar lived experiences was therapeutic. Furthermore, as supported in foundational research, engagement in a creative and collaborative activity was healing (Moxley et al., 2011).

These studies detail treatment with women with lower socioeconomic status, women who are homeless, working professionals, and college students and offer solid evidence for group therapy as a successful psychological treatment option for BAAW across different demographics. Furthermore, the infusion of Nguzo Saba has been consistent over time and implemented in different treatment settings with various therapeutic approaches. The Nguzo Saba provide a robust and comprehensible theoretical foundation for cultural adaptation as well as intervention strategies, topics, and themes. The Nguzo Saba also offers a plethora of themes to draw from, giving therapists the opportunity to utilize both traditional and nontraditional therapeutic approaches.

GROUP THERAPY TREATMENT PROCESS

Recruitment of Group Members

As mentioned in previous chapters (see Chapters 2, 3, 4 and 8), BAAW underutilize mental health services. Mental health disparities and incompetent care, cultural stigma and shame, and limited resources serve as reasons for this underutilization of care. These same issues can manifest within the group therapy setting. In general, mental health practitioners are undertrained in working with BAAW; this is also true of those working within a group context (Kohn et al., 2002). Although sister groups and collectivism are parts of the African American women experience for many, BAAW may struggle to enter and participate in group therapy due to cultural norms of strength and privacy. For fear of appearing weak or being judged for sharing "family business," they may feel apprehension in sharing personal and sensitive details about themselves with other BAAW or in therapy groups with diverse genders and ethnicities. Furthermore, even when BAAW are ready and willing to participate in group therapy, they may be challenged in finding a group therapy program that fits their needs. Given these issues, special consideration is needed for recruiting and retaining BAAW in group therapy.

Therapy group members can be recruited in several different ways depending on the treatment setting. In an agency setting, such as a community mental health center or a college counseling center, group referrals may come from in-house. After identifying a client as a good candidate for group therapy, group clients can be referred into group by intake counselors and/or individual counselors in the agency. When specialized or newly offered groups are introduced, such as those designed and adapted for BAAW, or when the participation of BAAW in traditional group therapy is low, recruitment efforts need to be made outside of the agency or counseling center. This means advertising for the group at locations that are well visited and recognized by BAAW. Due to simplicity, ability to specify, and wide reach, social media and email listservs may be primary resources in recruiting BAAW. However, it is recommended that a multitier recruitment plan be utilized to attract the greatest pool of BAAW (Stout et al., 2020), particularly those with little access to (or desired use of) technology. This includes more traditional forms of recruitment such as contacting civic organizations, social clubs and sororities, use of newspaper and ad prints, and placing group advertisements in churches, hair salons, coffee shops, and other gathering spaces.

In a private practice setting, group therapists would benefit from the same marketing strategy as an agency seeking members from outside the agency. In addition to groups and gathering places popular in the African American community, professional networks, and listservs for private practitioners in the local area would be helpful for generating referrals. Referrals from other clinicians may prove to be particularly helpful as such clients may have experience with therapy.

Clarity and simplicity are needed in recruitment initiatives. Successful recruitment efforts are targeted (as mentioned above), express the focus and benefits of the group, and provide clear detail about how members can contact the group coordinators and initiate group services. Furthermore, clinicians should also be mindful of stigma associated with mental health treatment for the African American community when recruiting and use language that is culturally relevant and free of bias.

Format and Group Type

As the literature indicates, a variety of types and formats for groups can be effective for BAAW. Some groups are open, taking in new members on a rolling basis, whereas others close membership once the group initiates, after growing to a certain number, or at a predetermined calendar date. Groups may be ongoing with no end date or may end after a set number of sessions. For example, Boyd-Franklin (1987) described ongoing psychotherapy groups for BAAW that meet continuously. Other groups such as Nia and Oh Happy Day offered a closed and structured manualized format (Kaslow et al., 2010; Ward & Brown, 2015).

Groups may be defined as support, psychoeducational, or therapy groups. Support groups function similarly to formats used in Alcoholics Anonymous or Narcotics Anonymous meetings. This format is less formal in nature and may even be peer-led rather than led by behavioral health professionals. Support groups may have different standards for confidentiality but maintain the goal of establishing sisterhood and support. Take, for example, a support group for Black women with depression. With little professional direction, women would have the opportunity to share their experiences and bond with other women with similar experiences. Psychoeducational groups are mostly instructional, functioning like a class. Using the previously mentioned group, a psychoeducation group would introduce psychoeducation on depression and provide tangible intervention aimed at insight building and perceptible change. Therapy groups found in the literature also have support and psychoeducation as dimensions yet differ in that they provide therapeutic interventions according to a theoretical approach. With the aforementioned group, it is now operationalized through attachment and feminist perspectives. Along with support and psychoeducation, trained group therapists are aiding group members in connecting themes and understanding relational patterns, challenging internalized and externalized manifestations of oppression, and using in-the-moment processing to foster growth and member development. The group type and format would ultimately be determined in advance by group leader(s) based on their training, theoretical orientation, and population needs.

Finally, groups differ in topical focus—general/interpersonal and focused/specific groups. General therapy groups would be open to members presenting with various concerns and needs. Although members are presenting with different concerns, ideally, the group creates space for all members' needs to be addressed. Take, for example, a college counseling group that includes members of different cultural backgrounds, ages, and genders, in which various members present with issues related to homesickness, test anxiety, relationship issues, and panic. Group leaders would work to create a safe environment conducive to addressing all needs. In focused groups, members connect through content or identity. Consider a college counseling group for African American graduate students or a racial trauma healing group for Black women. Although members in specified groups share an identity or experience, differences in individual identity still need to be recognized.

Pre-Group Screening and Entrance to Group

Once a potential group member has made contact, setting up a pre-group screening facilitates her entrance to group. Boyd-Franklin (1987) described important fears and concerns coming out during group screenings. She anticipated group members having difficulty expressing vulnerable emotions and planned for this with certain interventions. The purpose of a group screening is to build rapport between a group member and leaders, identify a client's goals for group, discuss group structure and expectations of members, and address concerns about starting group (Rutan & Stone, 2001).

Pack Brown et al. (1998) emphasized the pre-group meeting as an important time to demystify the process of therapy for African American woman with potential stigma or cultural mistrust associated with therapy. Transparency in a pre-group meeting would help to reduce fear and lessen anxiety about joining the group (Pack-Brown et al., 1998). Other important ground rules to cover would be confidentiality, expectations, and the process for leaving the group. A group that is primarily psycho-educational in nature and manualized group therapy may not require a pre-group screening. The clinicians may, however, establish exclusion criteria based on level of distress according to clinical measures (Ward & Brown, 2015).

The pre-group screening is used to determine clinical appropriateness for group depending on the type, format, and topical focus of the group. An individual who is unable to participate in the goals of the group due to logistical, intellectual, psychological, or interpersonal reasons would not be clinically appropriate (Yalom & Leszcz, 2005). Keeping in mind cultural context and experience, individuals with acute psychosis, severe personality disorders, recent trauma, and ongoing crises may require a more structured group setting or individual therapy (Pack-Brown et al., 1998). Once suitability has been determined, it is best to give feedback in the moment. It is important to be transparent about fit for group during a pre-group screening and to provide referrals or alternatives for treatment should group be deemed unsuitable for the potential member.

Challenges to Group Counseling

Having led groups for mixed-gender and BAAW-specific groups for over 10 years, this author can attest to perpetual recruitment challenges. In the author's previous work within the college counseling environment, general process groups and diagnosis-specific groups filled early into each semester, yet groups for African American students required constant recruitment efforts through referrals, community building, and advertising. Group therapists must remain intentional in addressing cultural barriers that dissuade BAAW from entering counseling, especially group therapy.

The stigma of seeking therapy in general, coupled with the fear of being judged by other SBW, may be barriers for BAAW seeking group. Attrition in group and premature termination are common problems in group therapy. Although situational factors may be at play (e.g., illness), Jones and Sam (2018) found decreasing attendance within the group over time to be a challenge for the group. They also asserted that group members may have unmet needs that come out in the group process. For example, the Strong Black Woman (SBW) archetype may be a barrier to full engagement in group for some BAAW. For fear of judgment, BAAW group members may struggle with the vulnerability required of active group participation. In the groups led by Boyd-Franklin (1987), underlying fears were addressed directly and made part of the group process.

During initial assessments, this author found potential group members often expressed a strong disliking of "drama" when group was recommended as a treatment option. Their perception and reticence may stem from stereotypes of BAAW fighting amongst themselves and/or lived negative experiences with other BAAW. The concern was addressed by emphasizing group ground rules facilitating safety. Potential members were also reminded of the value of improving their interpersonal and conflict resolution skills in real time with the support of group therapists.

More likely to be common in college settings and in small communities (i.e., churches, rural locations), preexisting relationships and issues of confidentiality may also impact BAAW participation in group. Black women may not feel open to sharing problems and concerns with other group members who have shared social spaces (clubs, organizations, classes, religious meetings). To minimize this issue, group leaders and members can create guidelines for addressing multiple relationships between members and readdress the importance of confidentiality and respecting each members' privacy.

CLINICAL ISSUES AND SKILLS

Group Facilitation Skill and Cultural Competence

A comprehensive discussion on format and theoretical orientation of groups is beyond what can be established in this chapter. However, group therapists leading groups with BAAW enter group with basic group leadership skills (i.e., active listening; ability to reflect, ask clarification and probing questions, encourage and support; tone-setting; linking;

coleadership) (Jacobs et al., 2016); advanced group leadership skills (i.e., focusing the group, cutting off and drawing out members, use of directive and processing exercises) (Jacobs et al., 2016); are well-versed in group psychological theory (i.e., cognitive behavioral therapy, person-centered, solution-focused therapy); and understand the challenges and needs presenting at different stages of group development. Group therapists leading groups with BAAW seek out ongoing training and professional development in group therapy skills and recognize group therapy as a specialty acknowledged by APA offering specific education and training (APA, 2018).

Group therapists working with BAAW also adhere to standard group guideline practices focused on integrating cultural competence in all stages of group. According the Association for Specialists in Group Work Multicultural and Social Justice Competence Principles for Group Workers (Singh et al., 2012), the multiculturally oriented group therapist continues to build awareness into their own identity and the identities of group members, operates using culturally competent strategies and skills in planning and performing in the group, and promotes social justice within and outside of the group. Furthermore, the multiculturally oriented group therapist needs to enter the group therapy process holding esteem, respect, and honor for BAAW.

Addressing Intense Emotion

BAAW present to group therapy with all the same concerns as their peers of different ethnic backgrounds. Group with BAAW is suitable for addressing issues related to mental health, relationships and family, self-esteem and identity concerns, and substance use. As well as the basic group facilitation skills needed to address these presenting concerns, group therapists working with BAAW require additional clinical skills specific to addressing the emotional expression of sadness, overwhelm, and anger. As previously mentioned, societal expectations, cultural norms, and internalized beliefs may stifle BAAW's expression of emotions considered weak, vulnerable, or incompetent. Given this, group leaders navigate the intricacies associated with safe emotional expression. As related to crying, Boyd-Franklin (1987) noted group members feeling most supported when other group members supported them silently or cried with them. The group leader's role would be holding space for strong emotions to be expressed and processed. It would be important for group members to debrief one's experience of crying in the group, as this typically facilitates group cohesiveness.

Similarly, group leaders address the complexities for BAAW of expressing anger. Frequently stereotyped as angry or aggressive, Black women may suppress anger because of stereotype threat (Kelly & Greene, 2010). Other Black women may lack role models for how to handle anger in constructive ways. In a group setting, anger and conflict are normal parts of the process. For example, in the group facilitated by Jones and Sam (2018), members would recognize and attend to anger in other members. Members were also able to express their angry toward those members who left group prematurely. Pack-Brown et al. (1998) observed that many group participants had anger just beneath the surface. Anger may reside just beneath the surface for BAAW due to a history of their emotional expression being criticized and invalidated. As well as helping group members resolve anger, group leaders are creating therapeutic environments that respect and validate anger held by BAAW.

Nontraditional Methods

The use of nontraditional methods, such as music and art, is commonplace for BAAW therapy groups (Jones & Sam, 2018; Pack-Brown et al., 1998). Ward and Brown (2015) and others offered meals during group times. The celebration of Kwanzaa is a celebration of the harvest, which is why it happens to mark the end of one year and the beginning of a new one. Kwanzaa celebrations typically involve a meal. Even when using nontraditional methods, it is important to set expectations and maintain appropriate boundaries for group. Having women share food with each other during a termination session or special purposes is done with alignment of overarching group goals.

Furthermore, inclusion of religion and spirituality may aid the group experience for some BAAW. As noted in other chapters (see Chapters 1 and 11), the prominence of the Black church has been well established in the African American community. Group leaders should remain open to various forms of religious and spiritual expression, such as verbal expression of gratitude or excitement (e.g., "Amen!" of "Thank the Lord!"). The Nguzo Saba are also reflective of spiritual values such as purpose and faith. Activities in group may involve a prayer or reflection of faith or spirituality.

Considerations for BAAW Group Leaders

The value of an all-BAAW group (both members and leaders identify as BAAW) in a therapeutic context has been explored empirically and anecdotally. The task for BAAW group leaders of balancing group leadership with membership may be particularly difficult due to the norm in many of the groups of sisterhood and connection. Thus, special considerations for African American women leading such groups with BAAW are warranted.

Self-disclosure for BAAW group leaders would need to be carefully considered. On the one hand, self-disclosure may be expected as a way of building connection and rapport between group leaders and members. The power difference may also be more neutral, especially in the face of mistrust of the mental health field among many people of color. On the other hand, African American therapists may assume they are more like their African American clients than they actually are (Kelly & Greene, 2010). Thus, it is important to be aware of the potential for BAAW to overidentify with members and miss important within-group differences. As well as the group format and setting helping to determine the appropriate group leader self-disclosure, operating group from a theoretical foundation that provides goals and sets ground rules for engagement can assist with staying task-oriented and preventing the group leader(s) from oversharing.

Furthermore, likely socialized with experiences similar to their BAAW group members, the group leaders would need to explore their own assumptions, biases, and attitudes related to BAAW. Similarly, Pack Brown et al. (1998) noted the relevance of racial identity development for BAAW group leaders. Optimally, the leaders would have internalized a positive racial identity and be able to recognize and empathize with group members working toward healthy internalization themselves.

To appropriately address countertransference and trigger responses, group coleaders are encouraged to debrief after each session (Pack-Brown et al., 1998), or single leaders need to seek appropriate consultation. It is also recommended for group leaders to consider their own therapeutic support to assist with maintaining healthy boundaries and protecting against burnout (Pack-Brown et al., 1998). The same self-care suggestions would apply to group leaders not identifying as BAAW.

Considerations for Non-BAAW Group Leaders

Jones and Sam (2018) posit it may be beneficial to have White or non-African American group leaders; however, the counselor must be invested in the well-being of the group members and be prepared to defer any hurt feelings stemming from hearing reactions to White or male supremacy. The group leader would be bound by ethical principles to respond appropriately and take in feedback that may be hard to receive. A non-African American female or an African American male group leader may be able to relate to some aspects of identity but not others. They may offer a unique perspective as members of a group with which some BAAW have difficulties, which may provide a corrective experience through healing or better understanding.

Regarding cultural competence, non-BAAW and male group leaders would need to engage in active self-reflection regarding perceptions, assumptions, and past experiences with BAAW that may play a role in how group members would be experienced and perceived. Group leaders need to identify any misguided efforts to "prove themselves" as being culturally competent by leading such a group (Jones & Sam, 2018). The needs and safety of group members would be the priority over the leader's own needs for acceptance or working through personal challenges. Another consideration related to majority group leaders is to practice humility and respect when utilizing nontraditional methods. For example, White female group leaders would need to consider potential conflicts and group member reactions related to the leader organizing and/or leading Kwanzaa activities.

Unique Group Variables

In literature and in the author's own experience leading groups with BAAW, the topics of strength, family, relationships, sexual orientation, skin color, and hair texture are ever present. Strength has already been discussed in this chapter, and other chapters detail family, relationship, and sexual orientation–related concerns. This section will focus on skin color and hair texture within a group context.

Skin Color. Identity and self-esteem of Black women have been influenced by perceptions held by self and others about their physical attributes. In particular, the prevalence of color gradation and attachment of social status to skin tones has been paramount in the Black community. Researchers and scholars, as well as artists, writers, and filmmakers, have covered "colorism" defined as "discrimination based on skin tone" by Hall (2017, 71). The author examined the influence of colorism on emotional well-being among African American women who self-identified as light-, medium-, dark- and very dark-skinned. Consistent with previous research, negative consequences were linked to being dark-skinned (perceived as less attractive, more aggressive, unintelligent), while light-skinned women were perceived as pretty, smart, and successful. The women identifying as medium had more neutral to positive experiences and felt accepted more broadly. Deeming the topic of colorism as sensitive in nature, Hall (2017) thought it essential to create more safety through homogeneous focus groups by matching the skin tone of group members and leaders. A therapeutic group of BAAW would most likely be diverse in skin tone, thus exploring issues related to colorism should be skillfully approached.

Another supposition of the research reviewed by Hall (2017) is that Black women have also been identified as the primary perpetuators of colorism. Indeed, the women in the study described how family members' comments and influence led to the internalization and perpetuation of colorism (Hall, 2017). In the context of the therapeutic relationship between a group therapist and member both identifying as BAAW, skin color dynamics are likely fertile ground for exploring the members' personal experiences (Kelly & Greene, 2010). Boyd-Franklin (1987) suggests bringing these issues forth directly, as a means of healing past hurts, challenging assumptions, and building connection.

Hair Texture. Hair texture, hair length, and style are often associated with ethnic identity, pride, and political leanings for African American women (Kelly & Greene, 2010). Hair styles such as dreadlocks or chemically straightened hair can elicit assumptions about the wearer of the style. The assumptions may have to do to with personal dimensions such as racial identity, political ideology, and economic status. Hair has been labeled as "good" if it is long, straight, or loosely curled and "bad" if it is short and tightly curled. The meaning and significance of hair texture and styles is typically discussed among BAAW.

Many authors describe deep-seated wounds and pain related to these issues (Hall, 2017; Kelly and Greene, 2010). Broaching these topics in casual settings may cause more wounds or leave issues unresolved. The BAAW group therapist is charged with the task of exploring these topics, perhaps using movies, songs, or poems as stimulus for the group (Pack-Brown et al., 1998). Moreover, the within-group differences with hair textures, lengths, and styles may offer the chance for healing and understanding past hurts as well as confronting assumptions about group leaders and members.

In the groups the author has led, simple acknowledgment and valida-tion of emotions and experiences related to complexion and hair produced cathartic moments for the group. BAAW want to discuss these issues, heal from pains related to color and hair, and refrain from passing these nega-tive messages on to their own daughters. Embracing all the beauty within the group created corrective emotional experiences that may only come in relationship with other BAAW.

CASE STUDY

A 10-session interpersonal process therapy group for BAAW was offered at a community counseling center that serves as a private prac-tice and training site for graduate students and professionals seeking licensure. Services are offered on a fee-for-service basis or a sliding-fee scale, while some clients use their insurance benefits to cover services. The group members were recruited through clinicians in the center as well as via a professional counseling listserv of the group leaders. Both group leaders identified as cisgender BAAW, and one identified as lesbian and the other as heterosexual.

As recommended in the literature, potential group members all attended a 30-minute prescreening to assess their fit for group. Of the eight poten-tial group members referred and screened, six women chose to partici-pate. There was one woman referred back to individual counseling due to ongoing life crisis events, and the other woman was unable to commit to the time of the group. The following group members were screened and selected to join the group:

1. Jada—32 years old. Adjustment to a recent move from out of state for a relationship that ended. Experiencing some symptoms of depres-sion and having difficulty establishing a social support network.

2. Trinity—26 years old. Single mother of one child experiencing conflict with child's father. Working full-time and attending school to become a nurse.
3. Gabby—35 years old. Recently married professional with a stressful and demanding job. One of few women of color on her job.
4. Brianna—38 years old. Transitioning out of a close-knit religious community, wanting to establish new connections, and build self-esteem.
5. Nikki—35 years old. Working in a male-dominated occupation as a law enforcement officer. In a relationship with a woman and caring for elderly mother who does not accept her sexual identity.
6. Kayla—22 years old. Dealing with social anxiety and was referred by individual therapist to work on social skills. Having trouble securing a job after graduation due to anxiety. Identifies as first-generation African American with parents born in Nigeria.

Initial Stage of Group, Sessions 1–2

The first sessions focused on group members and leaders' introductions. The members shared their reasons for joining group and discussed guidelines for group. Themes of the group included family conflict, feelings of social isolation, feeling misunderstood at work or in school due to identity as BAAW, and concerns about partner relationships. Gabby shared her recent nuptials, and Nikki stated she recently moved in with her partner. Group leaders were mindful to not make assumptions about members identities and mirrored members' language and pronouns. All members participated; however, Kayla was clearly the most reserved member.

Working Stage, Sessions 3–4

Over the next several group sessions, members went into more depth about their presenting concerns and goals for group. In session 3, Jada came to group visibly upset, and her mood was noticeably different. Group leaders interrupted Trinity, asking her permission to come back to her school issue after the group check-in with Jada. Once Trinity agreed, Brianna told Jada she was concerned to see her so upset and wanted to know what was wrong. Jada, at this point, began to cry and shared that her ex-boyfriend was in a new relationship. She had been putting on a brave face after moving to a new state for the relationship, which ended just after her move. Several other members became tearful as Jada shared feelings of loss, loneliness, and hopelessness. The group leaders checked in to explore her experience of sharing, and she noted it felt good to cry and receive support. Other members stated they appreciated her emotion as they had felt like crying in previous groups but did not know how the group would respond. The theme of loss was explored over the next several sessions, which resonated for other members.

Sessions 5–6

Several sessions later, Kayla asked Nikki about her job in law enforcement because Kayla had been considering law school. Group leaders explored Kayla's experience of checking in, and she stated Nikki was the other quiet group member. They were both able to explore reasons for being more reserved in the group. Other group members wanted to know more about Nikki's relationship. Gabby interrupted to say she felt Nikki was being targeted. Gabby expressed anger about group members asking invasive questions. Group leaders checked in with Nikki to hear her feelings on the situation. Nikki said it felt good to have someone stand up for her and thanked Gabby. Nikki said she liked having others show interest in her relationship. She came out to the group, stating she was sad her mother had not asked to meet her girlfriend. Kayla again related to Nikki, stating her parents are very traditional and she cannot share with them about dating and other concerns as she matures. The group leaders asked about Nikki's experience of coming out to the group. One group leader disclosed identifying as lesbian, which appeared to increase Nikki's comfort being out in the group.

Sessions 7–8

In subsequent groups, members showed vulnerability and took risks with one another. The leaders helped Gabby identify the source of her anger about Nikki being questioned, which stemmed from White coworkers constantly asking her about her personal life. Gabby was understandably guarded and private at work but felt she could not say no to inquiries fearing she may be overlooked for important projects and promotions or that she would be seen as hostile and unapproachable. All group members and leaders expressed similar feelings with head nods and affirming phrases and comments. The volume and energy in group were increased, with members giving examples of similar experiences.

Session 9

The theme of the next group was self-care practices in preparation for termination. Brianna expressed her use of prayer and spirituality to alleviate stress. Trinity previously did the same but felt she had been judged by members of the church when she had her child. Brianna and Trinity discussed pros and cons of being in tight-knit religious communities. Gabby noted her self-care was exercise via swimming. Another member stated that Gabby had "good hair," so it was easy for her to swim often. Gabby became withdrawn and stated other BAAW had made assumptions about her because of her hair texture and light skin. Jada validated her, stating something similar happened to her. Kayla stated she was criticized by family members and potential dates for having dark skin.

Brianna described wearing hairpieces that had caused damage to her hair. She expressed feeling angry and resentful of these negative messages. She now loves her short, curly hair. Group chimed in on liking her hairstyle, with some surprise about her past struggles. Group leaders commented on assumptions made about BAAW related to skin color and hair texture, and one group leader relayed a personal example.

Termination, Session 10

In the last session of the group, group members brought refreshments and reflected on themes from the group. In sharing about group experiences, Brianna reported being frustrated with not getting more direct feedback from group leaders. This led to a discussion of different opinions on the matter. Group leaders validated Brianna speaking up and checked in with her and other members about termination. The group ended with an exercise allowing group leaders and members to provide written feedback to one another on sheets of card stock given to each member by the leaders.

CONCEPTUALIZATION

1. Jada—Felt the need to be strong and not express her true feelings about the breakup. Allowing herself to be vulnerable in group paved the way for her to address her grief and make some initial progress in decreasing her depressive symptoms.
2. Trinity—Continues to seek balance of parenting responsibilities, work, and school. Able to identify how much she missed church for spiritual renewal and replenishment given her many roles. Trinity began looking for a new church where she would potentially find community with other single parents and feel more accepted.
3. Gabby—Hearing others' experiences of being the only BAAW at work and/or school was empowering. She was more mindful of sharing this stress with her husband instead of internalizing SBW concepts.
4. Brianna—Received affirmation on recent changes made to her appearance after rejecting standards of beauty that felt oppressive. Despite connections made, termination was triggering after leaving her religious community. However, challenging group leaders was another step toward building self-confidence and self-esteem.
5. Nikki—Although initially cautious, she was able to talk about her relationship with her girlfriend openly in group as a contrast to not being able to share with her mother. Received affirmation from group, especially through learning of group leader's identity as a sexual orientation minority. Left group with a desire to build additional affirming friendships.
6. Kayla—Able to practice initiating conversation and tolerating anxiety. Made progress in career plans and ability to express the

disconnect she feels with parents at times due to her being first-generation American.

7. Group—The process integrated interpersonal dynamics and curative factors of group such as universality and identification (Yalom & Lesczc, 2005), in addition to themes from the Nguzo Saba, especially Umoja—Unity, Ujima—Collective Work and Responsibility, Nia—Purpose, and Imani—Faith (Karenga, 2008).

CONCLUSION

The group members had many common and diverse experiences as BAAW. The group leaders were able to establish group cohesion, address difficult emotions, facilitate conflict in the group, and affirm group members' identities as BAAW. The group moved through phases of group work, and individual members progressed in their therapeutic goals. The benefits of group screenings helped group leaders navigate intense emotions and underlying fears. Group leaders were measured in their self-disclosure but used it as a tool to facilitate connection and individual members' progress. Also, group leaders were open to using music and sharing food as part of building community and sisterhood.

REFERENCES

American Psychological Association (APA). (2018, August). *Group psychology and group psychotherapy.* https://www.apa.org/ed/graduate/specialize/group-psychology-therapy

American Psychological Association (APA). (2019, October). *Psychotherapy: Understanding group therapy.* https://www.apa.org/topics/group-therapy

Bowser, Y. L., & Shulman, R. S. H. (Executive Producers). (1993–1998). *Living Single* [TV Series]. SisterLee Productions; Warner Brothers Television.

Boyd-Franklin, N. (1987). Group therapy for Black women: A therapeutic support model. *American Journal of Orthopsychiatry, 57*(3), 394–401. https://doi.org/10.1111/j.1939-0025.1987.tb03548.x

Carter, M. M., Sbrocco, T., Gore, K. L., Marin, N. W., & Lewis, E. L. (2003). Cognitive–behavioral group therapy versus a wait-list control in the treatment of African American women with panic disorder. *Cognitive Therapy and Research, 27*(5), 505–518. https://doi.org/10.1023/a:1026350903639

Grammer, K., Akil, M. B., & Hicks, R. Y. (Executive Producers). (2000–2008). *Girlfriends* [TV Series]. Paramount Network Television; CBS Paramount Network Television; Grammer Productions; Happy Camper Productions.

Hall, J. C. (2017). No longer invisible: Understanding the psychosocial impact of skin color stratification in the lives of African American women. *Health & Social Work, 42*(2), 71–78. https://doi.org/10.1093/hsw/hlx001

Hofmann, S. G., Asnaani, A., Vonk, I. J. J., Sawyer, A. T., & Fang, A. (2012). The efficacy of cognitive behavioral therapy: A review of meta-analyses. *Cognitive therapy and research, 36*(5), 427–440. https://doi.org/10.1007/s10608-012-9476-1

Jacobs, E. E., Schimmel, C. J., Masson, R. L., & Harvill, R. L. (2016). *Group counseling: Strategies and skills.* Boston, MA: Cengage.

Jones, M. K., & Sam, T. S. (2018). Cultural connections: An ethnocultural counseling intervention for Black women in college. *Journal of College Counseling, 21*(1), 73–86. https://doi.org/10.1002/jocc.12088

Karenga, M. (2008). *Kwanzaa: A celebration of family, community, and culture.* Los Angeles, CA: University of Sankore Press.

Kaslow, N. J., Leiner, A. S., Reviere, S., Jackson, E., Bethea, K., Bhaju, J., . . . & Thompson, M. P. (2010). Suicidal, abused African American women's response to a culturally informed intervention. *Journal of Consulting and Clinical Psychology, 78*(4), 449–458. https://doi.org/10.1037/a0019692

Kelly, J. F., & Greene, B. (2010). Diversity within African American, female therapists: Variability in clients' expectations and assumptions about the therapist. *Psychotherapy: Theory, Research, Practice, Training, 47*(2), 186–197. https://doi.org/10.1037/a0019759

Kohn, L. P., Oden, T., Munoz, R. F., Robinson, A., & Leavitt, D. (2002). Adapted cognitive behavioral group therapy for depressed low-income African American women. *Community Mental Health Journal, 38*, 497–504. http://dx.doi.org/10.1023/A:1020884202677

Lee, M. (Director). 2017. *Girls Trip* [Film]. Will Packer Productions; Perfect World Pictures.

Moxley, D. P., Feen-Calligan, H. R., Washington, O. G. M., & Garriott, L. (2011). Quilting in self-efficacy group work with older African American women leaving homelessness. *Art Therapy, 28*(3), 113–122.

Pack-Brown, S., Whittington-Clark, L., & Parker, W. (1998). *Images of me: A guide to group work with African-American women.* Needham Heights, MA: Allyn & Bacon.

Pickney, D. (1994, December). Afrocentric therapy. *Essence, 25*(8).

Rae, I., Penny, P., Rotenberg, M., Matsoukas, M., Becky, D., & Berry, J. (Executive Producers). (20016–present). *Insecure* [TV series]. HBO Entertainment; Issa Rae Productions; Penny for Your Thoughts Entertainment, Three Arts Entertainment.

Rutan, J., & Stone, W. (2001). *Psychodynamic group psychotherapy.* New York, NY: Guilford Press.

Singh, A., A., Merchant, N., Skudrzyk, B., & Ingene, D. (2012). *Association for specialists in group work: Multicultural and social justice competence principles for group workers.* https://c3c51c6c-8c32-4f6a-9af6-0d715ac3a752.filesusr.com/ugd/513c96_617884bff48f45b2827c7afc4e4e5b12.pdf

Stout, S. H., Babulal, G. M., Johnson, A. M., Williams, M. M., & Roe, C. M. (2020). Recruitment of African American and Non-Hispanic White older adults for Alzheimer disease research via traditional and social media: A case study. *Journal of Cross-Cultural Gerontology, 35*(3), 329–339.

Ward, E. C., & Brown, R. L. (2015). A culturally adapted depression intervention for African American adults experiencing depression: Oh Happy Day. *American Journal of Orthopsychiatry, 85*(1), 11–22. https://doi.org/10.1037/ort0000027

Whitaker, F. (Director). (1995). *Waiting to Exhale* [Film]. Twentieth Century Studios.

Yalom, I. D., & Leszcz, M. (2005). *The theory and practice of group psychotherapy* (5th ed.). New York, NY: Basic Books.

CHAPTER 11

Inpatient Treatment for African American Women

Stephanie N. Williams
Melissa G. Johnson

INTRODUCTION

This chapter discusses a range of issues regarding African American women who are hospitalized in a psychiatric inpatient unit. Psychiatric hospitalization, also referred to as inpatient treatment, is the typical remedy for acute psychiatric illnesses (Creed et al., 1990) and is the highest level of care available for people suffering from mental illness. Psychiatric patients enter into inpatient facilities on a voluntary or involuntary basis. Involuntary patients are placed in hospitals under their state's civil or forensic commitment statutes (Lutterman et al., 2017). The exact numbers of inpatient admissions each year is unclear, but a recent study reported that psychiatric inpatient hospitalizations accounted for approximately 6 percent of all hospitalizations in the United States in 2014; which represents a 20 percent increase from 2005 (McDermott, Elixhauser, & Sun, 2017). Mood disorders represent the eighth leading cause for all hospitalizations in the United States, while mood disorders and schizophrenia/psychotic disorders are ranked first and second respectively for hospital stays for the 18–44-year-old group (McDermott et al., 2017).

AFRICAN AMERICAN MENTAL HEALTH AND TREATMENT

Women worldwide continue to have higher rates of serious mental illness, depression, and post-traumatic stress disorder when compared to their male counterparts (Tolin & Foa, 2006; Weissman et al., 2015). Mental health disparities found in women are related to the fact that women endure more risk factors correlated with mental illness, including but not limited to income inequality, poverty, and violence (American Psychological Association, 2017). Approximately 50 percent of women with serious mental illness are mothers of dependent children and are at a higher risk of losing custody of their children as a result (Lacey et al., 2014; Seeman, 2012).

Although African American women have lower rates of mental illness when compared to other groups, they experience more persistent forms of mental illness and receive poorer levels of care (American Psychological Association, 2017; Wang, Berglund, & Kessler, 2000; Young et al., 2001). African American women's health is impacted by racism, with research showing that the experience of racism is correlated with anxiety (Maddox, 2013), disordered eating, depression, and other mental health disorders (Lacey et al., 2015; Perry, Harp, & Oser, 2013; Mays, 1995). Further complicating the issue of prevalent mental health factors with African American women is the misdiagnosis and/or under-diagnosis of their mental illness due to provider's lack of cultural understanding, and provider bias (Akinhanmi et al., 2018; APA, 2017; Gara et al., 2019; van Ryn & Burke, 2000).

African American women are more likely to be diagnosed with schizophrenia spectrum and psychotic disorders when compared to their White counterparts (Schwartz & Blankenship, 2014). African American women are overrepresented in inpatient settings and underrepresented in both outpatient settings and hospital associated case management services (Barrio et al., 2003; Snowden, Hastings, & Alvidrez, 2009), which may be attributed to misdiagnosis and lack of access to care in communities of color (Bailey, Blackmon, & Stevens, 2009). Research on mental health care for African American women is extremely limited (Coker, 2004). However, as a whole group, the literature indicates African Americans are usually hospitalized from various points of entry including but not limited to self-referral, referral from other sources (e.g., family, outpatient treatment centers, emergency room) (Bolden & Wicks, 2005; Delphin-Rittmon et al., 2015; Snowden & Cheung, 1990), and the criminal justice system (Pinals, Packer, & Fisher, 2004; Snowden & Cheung, 1990). However, the research on treatment etiology is polarized, with some researchers arguing that African American women tend to terminate treatment earlier and against medical advice despite receiving ratings of greater symptom severity at discharge (Delphin-Rittmon et al., 2015); while other researchers report that African American women are more likely than any other group to have longer lengths of stay in hospitals (Bolden & Wicks, 2005). Overall research has suggested that length of stay was associated with being female, having a psychotic disorder diagnosis, and being hospitalized in a larger hospital (Tulloch, Fearon, & David, 2011).

When it comes to treatment, African American women are more likely to receive older-phase medications (Kreyenbuhl et al., 2003; Puyat et al.,

2013) and are prescribed higher doses of antipsychotic medications when compared to their White peers (Chung, Mahler, & Kakuma, 1995; Glazer, Morgenstern, & Doucette, 1994; Segal, Bola, & Watson, 1996; Valenstein et al., 2001; Walkup et al. 2000). Furthermore, African American women received lower rates of follow-up and adequate treatment after discharge from inpatient hospitals (Carson et al., 2014).

CASE STUDY

This chapter has presented research on the mental health of African American women and the prevalent disparities within inpatient treatment. The chapter will now shift its focus to a case study that illustrates an African American woman presented to an inpatient facility and gives readers a sense of best practices when working with African American women in this unique setting.

Jessica is a 22-year-old, self-identified African American woman. She reported three maternal siblings and four paternal siblings. She noted that her parents separated when she was young and she predominantly "grew up in group homes." She is unmarried and does not have any children. She described a childhood history of emotional abuse by her parents, sexual abuse beginning at age nine by her stepfather, and physical violence by group home staff. Jessica specifically noted that while in foster care she was restrained in chairs alone for long periods of time. As an adult she reported experiencing intimate partner violence where she was both emotionally and physically abused; she stated that at 19 she was strangled and beaten by her partner, causing loss of consciousness.

Jessica completed the 11th grade, where she received special education services "because of my behavior." She noted an extensive history of school suspensions and expulsions. She later received her general education degree (GED) through a community adult educational program and completed one year of community college. Jessica does not have any formal work history but noted that she has participated in sexual services (i.e., prostitution) and receives social security disability supplemental income. Jessica reported previous diagnoses of schizophrenia, bipolar disorder, borderline personality disorder, attention deficit hyperactivity disorder, and anxiety disorder. She was prescribed several medications but was unable to recall them at the time of the interview.

According to documentation, Jessica has a significant history of alcohol, amphetamine, and cannabis abuse. She is positive for numerous head traumas including rolling out of a moving car, volitional head banging, seizures, and strangulation. Jessica has an extensive history of mental health services in both community outpatient and inpatient treatment facilities dating back to her childhood. She has a documented history of three suicide attempts, which resulted in three emergency room admissions. She has been involuntarily hospitalized for danger to self and others approximately 10 times.

Jessica's family history is positive for maternal bipolar disorder. During the clinical interview, Jessica endorsed difficulty with focusing, emotional regulation,

*and disorientation, which she described as "things moving too fast [in her envi-
ronment], I don't understand and my brain can't catch up. It's like my brain
shuts off or goes into psychosis." She also reported difficulty with her memory and
a history of anxiety. Chart review suggests that Jessica also experiences states of
depression that are characterized by depressed mood, fatigue, inability to concentrate, and suicidal ideation as well as states that include heightened irritability,
increased verbalizations, and distractibility.*

ASSESSMENT AND TRIAGE

To address the disparities with the treatment of African American
women within inpatient settings, clinicians should develop and utilize a
structured interview process, which has been shown to reduce provider
bias and increase diagnostic accuracy (Beach et al., 2006; McLaughlin,
2002). This structured interview should address several key clinical issues
and background information that specifically impact African American
women: suicide risk, trauma, family history, health concerns, and clinical
concerns. However, prior to any assessment and triage, clinicians should
have a strong foundation in the cultural implications of working with
African American women.

Cultural Understanding

When assessing African American women, clinicians need to have
an understanding of racial identity development (Cross, Parham, &
Helms, 1991; Helms, 1990) and specifically how identity development
can impact both the client's view of the questions being asked and the
clinician's interpretation of client responses. Understanding identity
development is uniquely important to the triage and assessment of African American clients in inpatient settings for two distinct reasons: 1) It
provides a foundation for understanding how bias can impact the outcome of clinical assessments; and 2) It can help build rapport. Research
has shown that African American clients respond better to clinicians
that integrate a sociohistorical context to treatment, and engage in interpersonal, collaborative, and/or psychoeducational approaches (Morris,
2001; Shorter-Gooden, 2009). Even though therapist–client matching
has shown positive outcomes in the therapeutic relationship (Cabral &
Smith, 2011; Maramba & Hall, 2002), it is important to note that even
if the clinician and the client both identify as African American, they
may not necessarily align with regard to their individual stages of racial
identity, which can impact the therapeutic relationship. So, in order to
improve treatment satisfaction, therapists should consider the importance of understanding racial bias and incorporate that understanding
into treatment when working with African American women (Meyer &
Zane, 2013).

Suicide Risk Assessment

All clinicians working within any inpatient setting should have a strong understanding of risk factors when working with acutely mentally ill inpatients. Researchers Chu et al. (2013) have suggested that there are three principles that influence suicide risk with persons of color. It has been reported that race and culture affect; 1) the types of stressors that lead to suicide; 2) one's tolerance for psychological pain as well as the subsequent acts of suicide; and 3) how thoughts, intentions, plans, and attempts are described. Although research suggests that African American women are the most protected group against suicide in the United States, this does not mean that they are not at risk for suicide. African American women experience more suicidal ideation due to issues surrounding poverty, racism, and sexism (Mengesha & Ward, 2012). Clinicians working with African American women should understand how social stressors (family discord and lack of social support); social status (educational attainment, homelessness, acculturative stress), and idioms of distress (i.e., what is seen as acceptable) impact suicide risk (Chu et al., 2013). As a result of the unique factors that impact African American women's suicide risk, clinicians should take a detailed approach to suicide risk assessment, examining cultural factors as well as protective variables such as adherence with familial and cultural prohibitions, to accurately assess a client's risk level (Chu et al., 2013) and how these factors are impacted while the client is residing in an inpatient unit.

Another area of assessment for clinicians when addressing suicide risk with African American women is whether they self-identify with the Strong Black Woman (SBW) archetype. This stereotype suggests that African American women are "naturally strong, resilient, self-contained, and self-sacrificing" (Donovan & West, 2015). However, research on the SBW archetype has suggested that it leads to poorer mental health outcomes for African American women and can increase depression and feelings of isolation (Donovan & West, 2015; West, Donovan, & Daniel, 2016) as well as have negative implications on overall emotional health (Jordan, 1997; Romero, 2000). An African American woman who engages in the behavior of "having it all together" or "directing their treatment" and/or "caring for others" is at the highest risk for poor outcomes associated with the SBW archetype. Treatment professionals should be vigilant to remind African American women to accept treatment without having to be the caretakers of others.

Trauma History

There is a high correlation between trauma and mental illness. Many clinicians do not properly assess for trauma in adults and/or African American women (Alim, Charney, & Mellman, 2006; Dougherty, 2004).

Furthermore, many laypersons may not actually understand what constitutes physical or emotional neglect and/or sexual abuse, so an in-depth and descriptive interview is imperative to fully assess trauma. Research shows that African American women experience higher rates of abuse when compared to other populations (Breiding et al., 2014). Although responses to trauma are unique and vary by person, many responses to trauma can encompass many symptoms that mirror other symptoms of mental illness and can lead to misdiagnosis, over diagnosis, and/or over pathologizing. Emotional reactions to trauma can include anger, anxiety, numbness and detachment, irritability and/or hostility, depression and mood swings, while the cognitive reactions include disorientation, racing thoughts, difficulty concentrating, memory problems, magical thinking, and suicidal thinking (Lacey et al., 2015; Substance Abuse and Mental Health Services Administration, 2014). The implications of inaccurate diagnosis include further destabilizing mood, unnecessary psychiatric prescriptions, and associated negative side effects. However, the biggest concern a clinician should be mindful of when overlooking the impact of trauma is how trauma responses can and may be reduced by the client's removal from their trauma-based environment and how reentry into the community may exacerbate symptoms that appear to be in remission while in an inpatient setting.

Family History

African American women are more likely to represent the head of household when compared to women of other ethnic and racial backgrounds (Anderson, 2016; Seeberger, 2019); as a result, clinicians should prioritize the client's homelife when assessing their level of functioning within the vacuum of inpatient treatment. It is very important to build an understanding of how to sustain outpatient treatment and prevent early termination within the framework of a woman's familial responsibilities. Factors to assess include whether the client cares for children, elderly parents, extended family, work schedule, and other unreported familial responsibilities. Understanding the familial responsibilities, scheduling concerns, and general access to resources (e.g., childcare) can support African American women in finding, securing, and engaging in ongoing outpatient treatment once released into the community.

Health Concerns

Mental health professionals have a required mandate to work within their scope; however, they should still be educated on the possible implications that medical issues have on mental illness. Although the scope of this chapter is for mental health professionals, it is harmful to practice within a vacuum not engaging in a holistic approach to health. Professionals should assess and/or educate themselves on the health concerns of their clients. Clinicians should ask about how clients manage their medical concerns in the community (successfully and/or unsuccessfully) and be made aware of how their client's medical symptoms may impact the functioning of their mental health. Some examples include asking an African American woman: *What happens when her blood sugar is unmanaged? Or Whether she is able to keep up with her thyroid medication? or What does she do to prevent her asthma from becoming aggravated?* Responses to these questions can then be used to help explain and educate African American women on the significant influence health issues have on a person's mental illness. Clinicians should also be aware of how medical problems can complicate the differential diagnosis of many mental health symptoms (McKee & Brahm, 2016). Ultimately, clinicians should understand that African American women simply do not receive the same quality of care as their White counterparts (Bridges, 2020) and need to understand the importance and prevalence of health disparity (Carter-Pokras & Baquet, 2002).

By addressing these issues in a clinical inpatient setting, the clinician can assist the patient in advocating with providers about how her medical care impacts her mental health. This assessment will allow the client autonomy in advocating appropriately for her future treatment as well as provide education on how medical health is often correlated with a person's mental health.

Clinical Concerns

Research has suggested that African Americans are described as experiencing more paranoia and skepticism when it comes to health care as a whole and more specifically mental health treatment (Kennedy, Mathis, & Woods, 2007; Powell et al., 2019; Whaley, 2004). A novice clinician may overlook this well-documented fact and inappropriately diagnose an African American woman as having delusions. Clinicians should take their time to define symptoms, ask about the client's experience with mental health care, and gain clarification regarding descriptors used because of the possible differences in class, linguistic expression, cultural norms, educational background, race, and age. Clinicians should have a strong understanding of the overrepresentation and/or sparse treatment of personality disorder (Males, 2018; McGilloway et al., 2010) as well as the overrepresentation of schizophrenia spectrum diagnoses within the African American population (Neighbors et al., 1989; Schwartz et al., 2019). As a result, clinicians should take the time to accurately assess for clinical criteria instead of "pulling forward" old or recorded diagnostic information. Clinicians should also be aware of cultural beliefs surrounding mental illness in the African American community and if and whether their specific client subscribes to any or all of the belief systems in order to build a bridge to ultimately provide better treatment and care.

Lastly, clinicians working with African Americans should understand that mental health treatment is often not considered due to the lack of open discussion of mental health issues and corresponding treatment in day-to-day life (McGoldrick, Giordano, & Garcia-Preto, 2005). As a result, clinicians should take care to broach any potential treatment with respectful understanding of any boundaries and/or defensiveness a client may experience during the course of inpatient treatment. Therapists should focus on building genuine rapport to assist in building trust while ensuring a good "first encounter" to ensure that any long-term treatment plans for mental health will not be sabotaged during the inpatient setting, hindering any future treatment the client may need.

THERAPEUTIC TREATMENT ISSUES

Studies evaluating the effectiveness of therapeutic treatments operating from a theoretical framework in inpatient settings are still in their infancy. However, current research on therapeutic outcomes has shown that the quality of therapeutic relationships is the strongest predictor of patient success, particularly relationships that allow for collaboration, patient feedback, flexibility, and responsiveness on the part of the provider (DeAngelis, 2019) irrespective of a specific treatment approach. This section will highlight the considerations required to provide ethical and culturally informed treatment to African American women, whether practicing from psychodynamic or cognitive behavioral perspective.

The two prevailing paradigms in modern psychology are psychodynamic and cognitive behavioral therapies. Psychodynamic theories have their roots in psychoanalysis, and this approach is mainly focused on addressing the intrapsychic conflicts and processing of emotions, existence of defenses, impact of childhood experiences, and personality development (Vinney, 2019). Conversely, cognitive behavioral therapy (CBT) theory is rooted in the concept that emotions and behaviors are the result of cognitive processes and requires examination of thoughts. In CBT, the therapist and client work closely to solve problems in order to reduce or eliminate negative states of emotion or behavior (Miller, 2012). Despite the prominence of these two approaches in practice, there is little research examining the utility and effectiveness of psychodynamic and/or cognitive behavioral treatments in acute inpatient treatment, and even less available regarding their effectiveness with African American women.

Psychodynamic Treatment

Psychodynamic treatment within inpatient settings has shown better clinical outcomes than medication alone (Ambresin et al., 2012), and a meta-analysis of psychodynamic treatments has shown that this modality of treatment is effective with a wide range of mental illness (Kösters et al., 2006). Clients that are most suitable for psychodynamic treatments are patients who have strong intellectual abilities, are insightful, and open to creating a strong therapeutic alliance. The biggest criticism of traditional psychodynamic psychotherapy with African American women is its exclusion of culture. Psychodynamic psychotherapy is highly individualistic, with emphasis on internal psychological states without regard to external factors and the environment. Traditional practices do not account for external experiences that can impact group consciousness and racially unique experiences of African American women. Specifically due to the fact that African American women are doubly oppressed (race and gender), these experiences must be accounted for in treatment. Dr. Greene (1997) found that African American women:

> are left with a range of interrelated psychological realities. Each of these realities brings particular tasks and stressors that may challenge, facilitate, or undermine certain aspects of their development (Greene, 1992b, 1996b; Jones, 1985). When these realities are viewed as spheres which overlap at different points, the point at which they converge may be seen as the presenting problem. The extent to which they overlap, when and where the overlap occurs, and the relative importance of each sphere will vary from client to client as will the initial and subsequent focus of treatment. (304)

When utilizing a psychodynamic approach with African American women in an inpatient setting, it is best to consider a short-term process that will assist the client in recognizing the feelings and/or thoughts that interfere with their daily functioning. These sessions should be an introduction of sorts, a time to help the client recognize the areas of improvement that are often hidden from themselves that highly influenced their trajectory to inpatient treatment as well as the obvious issues of race and gender.

Cognitive Behavioral Therapy

Cognitive behavioral therapy (CBT) has also shown significant clinical outcomes when compared to medication alone (Stuart & Thase, 1994). CBT has demonstrated effective treatment for recent onset psychotic patients (Haddock et al., 1999), and a meta-analysis suggested that CBT is beneficial with inpatients both as an initial treatment and as an adjunct to medication (Stuart & Bowers, 1995). The cultural adaptation of CBT for African American women suffering from emotional distress has shown an overall reduction in symptoms (Kohn et al., 2002; Ward & Brown, 2015). However, CBT is not without its own critiques. CBT's limited reliance on the therapeutic relationship may hinder the effectiveness when working with African American women due to the fact that African American clients prioritize relational approaches to treatment (Asnaani & Hofmann, 2012).

Furthermore, it is noted that many therapists that facilitate CBT techniques with clients have limited experience delivering the techniques when the antecedents of the distress are related to racial discrimination (Dale & Saunders, 2018). Yet, for those trained and skilled in culturally adapted CBT treatment for African American women, it is anticipated that the coupling of psychotherapy throughout inpatient stay supports client progress, and that treatment effects will have lasting value post-discharge when therapy is continued in the outpatient setting. African American women who have participated in culturally adapted CBT- based interventions report improvement in condition, increased quality of life, and improved understanding for mental condition (Khan et al., 2019). Thus, despite generalized resistance toward mental health services, culturally adapted CBT treatments are proving successful in efforts to resolve disparate outcomes identified in the literature. These efforts, however, are stifled by the continuing high frequency of mislabeling in the assessment phase, and unintentional exclusion of culture from the treatment phase that results in poor outcomes and perpetuates known mental health disparities.

CASE STUDY OUTCOME

Returning to the case of Jessica, the treating clinician completed a lengthy assessment and intake with Jessica lasting approximately six hours over the course of her first four days. Utilizing a structured clinical interview, objective measures, collateral information, and a detailed review of previous clinical records, the clinician determined that Jessica meets criteria for post-traumatic stress disorder, complex type, and alcohol use disorder, severe.

The clinician noted that Jessica regularly used euphemisms to describe her symptoms and clinical experiences that were inaccurately documented in her treatment records by other treating professionals. The clinician also noted that in addition to her mental health concerns, Jessica was diagnosed with diabetes and hypertension and reported that she was unable to regularly afford and/or adhere to her medication regimen. Jessica admitted that she was unfamiliar with the medical recommendations to maintain healthy insulin levels and/or blood pressure.

While working alongside Jessica, the clinician became aware that Jessica was very insightful and knowledgeable about the stressors African American women in her community faced when attempting to obtain adequate health care. She shared her beliefs about the poor treatment many African American women receive in the community and discussed how her lack of trust in the medical and mental health professions made it very difficult for her to adhere to treatment. Furthermore, she reported she did not feel a genuine connection with the treatment professional. Jessica reported that her main stressor was her lack of employment, which was directly related to 1) her psychiatric symptoms and 2) the time she spent securing and preserving her social services (e.g., food stamps, housing voucher, low-cost medical/psychiatric treatment). As a result of her primary goal of maintaining employment, Jessica agreed to work on her mental illness as it pertains to her interpersonal relationship and active symptoms of her mental illness.

Jessica was previously diagnosed with schizophrenia, bipolar disorder, borderline personality disorder, attention deficit hyperactivity disorder, and major anxiety; however, after a detailed interview, it was determined that her previously identified paranoia was actually culturally appropriate skepticism. Her unmanaged hypertension impacted her sleep and subsequent reporting of atypical visual aberrations that often occur in a sleeplike state. Similarly, her unmanaged diabetes caused fluctuating mood changes as well as fatigue, trouble thinking clearly, and anxiety. Additionally, it was determined that Jessica's inability to manage her health symptoms occasionally mirrored symptoms of psychosis.

The course of Jessica's inpatient treatment lasted approximately 10 days, with the first two days being focused on crisis and symptom stabilization. Once Jessica achieved baseline functioning, she participated in a time limited dynamic psychotherapy (TLDP) (Strupp & Binder, 1984) which is a short-term form of psychodynamic therapy. Meeting with Jessica daily for approximately 30-minute sessions, the therapist focused on addressing Jessica's maladaptive interpersonal style in order to help her learn how to build positive relationships and address her pattern of self-sabotage; specifically as it relates to her mental health treatment. The therapist focused on identifying cyclic patterns, areas where Jessica was interpersonally inflexible, as well as some of her negative self-appraisals. The therapist helped her learn how to independently identify these maladaptive behaviors and provided her with tools to address them or at a minimum acknowledge that they were happening. By utilizing TLDP, the therapist was able to help Jessica pinpoint where her biggest concerns were regarding her overall health and come up with a plan to address them. Furthermore, the therapeutic modality used allowed the therapist to address the many "isms" that Jessica noted that impacted her overall mental health on a daily basis (i.e., sexism, racism, colorism, classism). TLDP helped Jessica incorporate how her past and current relationships were impacted by her negative appraisals of life stressors while addressing her maladaptive way of being heard in her community. Specifically, Jessica was able to learn appropriate boundaries to assist with the management of her day-to-day life.

Jessica also participated in a CBT-driven, evidence-based group therapy treatment entitled Seeking Safety (Najavits, 2002). This treatment approach was developed specifically for co-occurring PTSD and substance abuse., with a focus on establishing safety (i.e., harmful relationships, symptoms of dissociation). The program focuses on teaching "safe coping skills" that apply to symptoms of both substance abuse and PTSD.

The novelty of this program is that although the lessons are structured, they can be conducted in any order and utilized in different formats and settings, which is ideal for inpatient treatment. Group therapy occurred three times a week and lasted approximately 90 minutes. Due to the open format, Seeking Safety was an ideal choice for addressing some of Jessica's clinical needs. However, other ideal treatments on inpatient units include trauma-focused CBT, 12-step programs, and matrix model.

Aftercare was initiated by the treatment team, and Jessica was referred to a short-term CBT-based program that would focus on resolving one "issue" at a time, with the first concern being her regular adherence to her medical issues. This plan for treatment was developed solely by Jessica with assistance from her inpatient therapist utilizing a detailed step-by step process that would help ensure short-term success following her discharge from the unit. Jessica worked with the clinician to determine how often she would be able to attend sessions due to her financial limitations and need to use public transportation. The clinician assisted Jessica with seeking out a qualified mental health professional that would take her state-provided medical insurance and who self-identified as female. Although Jessica ideally wanted a young African American therapist, there were none within her insurance that were accepting new clients; so, Jessica agreed to work alongside a Latina therapist after processing her disappointment with her therapist utilizing a psychodynamic approach. Additionally, Jessica was provided with detailed information regarding her diagnosis, possible treatments, and long-term outcomes that were tailored to African American women. She was provided with information regarding the typical course of treatment for post-traumatic stress disorder, and alcohol use disorder as well as a realistic representation of the highs and lows of therapy.

Jessica was referred to a psychiatrist for follow-up within five days to keep the momentum utilizing telepsychiatry due to her limited ability to find reliable transportation. She was also set up with an aftercare appointment with the inpatient social worker to follow up on appointment compliance and treatment adherence via telephone. These support resources have been shown to significantly increase treatment compliance with long-term success for African American women.

REFERENCES

Akinhanmi, M. O., Biernacka, J. M., Strakowski, S. M., McElroy, S. L., Balls Berry, J. E., Merikangas, K. R., Assari, S., McInnis, M. G., Schulze, T. G., LeBoyer, M., Tamminga, C., Patten, C., & Frye, M. A. (2018). Racial disparities in bipolar disorder treatment and research: A call to action. *Bipolar Disorders*, *20*(6), 506–514. https://doi.org/10.1111/bdi.12638

Alim, T. N., Charney, D. S., & Mellman, T. A. (2006). An overview of posttraumatic stress disorder in African Americans. *Journal of Clinical Psychology*, *62*(7), 801–813.

Ambresin, G., Desplan, J. N., Preisig, M., & de Roten, Y. (2012). Efficacy of an adjunctive brief psychodynamic psychotherapy to usual inpatient treatment of depression: Rationale and design of a randomized controlled trial. *BMC Psychiatry, 12*(182). http://www.biomedcentral.com/1471-244x/12/182

American Psychological Association (APA). (2017). *African Americans have limited access to mental and behavioral health care.* https://www.apa.org/advocacy /civil-rights/diversity/african-american-health

Anderson, J. (2016). *Breadwinner mothers by race/ethnicity and state.* https://iwpr .org/iwpr-issues/employment-and-earnings/breadwinner-mothers-by-race -ethnicity-and-state/

Asnaani, A., & Hofmann, S. G. (2013). Collaboration in culturally responsive ther-apy: Establishing a strong therapeutic alliance across cultural lines. *Journal of Clinical Psychology, 68*(2), 187–197. https://doi.org/10.1002/jclp.21829

Bailey, R. K., Blackmon, H. L., & Stevens, F. L. (2009). Major depressive disorder in the African American population: Meeting the challenges of stigma, misdi-agnosis, and treatment disparities. *Journal of the National Medical Association, 101*(11), 1084–1089.

Barrio, C., Yamada, A., Hough, R. L., Hawthorne, W., Garcia, P., & Jeste, D. V. (2003). Ethnic disparities in use of public mental health case management services among patients with schizophrenia. *Psychiatric Services, 54*(9), 1264–1270. https://doi.org/10.1176/appi.ps.54.9.1264

Beach, M. C., Gary, T. L., Price, E. G., Robinson, K., Gozu, A., Palacio, A., Smarth, C., Jenckes, M., Feuerstein, C., Bass, E. B., Powe, N. R., & Cooper, L. A. (2006). Improving health care quality for racial/ethnic minorities: A systematic review of the best evidence regarding provider and organization interven-tions. *BMC Public Health, 6*(104). https://doi.org/10.1186/1471-2458-6-104

Bolden, L., & Wicks, M. N. (2005). Length of stay, admission types, psychiatric diagnoses, and the implications of stigma in African Americans in the nationwide inpatient sample. *Issues in Mental Health Nursing, 26*(10), 1043–1059. https://doi.org/ 10.1080/01612840500280703

Breiding, M. J., Smith, S. G., Basile, K. C., Walters, M. L., Chen, J., & Merrick, M. T. (2014). Prevalence and characteristics of sexual violence, stalking, and inti-mate partner violence victimization—National Intimate Partner and Sexual Violence Survey, United States, 2011, *MMWR Surveill Summ., 63*(8), 1–18.

Bridges, K. (2020). Implicit bias and racial disparities in healthcare. *Human Rights Magazine, 43*(3). https://www.americanbar.org/groups/crsj/publications /human_rights_magazine_home/the-state-of-healthcare-in-the-united-states /racial-disparities-in-health-care/

Cabral, R. R., & Smith, T. B. (2011). Racial/ethnic matching of clients and thera-pists in mental health services: A meta-analytic review of preferences, per-ceptions, and outcomes. *Journal of Counseling Psychology, 58*(4), 537–554. https://doi.org/10.1037/a0025266

Carson, N. J., Vesper, A., Chen, C. N., & Lê Cook, B. (2014). Quality of follow-up after hospitalization for mental illness among patients from racial-ethnic minority groups. *Psychiatric Services* (Washington, D.C.), *65*(7), 888–896. https://doi.org/10.1176/appi.ps.201300139

Carter-Pokras, O., & Baquet, C. (2002). What is a "health disparity"? *Public Health Reports* (Washington, DC: 1974), *117*(5), 426–434. https://doi.org/10.1093 /phr/117.5.426

Chu, J., Floyd, R., Diep, H., Pardo, S., Goldblum, P., & Bongar, B. (2013). A tool for the culturally competent assessment of suicide: The Cultural Assessment of

Risk for Suicide (CARS) Measure. *Psychological Assessment, 25*(2), 424–434. https://doi.org/10.1037/a0031264

Chung, H., Mahler, J. C., & Kakuma, T. (1995). Racial differences in treatment of psychiatric inpatients. *Psychiatric Services, 46*(6), 581–591.

Coker, A. (2004). Counseling African American women: Issues, challenges, and intervention strategies. In G. Walz, & R. Yep (Eds.), *VISTAS: Perspectives and counseling* (pp. 129–136). Alexandria, VA: American Counseling Association and Counseling Outfitters/CAPS Press.

Creed, F., Black, D., Anthony, P., Osborn, M., Thomas, P., & Tomenson, B. (1990). Randomised controlled trial of day patient versus inpatient psychiatric treatment. *BMJ, 300*, 1033–1037. https://doi.org/10.1136/bmj .300.6731.1033

Cross, W. E., Jr., Parham, T. A., & Helms, J. E. (1991). The stages of Black identity development: Nigrescence models. In R. L. Jones (Ed.), *Black Psychology* (pp. 319–338). Oakland, CA: Cobb & Henry Publishers.

Czekalinsk, S. (2012). *Black women key to easing military suicides?* https://www .nationaljournal.com/s/114480

Dale, S. K., & Saunders, S. (2018). *Using cognitive behavioral therapy to assist individuals facing oppression.* http://www.societyforpsychotherapy.org/using -cognitive-behavioral-therapy-to-assist-individuals-facing-oppression

DeAngelis, T. (2019). Better relationships with patients lead to better outcomes. *American Psychological Association, 50*(10), 38.

Delphin-Rittmon, M. E., Flanagan, E. H., Andres-Hyman, R., Ortiz, J., Amer, M. M., & Davidson, L. (2015). Racial-ethnic differences in access, diagnosis, and outcomes in public-sector inpatient mental health treatment. *Psychological Services, 12*(2), 158–166. https://doi.org/10.1037 /a0038858

Donovan, R. A., & West., L. M. (2015). Stress and mental health: Moderating role of the Strong Black Woman stereotype. *Journal of Black Psychology, 41*(4), 384–396. https://doi.org/10.1177/0095798414543014

Dougherty, R. H., & American College of Mental Health Administration. (2004). Reducing disparity in behavioral health services: A report from the American College of Mental Health Administration. *Administration and Policy in Mental Health and Mental Health Services Research, 31*(3), 253–263. https:// doi.org/10.1023/b:apih.0000018833.22506.fc

Gara, M. A., Minsky, S., Silverstein, S. M., Miskimen, T., & Strakowski, S. M. (2019). A naturalistic study of racial disparities in diagnoses at an outpatient behavioral health clinic. *Psychiatric Services, 70*(2), 130–134. https:// doi.org/10.1176/appi.ps.201800223

Glazer, W. M., Morgenstern, H., & Doucette, J. (1994). Race and tardive dyskinesia among outpatients at a CMHC. *Hosp Community Psychiatry, 45*(1), 38–42. https://doi.org/10.1176/ps.45.1.38

Greene, B. (1997). Psychotherapy with African American Women: Integrating feminist and psychodynamic models. *Smith College Studies in Social Work, 67*(3), 299–322.

Haddock, G., Tarrier, N., Morrison, A., Hopkins, R., Drake, R., & Lewis, S. (1999). A pilot study evaluating the effectiveness of individual inpatient cognitive-behavioural therapy in early psychosis. *Social Psychiatry and Psychiatric Epidemiology, 34*, 254–258. https://doi.org/10.1007/s001270050141

Helms, J. E. (Ed.). (1990). *Contributions in Afro-American and African studies, No. 129. Black and White racial identity: Theory, research, and practice.* Westport, CT: Greenwood Press.

Jordan, J. M. (1997). Counseling African American women from a cultural sensitivity perspective. In C. Lee (Ed.), *Multicultural issues in counseling: New approaches to diversity* (pp. 109–121). Alexandria, VA: American Counseling Association.

Kennedy, B. R., Mathis, C. C., & Woods, A. K. (2007). African Americans and their distrust of the health care system: Healthcare for diverse populations. *Journal of Cultural Diversity, 14*(2), 56–60.

Khan, S., Lovell, K., Lunat, F., Masood, Y., Shah, S., Tomenson, B., & Husain, N. (2019). Culturally-adapted cognitive behavioural therapy based intervention for maternal depression: A mixed-methods feasibility study. *BMC Women's Health, 19*(21). https://doi.org/10.1186/s12905-019-0712-7

Kohn, L. P., Oden, T., Munoz, R., Robinson, A., and Leavitt, D. (2002). Brief Report: Adapted cognitive behavioral group therapy for depressed low-income African American women. *Community Mental Health Journal, 38*(6), 497–504.

Kösters, M., Burlingame, G. M., Nachtigall, C., & Strauss, B. (2006). A meta-analytic review of the effectiveness of inpatient group psychotherapy. *Group Dynamics: Theory, Research, and Practice, 10*(2), 146–163. https://doi.org/10.1037/1089-2699.10.2.146

Kreyenbuhl, J., Zito, J. M., Buchanan, R. W., Soeken, K. L., & Lehman, A. F. (2003). Racial disparity in the pharmacological management of schizophrenia. *Schizophrenia Bulletin, 29*(2), 183–194. https://doi.org/10.1093/oxfordjournals.schbul.a006996

Lacey, K. K., Parnell, R., Mouzon, D. M., Matusko, N., Head, D., Abelson, J. M., & Jackson, J. S. (2015). The mental health of US Black women: The roles of social context and severe intimate partner violence. *BMJ Open, 5*(10), e008414.

Lacey, K. K., Sears, K. P., Matusko, N., & Jackson, J. S. (2015). Severe physical violence and Black women's health and well-being. *American Journal of Public Health, 105*(4), 719–724. https://doi.org/10.2105/AJPH.2014.301886

Lacey, M., Paolini, S., Hanlon, M. C., Melville, J., Galletly, C., & Campbell, L. E. (2014). Parents with serious mental illness: Differences in internalized and externalized mental illness stigma and gender stigma between mothers and fathers. *Psychiatry Research, 225*(3), 723–733.

Lutterman, T., Shaw, R., Fisher, W. H., & Manderscheid, R. (2017). *Trend in psychiatric inpatient capacity, United States and each state, 1970 to 2014.* Alexandria, VA: National Association of State Mental Health Program Directors. https://www.nasmhpd.org/sites/default/files/TACPaper.2.Psychiatric-Inpatient-Capacity_508C.pdf

Maddox, T. (2013). Professional women's well-being: The role of discrimination and occupational characteristics. *Women & Health, 53*(7), 706–729. https://doi.org/10.1080/03630242.2013.822455

Males, M. (2018). Racial implications of the narcissistic personality inventory reinterpreting popular depictions of narcissism trends. *Journal of Psychology and Psychiatry, 2.* https://doi.org/10.15761/JPP.1000106

Maramba, G. G., & Nagayama Hall, G. C. (2002). Meta-analyses of ethnic match as a predictor of dropout, utilization, and level of functioning. *Cultural Diversity and Ethnic Minority Psychology, 8*(3), 290–297.

Mays, V. M. (1995). Black women, women, stress, and perceived discrimination: The focused support group model as an intervention for stress reduction. *Cultural Diversity Mental Health, 1*(1), 53–65.

McDermott, K. W., Elixhauser, A., & Sun, R. (2017). *Trends in hospital inpatient stays in the United States, 2005–2014.* HCUP Statistical Brief #225. June 2017. Agency for Healthcare Research and Quality, Rockville, MD. https://www.hcup-us.ahrq.gov/reports/statbriefs/sb225-Inpatient-US-Stays-Trends.pdf

McGilloway, A., Hall, R. E., Lee, T., & Bhui, K. S. (2010) A systematic review of personality disorder, race and ethnicity: Prevalence, aetiology and treatment. *BMC Psychiatry, 10*(33). https://doi.org/10.1186/1471-244X-10-33

McGoldrick, M., Giordano, J., & Garcia-Preto, N. (Eds.). (2005). *Ethnicity and family therapy* (3rd ed.). New York, NY: Guilford Press.

McKee, J., & Brahm, N. (2016). Medical mimics: Differential diagnostic considerations for psychiatric symptoms. *Mental Health Clinician, 6*(6), 289–296. https://doi.org/10.9740/mhc.2016.11.289

McLaughlin, J. E. (2002). Reducing diagnostic bias. *Journal of Mental Health Counseling, 24*(3), 256–269.

Mengesha, M., & Ward, E. C. (2012). Psychotherapy with African American women with depression: Is it okay to talk about their religious/spiritual beliefs? *Religions, 3*(1), 19–36.

Meyer, O. L., & Zane, N. (2013). The influence of race and ethnicity in clients' experiences of mental health treatment. *Journal of Community Psychology, 41*(7), 884–901. https://doi.org/10.1002/jcop.21580

Miller, A. (2012). *Instructor's manual for Aaron Beck on cognitive therapy with Aaron Beck, M.D.* Psychotherapy.net.

Morris, E. F. (2001). Clinical practices with African Americans: Juxtaposition of standard clinical practices and Africentricism. *Professional Psychology: Research and Practice, 32*(6), 563–572. https://doi.org/10.1037/0735-7028.32.6.563

Najavits, L. M. (2002). *Seeking safety: A treatment manual for PTSD and substance abuse.* New York, NY: Guilford Press.

Neighbors, H. W., Jackson, J. S., Campbell, L., & Williams, D. (1989). The influence of racial factors on psychiatric diagnosis: A review and suggestions for research. *Community Mental Health Journal, 25*(4), 301–311.

Perry, B. L., Harp, K. L. H., & Oser, C. B. (2013). Racial and gender discrimination in the stress process: Implications for African American women's health and well-being. *Sociological Perspectives, 56*(1), 25–48.

Pinals, D., Packer, I., & Fisher, W. (2004). Relationship between race and ethnicity and forensic clinical triage dispositions. *Psychiatric Services, 55*(8), 873–878. https://doi.org/10.1176/appi.ps.55.8.873

Powell, W., Richmond, J., Mohottige, D., Yen, I., Joslyn, A., & Corbie-Smith, G. (2019). Medical mistrust, racism, and delays in preventive health screening among African-American men. *Behavioral Medicine, 45*(2), 102–117. https://doi.org/10.1080/08964289.2019.1585327

Puyat, J. H., Daw, J. R., Cunningham, C. M., Law, M. R., Wong, S. T., Greyson, D. L., & Morgan, S. G. (2013). Racial and ethnic disparities in the use of antipsychotic medication: A systematic review and meta-analysis. *Social Psychiatry and Psychiatric Epidemiology, 48*(12), 1861–1872. https://doi.org/10.1007/s00127-013-0753-4

Romero, R. E. (2000). The icon of the Strong Black Woman: The paradox of strength. In L. C. Jackson & B. Greene (Eds.), *Psychotherapy with African American women: Innovations in psychodynamic perspective and practice* (pp. 225–238). New York, NY: Guilford Press.

Schwartz., E. K., Docherty, N. M., Najolia, G. M., & Cohen, A. S. (2019). Exploring the racial diagnostic bias of schizophrenia using behavioral and clinical-based measures. *Journal of Abnormal Psychology, 128*(3), 263–271. https://doi .org/10.1037/abn0000409

Schwartz, R. C., & Blankenship, D. M. (2014). Racial disparities in psychotic disorder diagnosis: A review of empirical literature. *World Journal of Psychiatry, 4*(4), 133–140. https://doi.org/10.5498/wjp.v4.i4.133

Seeberger, C. (2019). *Nearly two-thirds of mothers continue to be family breadwinners, Black mothers are far more likely to be breadwinners.* https://www .americanprogress.org/press/release/2019/05/10/469660/release-nearly-two -thirds-mothers-continue-family-breadwinners-black-mothers-far-likely -breadwinners

Seeman, M. (2012). Intervention to prevent child custody loss in mothers with schizophrenia. *Schizophrenia Research and Treatment, 2012*, 1–6. https://doi.org /10.1155/2012/796763

Segal, S. P., Bola, J., & Watson, M. (1996). Race, quality of care, and antipsychotic prescribing practices in psychiatric emergency services. *Psychiatric Services, 47*(3), 282–286.

Shorter-Gooden, K. (2009). Therapy with African American men and women. In H. A. Neville, B. M. Tynes, & S. O. Utsey (Eds.), *Handbook of African American psychology* (pp. 445–458). Thousand Oaks, CA: Sage.

Snowden, L. R., & Cheung, F. K. (1990). Use of inpatient mental health services by members of ethnic minority groups. *American Psychologist, 45*(3), 347–355. https://doi.org/10.1037/0003-066X.45.3.347

Snowden, L. R., Hastings, J. F., & Alvidrez, J. (2009). Overrepresentation of Black Americans in psychiatric inpatient care. *Psychiatric Services, 60*(6), 779–785. https://doi.org/10.1176/appi.ps.60.6.779

Strupp, H. H., & Binder, J. L. (1984). *Psychotherapy in a new key.* New York, NY: Basic Books.

Stuart, S., & Bowers, W. A. (1995). Cognitive therapy with inpatients: Review and meta-analysis. *Journal of Cognitive Psychotherapy, 9*(2), 85–92.

Stuart, S., & Thase, M. (1992). Inpatient applications of cognitive-behavioral therapy: A review of recent developments. *Journal of Psychotherapy Practice and Research, 3*(4), 284–299.

Substance Abuse and Mental Health Services Administration (SAMHSA). (2014). *Trauma-informed care in behavioral health services.* Treatment Improvement Protocol (TIP) Series 57. HHS Publication No. (SMA) 13-4801. Rockville, MD: Substance Abuse and Mental Health Services Administration.

Tolin, D. F., & Foa, E. B. (2006). Sex differences in trauma and posttraumatic stress disorder: A quantitative review of 25 years of research. *Psychological Bulletin, 132*(6), 959–992. https://doi.org/10.1037/0033-2909.132.6.959

Tulloch, A. D., Fearon, P., & David, A. S. (2011). Length of stay of general psychiatric inpatients in the United States: Systematic review. *Administration and Policy in Mental Health, 38*, 155–168. https://doi.org/10.1007 /s10488-010-0310-3

Valenstein, M., Copeland, L., Owen, R., Blow, F., & Visnic, S. (2001). Delays in adopting evidence-based dosages of conventional antipsychotics. *Psychiatric Services, 52*(9), 124–1244. https://doi.org/10.1176/appi.ps.52.9.1242

Van Ryn, M., & Burke, J. (2000). The effect of patient race and socio-economic status on physicians' perceptions of patients. *Social Science & Medicine, 50*(6), 813–828. https://doi.org/10.1016/s0277-9536(99)00338-x

Vinney, C. (2019). *Psychodynamic theory: Approaches and proponents.* ThoughtCo. https://www.thoughtco.com/psychodynamic-theory-4588302

Walkup, J. T., McAlpine, D. D., Olfson, M., Labay, L. E., Boyer, C., & Hansell, S. (2000). Patients with schizophrenia at risk for excessive antipsychotic dosing. *Journal of Clinical Psychiatry, 61*(5), 344–348.

Wang, P. S., Berglund, P., & Kessler, R. C. (2000). Recent care of common mental disorders in the United States: Prevalence and conformance with evidence-based recommendations. *Journal of General Internal Medicine, 15*(5), 284–292. https://doi.org/10.1046/j.1525-1497.2000.9908044.x

Weissman., J. F., Pratt, L. A., Miller, E. A., & Parker, J. D. (2015). Serious psychological distress among adults: United States, 2009–2013. *NCHS Data Brief, 203,* 1–8.

West, L. M., Donovan, R. A., & Daniel, A. R. (2016). The price of strength: Black college women's perspectives on the Strong Black Woman stereotype, *Women & Therapy, 39*(3–4), 390–412. https://doi.org/10.1080/02703149.2016.1116871

Whaley, A. L. (2004). Ethnicity/race, paranoia, and hospitalization for mental health problems among men. *American Journal of Public Health, 94*(1), 78–81. https://doi.org/10.2105/ajph.94.1.78

Ward, E., & Brown, R. L. (2015). A culturally adapted depression intervention for African American adults experiencing depression: Oh Happy Day. *American Journal Orthopsychiatry, 85*(1), 11–22. https://doi.org/10.1037/ort0000027

Young, A. S., Klap, R., Sherbourne, C. D., & Wells, K. B. (2001). The quality of care for depressive and anxiety disorders in the United States. *Archives of General Psychiatry, 58*(1), 55–61.

CHAPTER 12

Sexual Orientation and Gender Identity Minorities

Danielle Simmons

MEET BEATRICE

Beatrice, a 56-year-old Black woman, sought counseling to address anxiety and sexuality-related concerns. After 25 years of marriage to the father of her four children, Beatrice is divorced and in a nine-year romantic relationship with a woman named Sheila. Both Beatrice and Sheila are active members of the same church and struggle with their romantic connection due to their conservative upbringings, dogmatic Christian beliefs, and fears of the implications of openly being together. Beatrice is only out to Sheila. They do not identify as being lesbian lovers, but rather as best friends who fell in love. Sheila is still married to her husband of several decades and has expressed no plans of divorcing him. Although he knows Beatrice and Sheila spend a great deal of time together, he does not know about their hand-holding, cuddling, and deep love and affection toward each other. Beatrice feels conflicted about being in a relationship with a married woman and has expressed feeling great sadness and anxiety. She wants to use counseling to feel better emotionally and gain more understanding of her attraction to women.

Beatrice indicated she must work with a Black female therapist to address her sexual identity–related concerns. Although it was previously recommended by a friend, she refused pastoral counseling due to fears of being misunderstood or condemned. Also, despite there being non-Black therapists closer to her home and work, she expressed a willingness to travel to see the right provider. After months of searching provider directories, she identified me on the directory Therapy for Black Girls.

INTRODUCTION

Beatrice's story demonstrates many challenges faced by queer women of color (QWOC), including narratives related to coming out; experiences navigating society, culture, and religion; and complexities managing familial, peer, and romantic entanglements. As a Black queer therapist, married to a trans-identified man, I am personally and professionally invested in the advancement of lesbian, gay, bisexual, transgender, and queer (LGBTQ) communities. With 15 years of clinical experience in a large metropolitan city, I maintain a caseload largely comprised of Black and Brown queer and transgender clients. Although some of my clients seek therapy to address matters pertaining to their sexual orientations and gender identities, many also report experiencing common clinical concerns such as anxiety, depression, career and relationship issues, which may or may not be related to their sexual orientation and gender identity. In many cases, I am sought out by queer and trans individuals of color because of our shared identities and my clinical expertise and reputation in providing client-centered, affirming therapy to members of marginalized groups.

In this chapter, queer is an umbrella term used to encompass a wide variety of sexual orientations, including gay, lesbian, bisexual, and pansexual. Although historically a derogatory term, queer has been reclaimed and rebranded by some members of LGBTQ communities to expand and redefine their sexual and gender identities (Bieschke, Perez, & DeBord, 2007). Some queer and trans people of color (QTPOC), or for the purposes of this chapter, Black queer and trans women (BQTW), may feel comfortable using or being referred to as queer, while others may not. Although LGBTQ are more commonly named sexual and gender identities, some intersex (I) and asexual (A) individuals also identify as queer (Kort, 2018). It would be nearly impossible to represent all sexual and gender markers; as a result, queer and LGBTQ are used as shorthand. It is important to keep in mind that nomenclature is living and ever evolving. If you are seeking additional resources on term definitions created by QTBIPOC, you can find them at www.artforourselves.org/glossary.html.

Given the varied experiences of Black and African American queer and trans women, this chapter will not be an exhaustive overview, but rather a summary of some of the experiences BQTW may face in their communities, families, and therapy. Throughout this chapter we will revisit Beatrice's case, and I will review affirmative clinical care and treatment recommendations for working with BQTW.

Navigating Complexities of Identities and Systems

There is a paucity of research documenting the clinical experiences of BQTW. Much of the LGBTQ research uses primarily White participants, while much of the literature on Black experiences is about, or assumed to be about, heterosexual individuals (Barnett et al., 2019; Parks, Hughes, & Matthews, 2004). BQTW's intersecting marginalized identities are unique because of the increased risks and vulnerabilities associated with moving through life as gender, racial, and sexual minorities. For many, this means greater exposure to discrimination and harassment, such as educational, housing and job discrimination, and decreased feelings of safety and security due to increased experiences of verbal and physical assault, and murder (Bowleg et al., 2003; Follins, Walker, & Lewis, 2014; Greene, 1994, 2000; Singh, Hays, & Watson, 2011). Furthermore, BQTW may experience conflicts between their racial/ethnic and sexual orientation and gender identities, as evidenced by the simultaneous feelings of pride in one's racial/ethnic identity, internalized homophobia and/or transphobia, internalized racism, and/or feelings of being an outsider within predominately White queer and trans spaces (Greene, 1994, 2000; Moore, 2011; Sarno et al., 2015).

Mental Health Concerns

Given the stress of living with multiple marginalized identities, BQTW experience disproportionate rates of mental and physical health issues (Griffith, Jones, & Stewart, 2018; Hughes, Smith, & Dan, 2013; Omoto & Kurtzman, 2006). For many there is a direct correlation between increased exposure to abuse and trauma, decreased self-esteem and feelings of self-worth, and increased use of maladaptive strategies to cope, including engagement in self-harming behaviors and increased substance abuse (Kerr & Oglesby, 2017; Kort, 2018; Ritter & Terndrup, 2002; Szymanski & Gupta, 2009). BQTW also experience higher suicide rates (Blosnich et al., 2016; Griffith, Jones, & Stewart, 2018; Hughes, Smith, & Dan, 2013). Despite experiencing increased symptoms of anxiety and depression, BQTW face real barriers and psychological hurdles to seeking mental health support (i.e., being refused care), which unfortunately results in underutilization of counseling and psychiatric services among members of these vulnerable populations (Corrigan, 2004; Greene, 1994; Griffith, Jones, & Stewart, 2018).

The minority stress model denotes that stigma, prejudice, and discrimination produce a hostile and stressful social environment for people of color and sexual and gender minorities, which leads to poor mental health, and with prolonged exposure, diminished physical health (Balsam et al., 2011). This minority stress model acknowledges it is not the BQTW who are ill or problematic but rather anti-Black, antigay, transphobic systems that are the problem. It takes some of the psychological burden off the client and places the onus where it belongs—on systems of oppression that need to be dismantled. As multiculturally sensitive providers, we are not here to police or pathologize clients, but instead help them cultivate and access internal strengths, capabilities, and resilience to effectively overcome barriers to their mental, emotional, physical, and social wellness. Through strong collaborative therapeutic bonds, therapists assist clients in learning to adaptively manage stress related to their oppressed identities and find what they need to live authentically.

Whether engaged in counseling or not, BQTW are successfully forming healthy, loving, and lasting peer and romantic relationships with others who support, accept, and affirm them. They are active community leaders, successfully managing families and businesses. Although the bias, prejudice, discrimination, and oppression of queer and trans individuals are undeniable, many queer and trans-identified people are happy, thriving, and demonstrate resilience, strength, and courage while living fulfilling lives. By focusing solely on the negative aspects of their lives, we fail to see and appreciate a full picture of Black queer and trans lives (Akerlund & Cheung, 2000; Riggle et al., 2008).

THE LIVED EXPERIENCES OF BLACK QUEER AND TRANS WOMEN

Sexuality in Black Queer Women

Heteronormativity, gender and cultural norms, and pressure to adhere to them complicate the process of exploration and expression of healthy sexuality for queer and trans folks (Balsam et al., 2011). For many BQTW, sexual and gender identity development is peripheral to several other concerns related to racism, genderism/sexism, classism, and other sociopolitical factors, prompting suppression of desires or exploration being done privately (Battle & Barnes, 2010; Greene, 1994). When Black women have enough emotional bandwidth to turn their gaze inward and explore their gender and sexuality, they are often confronted with explicit and internalized messages that signal they are doing something wrong or taboo. For example, I have had cisgender female clients recall childhood experiences of being forced to wear dresses because their parents thought their look was too masculine or butch. This perceived failure to adhere to gender norms can result in severe consequences, including ruptured relationships, harassment, and physical violence (Bostwick et al., 2019; Moore, 2011).

The process of developing healthy self-expression and sexuality for Black women is further complicated by the historical lack of acceptance of queerness in communities of color. Women, most notably women of color, are expected to follow a strict set of rules centered on taking care of others and prioritizing the White community over self (Crenshaw, 1990; Greene & Boyd-Franklin, 1996). BQTW may spend many years internally grappling with what it means for them to be queer, and for some, the process of coming to accept themselves and the legitimacy of their feelings happens years before they ever communicate this part of themselves to another person (Jensen, 1999; Patton & Simmons, 2008).

As BQTW are navigating their sexual and/or gender identities, they may form a deep emotional connection with another woman, and sometimes emotional intimacy grows and blossoms into romantic intimacy (Johnson, 2018; Larkin, 1999), as was the case with Beatrice and Sheila. Sexuality is fluid, expansive, and exists on a continuum rather than immutable binary categories of gay or straight. Some women feel romantic, sexual, and/or emotional attractions to women and describe themselves as gay, lesbian, bisexual, queer, pansexual, or questioning, whereas others do not use labels. People have the right to self-identify and evolve. Unfortunately, for many queer and trans-identified individuals, the developmental process of exploration is confined by rigid societal ideologies and expectations of sexuality and gender, which pathologizes exploration as confusion (Battle & Barnes, 2010).

Unique Experiences of Trans Women

Similar to sexuality, genders also exist on a continuum rather than only dichotomous categories of male and female (American Psychological Association, 2015). However, T for transgender, although routinely tagged on to the LGB acronym, is often treated as an afterthought and can be overlooked by service providers attempting to be inclusive. This means affirming care for LGB individuals may not reflect the distinct needs of gender-variant and trans populations (Fassinger & Arseneau, 2007; Singh, Hays, & Watson, 2011). In fact, trans individuals may be misunderstood and discriminated against even by some members of LGB communities; therefore, increasing the need for advocacy for trans community members, such as enhancing access to affordable health care and gainful employment (Fassinger & Arseneau, 2007; Glynn et al., 2016; Singh et al., 2011). Transphobia and transprejudice manifest in the neglect, objectification, misunderstanding, and pathologizing of individuals who identify as trans (Glynn et al., 2016). For example, in many states, trans people have to "admit" to being born in the wrong body for access to services.

Anti-LGBT laws lead to widespread systemic oppression, injustices, and discrimination against queer and trans people. Given our current social and political climate, white cisgender heterosexual men in government are responsible for creating and changing policies in schools, bathrooms, and other aspects of public and private life for trans people. Moreover, society is not welcoming for trans women at any stage of their transition, especially for those who defy gender stereotypes. Trans folks are judged on how well they "pass" within society's binary imposition of gender identity and expression (Bess & Stabb, 2009). Passing is a complex concept that demonstrates the interconnection between external influences and internal processes, and trans people respond in various ways including aspirations to pass, deliberately pushing back, and/or moving back and forth. Motivations to pass vary and may include the unfortunate reality that passing may lessen discrimination and harassment (Singh, 2013; Singh, Hays, & Watson, 2011). Many trans people, particularly those who begin to pass more consistently, have anxiety about the potential outcomes of involuntary disclosure (being outed, someone finding out) throughout their lives and relationships. Because of binary constraints, trans people may live in constant fear of others' negative responses to their trans identity, which may occur through violence.

Violence against Black Trans Women. "The paradox of visibility" is a theoretical phrase that seeks to explain the ways some aspects of existence are accepted, narrated, and sometimes lauded, while other aspects in the same individual or community are left underrepresented or invisible (Berberick, 2018). In regard to trans visibility, this paradox can be seen in the increased number of trans people in the media, on TV shows such as *Orange Is the New Black* and *Pose* and, at the same time, invisibility and lack of media coverage of worldwide murders of trans people of color, mostly Black and Brown trans women. However, some Black transgender women of color in the spotlight such as Janet Mock, Laverne Cox, and Angelica Ross use their platform to bring more awareness and visibility to the equity and safety issues faced by TWOC.

While there is growing visibility, trans women of color are at a disproportionate risk for severe hate crimes in their daily lives (National Coalition of Anti-Violence Programs, 2016). Of the transgender individuals murdered in 2019, all but one was a woman of color (Ring, 2020), and the majority of them were Black. Not to suggest that any form of violence is acceptable; however, the violence and murder of Black trans women represent a distinct level of brutality. In 2019, with bystanders watching (and some cheering), 23-year-old Muhlaysia Booker was beaten in broad daylight by a mob of men; one reportedly offered $200 to beat the trans woman (Dart, 2019). A month later, Muhlaysia was found dead in the street from a gunshot wound. In Florida, 23-year-old Bee Love Slater's body was found burned beyond recognition (Ring, 2020). And the reports go on. Too many Black trans women are being killed due to people's ignorance, bias, and fear of what attraction to trans women may mean for them. In an interview aired on BuzzFeed News, Cox, understanding the systemic and societal influences said, "Your attraction to me as a trans woman is not a reason to kill me" (Blackmon, 2019).

Medically Transitioning. For trans people, curiosity and questions about genitals are commonplace. Trans people are repeatedly asked detailed questions about their decisions concerning their bodies, surgeries, and hormonal treatments without much regard for their privacy or recognition that there is no prescribed way to be trans (Bess & Stabb, 2009; Erickson-Schroth, 2014; Singh, 2013). This preoccupation with trans bodies contributes to the perpetuation of the view of trans people as "others" rather than as legitimate and valued members of society (Bess & Stabb, 2009; Glynn et al., 2016). There are many ways to transition, for example from male to female (MtF) or female to male (FtM). Some identify as genderqueer, nonbinary, and/or gender nonconforming. Although hormones and gender-aligning surgeries may be a part of transitioning, this medicalized perspective does not include all trans people's experiences.

For those who seek to medically transition, there are many considerations including expenses and long-term effects, not to mention the long and arduous nature of the process. The challenges of these processes are exacerbated by difficulties accessing hormones and requiring letters of support from mental health professionals to validate the needs of trans women. This gatekeeping role is pathologizing and invalidating and may create additional obstacles to trans communities gaining access to adequate health care (Chang, Singh, & dickey, 2019). To eliminate barriers, the World Professional Association for Transgender Health (WPATH) Standards of Care (2012) advocates for an informed consent model allowing clients to access hormone treatments and surgical interventions without undergoing a mental health evaluation. With this model, clients are provided autonomy to make informed decisions about their care, similar to other health-care choices.

Importance of Community

Engagement in affirming communities is an integral part of identity formation for queer and trans individuals, and is a necessary part of survival (Donovan, Heaphy, & Weeks, 2003; Singh, 2013). Through building accepting communities, BQTW create buffers to counterbalance the pervasiveness of heterosexism and trans oppression in their lives (Bowleg, Craig, & Burkholder, 2004). By attending and participating in queer events and organizations, BQTW can see reflections of themselves and feel part of something designed just for them. In this day of social media, women can also log onto sites such as Instagram, Twitter, or Facebook to see examples and engage with other BQTW. On and off-line BQTW are creating affirming spaces to explore their identities, dating, coming out, and day-to-day circumstances.

Routinely, Black people rely on talking to friends or family or are encouraged to deepen their spiritual or religious practices when managing distress. Although prayer and meditation can be wonderful resources for some trans and queer folks, the long-standing history of antigay teachings by many traditional religions has caused a significant rift, making these potential sanctuaries feel unsafe (Walker & Longmire-Avital, 2013). Queerness is ignored or openly condemned in some traditional places of worship, so being a queer person of color with a strong faith base can be fraught with turmoil, including the potential loss of religion or access to religious communities (Burke, Chauvin, & Miranti, 2005). Some Black queer–identified individuals are emotionally struggling to challenge teachings that there is something sinful and wrong about being queer. It often takes many years to challenge and change these deeply ingrained beliefs. For many, it is not until they develop a relationship with another queer or trans person or become involved in an affirming community of support that they can begin to reconcile the tension of holding several, sometimes seemingly opposing, identities (Donovan, Heaphy & Weeks, 2003).

In Beatrice's case, she stopped attending her church since she felt like a hypocrite the more she explored her queer identity. Therapy provided an opportunity for her to grieve the loss of her connection to church, although she continued to regularly pray and read the Bible. Time in therapy was also devoted to exploring additional options for spiritual, emotional, and social support because she had derived so much of that from attending her home church. While empathizing with and validating her feelings of loss, we also spent time exploring positive aspects of being queer. Some positive aspects include demonstrating resilience and developing kinship and the opportunities for disclosure and vulnerability that come from engagement with affirming social networks (Bowleg, Craig, & Burkholder, 2004; Riggle et al., 2008).

Through community, queer and trans individuals develop great insight into and empathy for themselves and others, and experience liberation and freedom from societal definitions of roles (Riggle et al., 2008). Being a member of Black queer populations gives access to a world that challenges the status quo, where individuals can create and redefine their realities. Differences become strengths. Not fitting into society's small boxes of who and how people should be and live is liberating and allows for more authentic self-expression. Self-validation and the validation of others who see, sympathize, and accompany them on their journey are invaluable.

For Beatrice, this came in the form of joining a Black queer women's support group at the local LGBT community center. She also started regularly attending Codependence Anonymous groups for increased social support and to deepen her understanding of ways she has neglected her own needs by focusing on the needs of others. Throughout our time working together, she explored various self-reflective practices such as journaling and meditating. Although she was deeply in love with Sheila, Beatrice admitted there were ways she felt hurt and inhibited in this relationship. The idea of leaving this relationship was agonizing as she knew Sheila would not likely leave her husband.

As their relationship deepened, Beatrice felt tempted to ask Sheila to leave her marriage. Although they sometimes imagined what life could be like together as primary partners, they both worried about the impacts this could have on their children and acceptance within their families. Further, Sheila did not identify as queer. She viewed her love for Beatrice as an isolated event and expressed having no other attractions to women.

Beatrice worked very hard to become familiar with the barriers to seeking partnership aligned with her wants and needs. She expressed concern that if she began dating someone else, she would not be fully available to them because of her relationship with Sheila. Using attachment theory (Levine & Heller, 2012), we explored how her attachments within her family system may impact her romantic attachments.

Black Queer and Trans Women in Families

The necessity of the Black family unit is well documented (Evans, Bell, & Burton, 2017; Greene & Boyd-Franklin, 1996; Moore, 2011) and is "the primary social unit and most prominent source of emotional and material support for most, but certainly not all, African American lesbians" (Greene, 2000, p. 245). Family can provide a foundation of love and support and can also be a source of great pain when sexual and gender exploration and expression are prohibited, ignored, and shamed. Often queer and trans individuals are motivated to come out to gain support that buffers against homophobia and transphobia outside of the home, but this cannot happen when the family is also a source of abuse. For members of LGBTQ communities, authentic self-expression can come with significant repercussions, including being ostracized, put out of their homes, disowned by their families, and even worse, beaten or killed.

LGBTQ individuals usually want to share aspects of their sexuality and gender journeys with their family members to be closer to them (Kort, 2018). Before such disclosures, relationships may feel distant and strained because relatives are not privy to key parts of queer and trans individuals' lives, such as crushes, anniversaries, and milestones they experience in romantic relationships. When speaking with relatives about dating and partnership, queer family members may deny their relationships and use gender-neutral pronouns to avoid making relatives uncomfortable or emboldened to make hurtful comments. When disparaging views are shared, it can be disappointing and exhausting for courageous queer and trans individuals, and allies, to interrupt problematic behavior.

TREATMENT CONSIDERATIONS AND RECOMMENDATIONS

Affirmative Therapy with Black Queer and Trans Women

What Is Affirmative Care? Chernin and Johnson (2003) define affirmative therapy as clinical work that validates and advocates for the needs of sexual and gender minority clients. Affirmative care is ethical care. Adhering to the Guidelines for Psychological Practice with Transgender and Gender Nonconforming People (APA, 2015), affirming practitioners must demonstrate an understanding of the aforementioned pathologizing and punishing cultural context toward sexual and gender variance. We also need to be mindful of the protective factors, such as community engagement and family support, that can buffer the impacts of systemic oppression for BQTW. Multiculturally sensitive affirmative therapy embraces, celebrates, and advocates for the authenticity, integrity, and truth of our clients and their relationships (Ritter & Terndrup, 2002; Tozer & McClanahan, 1999). By treating queer and trans clients as self-determined individuals who are knowledgeable of their own experiences and needs, we promote agency and honor their humanity.

Providers can work across theoretical approaches to model an affirmative stance toward all clients, particularly those who identify as BQTW. On a very basic level, LGBTQ-affirming therapists need to distinguish the differences between sexual orientation, assigned sex, gender identity, and gender expression and recognize these concepts as complex, related, and separate (Burnes et al., 2010). We understand sexuality and gender as social constructs and are genuinely curious about the manifestations of these concepts in our clients' lives. We learn and use the names, pronouns, and labels our clients use in describing their experiences, recognizing that labels only provide basic information and can mean many different things to individuals. Queer and gender-affirming therapists may choose to introduce their pronouns to demark therapy as a safe space to discuss gender and sexuality. Other affirming practices include using more than male/female or single/married markers on paperwork and allowing for self-identification so as not to assume that all clients are cisgender and heterosexual. This includes the use of "they" and "their" pronouns in the singular. We are intentional with our questions and interventions to ensure we are not perpetuating heteronormative binary thinking.

Microaggressions are subtle offenses or insults, often unconscious and unintentional, that invalidate client realities and foster a sense of marginalization (Shelton & Delgado-Romero, 2013; Sue, 2010). Asking trans clients about their deadnames or accusing individuals who come out later in life as "living a lie" are examples of microaggressions on the part of therapists. These are common occurrences in and outside of therapy, and affirming therapists, even the most talented ones, will commit microaggressions; it is inevitable. By practicing humility and being honest about our strengths and areas of growth as affirming providers, we can acknowledge the impact of our missteps without overstating our intentions. For example, if we misgender someone, we can apologize, correct ourselves, and move on with the interactions, deliberately and mindfully as not to commit the offense again. Clients do not need to hear explanation or justification for the misstep; instead, they need to know we can tolerate being challenged and contain our emotions to fully tend to them. We can invite BQTW clients to call us out when there are future missteps, create space for them to name their feelings, and actively listen to them when they share the impacts our words and actions have on them.

Affirming therapists work to neutralize the power differential inherent in therapeutic relationships by being transparent. Our willingness to humble ourselves to learning processes and respond appropriately when such offenses are pointed out strengthens therapeutic relationships, establishes open dialogue, and promotes healthy rapport. Failure to acknowledge ruptures caused by microaggressions will diminish a client's trust in the therapeutic process and also reveals a lack of awareness on the part of the therapist (Shelton & Delgado-Romero, 2013). This also contributes to underutilization of counseling and premature termination (Sue, 2010). Affirming therapy can provide a safe place for BQTW clients to practice using their voice, naming their emotions, honoring their existence, and unapologetically taking up space. As they gain comfort and prowess with these socio-emotional skills in session, they can practice and gain confidence using them in other contexts and relationships.

Beyond basic care, affirming practitioners are knowledgeable about the legal, political, and clinical developments that may impact our clients. This includes remaining current with local and national policies impacting BQTW, as well as skill in treatment strategies introduced by the WPATH Standards of Care (2012); the APA Guidelines for Psychological Practice with Lesbian, Gay, and Bisexual Clients (APA, 2012); and the APA Guidelines for Psychological Practice with Transgender and Gender Nonconforming People (APA, 2015). Although queer and trans individuals are often quite knowledgeable about new developments that impact them, clinicians are obliged to do their own research.

Affirmative Care with Beatrice. When applying an affirming multicultural lens to my work with Beatrice, I needed to understand what it meant for her as a Black, Christian, mother questioning her sexuality and choosing to seek counseling to do so. Due to the impacts of these intersecting and overlapping identities, there were many internal and external pressures she felt to suppress her romantic and sexual desires, and this brought about great anxiety and feelings of being a defective human. For these reasons, our work centered on further exploring the emotional toll of maneuvering cultural contexts with limited social and emotional support. We also worked on validating and normalizing her sexual identity development process, recognizing the conflicts she may need to reconcile between deeply internalized belief structures and her current desires. One area of considerable consternation for Beatrice was related to her romantic attractions to women and her historical attraction to her husband.

In session, Beatrice disclosed she was no longer interested in dating men. She spent some time questioning the legitimacy of her romantic feelings toward her ex-husband and acknowledged their connection was more emotional than sexual. She acknowledged having loved him very deeply throughout their marriage, but said she also felt like something was missing. In one session as we explored her past and present sexual encounters, Beatrice revealed she had not experienced an orgasm during sex with her husband. It was not until she slept with Sheila that she felt sexually satisfied. We spent time discussing the differences in emotional, physical, romantic, and sexual attractions, and this was both illuminating and normalizing for Beatrice.

As Beatrice felt more comfortable and continued to open up, she disclosed her history of same-sex attractions and sexual relationships with at least two women before Sheila, but she never considered herself queer. One of the affairs with a woman happened within her first few years of marriage. Although she told her ex-husband about the affair and expected him to leave her, he begged her to stay. They decided to become more heavily involved with their church and spend more time with other heterosexual married couples; Sheila is the wife in one of those married couples.

Therapist Self-Awareness. Providers must increase their understanding of attitudes, values, assumptions, and biases that may impact their willingness to be affirming, multiculturally informed, and flexible in their work with diverse populations (APA, 2012; Bieschke, Perez, & DeBord, 2007; Johnson, 2012; Pope & Dworkin, 2014; Sue, 2010). By increasing our self-awareness, clinicians can address the limitations of our support and work to develop strategies designed to attract and keep BQTW in counseling (Bridges, Selvidge, & Matthews, 2003; Coker, 2004). We have to be brutally honest in recognizing and dismantling our own heteronormativity, transphobia, racial privilege, and limitations of providing affirmative care to BQTW.

Additionally, BQTW need support in response to ongoing injustices; therefore, affirming therapists can engage in social justice–oriented work by exploring social movements and activist groups to promote systemic change. To consciously do this work, providers have to interrogate their values to see how implicit bias may influence the support offered. This continuous examination of therapists' ideologies and competencies also informs providers of when they may benefit from consultation and/or referring clients to providers who may be a better fit. Table 12.1 provides a list of reflexive questions for additional self-reflection.

Access to Care. For BQTW looking for affirmative care, there are many challenges to finding a provider who is multiculturally sensitive and knowledgeable regarding the issues queer and trans folks face. Even in large cities, there is often a scarcity of providers who specialize with and/or identify as queer women of color, and even fewer who are Black. Due to the power of word of mouth, when such providers are present, their practices tend to fill, limiting their capacity to accept new referrals. Recognizing that the number of individuals seeking affirming care exceeds the number of slots a few queer providers of color can fill, all counselors,

Table 12.1
Reflexive Processing Questions

1. What do I know about BQTW?

2. How did I learn about BQTW?

3. What prior personal and professional experiences do I have with BQTW?

4. How will these experiences, or lack thereof, impact my clinical work with BQTW?

5. What personal values do I hold that may both positively and negatively impact/influence my work with BQTW?

6. How might I impose my beliefs and value systems onto BQTW?

7. What might interfere with my ability to affirmatively support BQTW?

8. What are my areas of continued growth and development related to understanding and supporting members of BQTW?

9. How open and willing am I to admit to missteps in my work?

10. What are some past clinical ruptures and how did I move through them?

11. What fears and insecurities do I have regarding clinical work with BQTW?

especially other providers of color, need to be able to assist in meeting the needs of BQTW. It is important to note that being queer and/or trans does not necessarily make one an expert on queer and gender issues; however, many clients desire to and prefer working with providers who share their identities. This is due to comfort being in a familiar presence, clients' desire to build community, and wanting a provider who will *get* them.

Unfortunately, clinicians are not well trained to work with BQTW due to insufficient multicultural training in academic programs and professional workshops (Bidell, 2016; Burckell & Goldfried, 2006; Lyons et al., 2010). Even when such training is made available, it may be costly and is not required by licensure boards; therefore, some providers may opt out of this important training. As a result, many well-meaning providers are unintentionally harming clients by engaging in practices rooted in bias and ignorance. When this happens, BQTW are tasked with educating their providers and may opt out of therapy due to fear of being mistreated or having their care mishandled by clinicians or their front desk staff. Ideally, clinicians and all staff who interface with clients would receive training to provide multiculturally sensitive care rooted in unconditional positive regard, acceptance, and affirmation of clients' self-identification regarding their sexual orientation and gender (Crisp, 2006; National LGBT Health Education Center, 2016).

Family and Couple Counseling. In therapy, BQTW can explore their feelings of frustration and powerlessness within their family systems. I often work both to validate clients' feelings and to help create empathy for their relatives' lack of knowledge. In many cases it is lack of knowledge, not malicious intent, that leads to lack of support. Timing and intentionality with these interventions are crucial because it can be harmful if therapists invalidate clients' experiences in attempts to normalize what may be happening for relatives. When providing affirmative therapy to BQTW, it is not uncommon for them to want to include members of their support network in their care. Clients may request or the therapists can suggest clients bring members of their family of origin, chosen family, or romantic partners into sessions to assist in restating needs and boundaries and to address unresolved concerns. If joint sessions are not possible, either due to inability or unwillingness, letter writing or role play in sessions may be helpful for processing emotions and exploring ways to use what clients learn in counseling outside of therapy.

To promote growth, development of boundaries, and practices of self-love and preservation, I routinely explore with clients what to keep, release, and alter in the family system. For example, if Sunday dinners are meaningful family traditions, some BQTW choose to keep attending, but when made to feel uncomfortable, we practice ways they can excuse themselves. It can be very affirming for BQTW to hear they have the right to set boundaries or sever ties with problematic relatives, especially when their health and well-being are in jeopardy. In communities of color, there may be messages that challenge and shame such boundary setting, but in affirming care, we explore all possible options to promote wellness. If a relationship or situation is hurtful, BQTW may need therapists to validate their decision to temporarily, or permanently, walk away.

In therapy with BQTW, our work centers on enhancing access to quality social support because the absence of a caring community can have devastating effects. Through the exploration of factors that contribute to strained family relationships, BQTW routinely name a lack of adequate support from family leading to feelings of inadequacy, degradation, and social and emotional isolation. This is why access to affinity groups and chosen families are necessary for survival and invaluable for BQTW. Even when members of the family of origin are accepting, affirming, and nurturing of self-exploration and expression, there remains a need for camaraderie, witnessing, and mirroring for queer and trans-identified individuals (Patton & Simmons, 2008; Singh, 2013).

With relatives and loved ones of QTPOC, our work focuses on ways to increase understanding of queer and trans experiences and needs. Individual, couples, and family therapy are places in which all parties can gain support; process their reactions to being in community with queer and trans loved ones; and process how loving queer and trans individuals often means letting go of preconceived notions to see and accept them, truly and authentically. While recognizing that it takes time to come to terms with someone's sexual orientation or gender identity, it is often very painful for LGBTQ individuals when relatives are dismissive of transitions, refuse to educate themselves, and/or justify hurtful actions. Over time, relatives learn that they cannot avoid, manipulate, or control decisions about identification and expression because ultimately people are self-determined. Referrals to organizations such as Parents, Families, and Friends of Lesbians and Gays (PFLAG) can provide additional support.

Support for Gender-Affirming Interventions. The World Professional Association for Transgender Health (WPATH) Standards of Care for the Health of Transsexual, Transgender, and Gender Nonconforming People (2012) sets guidelines for medical and behavioral health providers. As previously mentioned, operating from an informed consent model, trans individuals seeking gender-affirming interventions such as hormone replace therapy (HRT) and surgeries can directly access care from medical professionals. However, many health-care providers continue to require documentation from mental health professionals prior to provision of HRT or surgery, and affirming therapists can provide such support letters. They should keep in mind that the purpose of the letter is not to prove or establish how "trans" the individual is, rather to provide documentation of the client's ability to make informed decisions regarding their medical care. Documentation might include a formal diagnosis of gender dysphoria, current symptoms, and other diagnoses and their effects on daily functioning, information about treatment history, and the provider's professional assessment justifying the necessity of medical interventions. An example of a support letter is provided in Appendix A.

Affirming therapists help to support hormonal and medical transitions in providing a space to process physical and hormonal changes a client is experiencing. This requires therapists to be knowledgeable of the impact of hormonal interventions, potentially working closely with the prescribing medical professional. Affirming therapy will also involve support around social transitions associated with physical change, including helping clients explore ways physical changes may impact others' perceptions of and engagement with them.

SUMMARY

Affirming therapy for BQTW enhances clinical and social justice–oriented work. Mental health professionals can benefit from developing a nuanced understanding of the unique needs of members of these communities, particularly as they relate to family, community, and therapy engagement. Historically, counselors are positioned as experts and gatekeepers despite the limited training they receive for providing culturally sensitive counseling to members of disenfranchised communities. To improve the quality of care, we have to engage in ongoing self-exploration, supplement our knowledge through diversity trainings, build rich referral networks, and actively seek consultation.

REFERENCES

Akerlund, M., & Cheung, M. (2000). Teaching beyond the deficit model: Gay and lesbian issues among African Americans, Latinos, and Asian Americans. *Journal of Social Work Education, 36*(2), 279–292.

American Psychological Association (APA). (2012). Guidelines for psychological practice with lesbian, gay, and bisexual clients. *American Psychologist, 67*(1), 10–42.

American Psychological Association (APA). (2015). Guidelines for psychological practice with transgender and gender nonconforming people. *American Psychologist, 70*(9), 832–864.

Balsam, K. F., Molina, Y., Beadnell, B., Simoni, J., & Walters, K. (2011). Measuring multiple minority stress: The LGBT People of Color Microaggressions Scale. *Cultural Diversity and Ethnic Minority Psychology, 17*(2), 163–174.

Barnett, A., del Río-González, A., Parchem, B., Pinho, V., Aguayo-Romero, R., Nakamura, N., . . . & Zea, M. (2019). Content analysis of psychological research with lesbian, gay, bisexual, and transgender people of color in the United States: 1969–2018. *American Psychologist, 74*(8), 898–911.

Battle, J., & Barnes, S. L. (2010). *Black sexualities: Probing powers, passions, practices, and policies.* New Brunswick, NJ: Rutgers University Press.

Berberick, S. N. (2018). The paradox of trans visibility: Interrogating the "year of trans visibility." *Journal of Media Critiques, 4*(13), 123–144.

Bess, J., & Stabb, S. (2009). The experiences of transgendered persons in psychotherapy: Voices and recommendations. *Journal of Mental Health Counseling, 31*(3), 264–282.

Bidell, M. P. (2016). Mind our professional gaps: Competent lesbian, gay, bisexual, and transgender mental health services. *Counselling Psychology Review, 31*(1), 67–76.

Bieschke, K. J., Perez, R. M., & DeBord, K. A. (2007). *Handbook of counseling and psychotherapy with lesbian, gay, bisexual, and transgender clients.* Washington, DC: American Psychological Association.

Blackmon, M. (2019). *Laverne Cox opened up on the epidemic of Black trans women being murdered in the US.* https://www.buzzfeednews.com/article /michaelblackmon/laverne-cox-black-trans-women-murders

Blosnich, J. R., Nasuti, L. J., Mays, V. M., & Cochran, S. D. (2016). Suicidality and sexual orientation: Characteristics of symptom severity, disclosure, and timing across the life course. *American Journal of Orthopsychiatry, 86*(1), 69–78.

Bostwick, W. B., Hughes, T. L., Steffen, A., Veldhuis, C. B., & Wilsnack, S. C. (2019). Depression and victimization in a community sample of bisexual and lesbian women: An intersectional approach. *Archives of Sexual Behavior, 48*(1), 131–141.

Bowleg, L., Craig, M. L., & Burkholder, G. (2004). Rising and surviving: A conceptual model of active coping among Black lesbians. *Cultural Diversity and Ethnic Minority Psychology, 10*(3), 229–240.

Bowleg, L., Huang, J., Brooks, K., Black, A., & Burkholder, G. (2003). Triple jeopardy and beyond: Multiple minority stress and resilience among Black lesbians. *Journal of Lesbian Studies, 7*(4), 87–108.

Bridges, S. K., Selvidge, M. M. D., & Matthews, C. R. (2003). Lesbian women of color: Therapeutic issues and challenges. *Journal of Multicultural Counseling and Development, 31*(2), 113–130.

Burckell, L. A., & Goldfried, M. R. (2006). Therapist qualities preferred by sexual-minority individuals. *Psychotherapy: Theory, Research, Practice, Training, 43*(1), 32–49.

Burke, M. T., Chauvin, J. C., & Miranti, J. G. (2005). *Religious and spiritual issues in counseling: Applications across diverse populations.* New York, NY: Brunner-Routledge.

Burnes, T. R., Singh, A. A., Harper, A. J., Harper, B., Maxon-Kann, W., Pickering, D. L., Moundas, S., Scofield, T. R., Roan, A., & Hosea, J. (2010). American Counseling Association: Competencies for counseling with transgender clients. *Journal of LGBT Issues in Counseling, 4*(3–4), 135–159.

Chang, S. C., Singh, A. A., & dickey, l. m. (2018). *A clinician's guide to gender-affirming care: Working with transgender and gender nonconforming clients.* Oakland, CA: New Harbinger.

Chernin, J. N., & Johnson, M. R. (2003). *Affirmative psychotherapy and counseling for lesbians and gay men.* Thousand Oaks, CA: Sage.

Coker, A. (2004). Counseling African American women: Issues, challenges, and intervention strategies. *VISTAS: Perspectives on Counseling,* 129–136.

Corrigan, P. (2004). How stigma interferes with mental health care. *American Psychologist, 59*(7), 614–625.

Crenshaw, K. (1990). Mapping the margins: Intersectionality, identity politics, and violence against women of color. *Stanford Law Review, 43*(6), 1241–1299.

Crisp, C. (2006). The Gay Affirmative Practice Scale (GAP): A new measure for assessing cultural competence with gay and lesbian clients. *Social Work, 51*(2), 115–126.

Dart, T. (2019, May 21). *Muhlaysia Booker: An advocate against trans violence is mourned in Texas.* https://www.theguardian.com/us-news/2019/may/21/muhlaysia-booker-trans-woman-death-texas-dallas-mourns-activist

Donovan, C., Heaphy, B., & Weeks, J. (2003). *Same sex intimacies: Families of choice and other life experiments.* New York, NY: Routledge.

Erickson-Schroth, L. (Ed.). (2014). *Trans bodies, trans selves: A resource for the transgender community.* New York, NY: Oxford University Press.

Evans, S. Y., Bell, K., & Burton, N. K. (2017). *Black women's mental health: Balancing strength and vulnerability.* Albany, NY: SUNY Press.

Fassinger, R. E., & Arseneau, J. R. (2007). "I'd rather get wet than be under that umbrella": Differentiating the experiences and identities of lesbian, gay, bisexual, and transgender people. In K. J. Bieschke, R. M. Perez, & K. A. DeBord (Eds.), *Handbook of counseling and psychotherapy with lesbian, gay, bisexual, and transgender clients* (2nd ed., pp. 19–49). Washington, DC: American Psychological Association.

Follins, L. D., Walker, J. N. J., & Lewis, M. K. (2014). Resilience in Black lesbian, gay, bisexual, and transgender individuals: A critical review of the literature. *Journal of Gay & Lesbian Mental Health, 18*(2), 190–212.

Glynn, T. R., Gamarel, K. E., Kahler, C. W., Iwamoto, M., Operario, D., & Nemoto, T. (2016). The role of gender affirmation in psychological well-being among transgender women. *Psychology of Sexual Orientation and Gender Diversity, 3*(3), 336–344.

Greene, B. (1994). Ethnic-minority lesbians and gay men: Mental health and treatment issues. *Journal of Consulting and Clinical Psychology, 62*(2), 243–251.

Greene, B. (2000). African American lesbian and bisexual women. *Journal of Social Issues, 56*(2), 239–249.

Greene, B., & Boyd-Franklin, N. (1996). African American lesbian couples: Ethnocultural considerations in psychotherapy. *Women & Therapy, 19*(3), 49–60.

Griffith, E. E. H., Jones, B. E., & Stewart, A. J. (Eds.). (2018). *Black mental health: Patients, providers, and systems*. Washington, DC: American Psychiatric Association Publishing.

Hughes, T., Smith, C., & Dan, A. (2013). Sexual minorities seeking services: A retrospective study of the mental health concerns of lesbian and bisexual women. In *Mental Health Issues for Sexual Minority Women: Redefining Women's Mental Health* (pp. 147–166). New York, NY: Routledge.

Jensen, K. L. (1999). *Lesbian epiphanies: Women coming out in later life*. New York, NY: Harrington Park Press.

Johnson, E. P. (2018). *Black. Queer. Southern. Women.: An Oral History*. Charlotte, NC: UNC Press Books.

Johnson, S. D. (2012). Gay affirmative psychotherapy with lesbian, gay, and bisexual individuals: Implications for contemporary psychotherapy research. *American Journal of Orthopsychiatry, 82*(4), 516–522.

Kerr, D. L., & Oglesby, W. H. (2017). LGBT populations and substance abuse research: An overview. In *Research Methods in the Study of Substance Abuse* (pp. 341–355). New York, NY: Springer.

Kort, J. (2018). *LGBTQ clients in therapy: Clinical issues and treatment strategies*. New York: New York, NY: W.W. Norton.

Larkin, J. (Ed.) (1999). *A woman like that: Lesbian and bisexual writers tell their coming out stories*. New York, NY: Avon Books.

Levine, A., & Heller, R. (2012). *Attached: The new science of adult attachment and how it can help you find—and keep—love*. New York, NY: Penguin.

Lyons, H. Z., Bieschke, K. J., Dendy, A. K., Worthington, R. L., & Georgemiller, R. (2010). Psychologists' competence to treat lesbian, gay and bisexual clients: State of the field and strategies for improvement. *Professional Psychology: Research and Practice, 41*(5), 424–434.

Moore, M. (2011). *Invisible families: Gay identities, relationships, and motherhood among Black women*. Berkeley, CA: University of California Press.

National Coalition of Anti-Violence Programs (NCAVP). (2016). *Lesbian, gay, bisexual, transgender, queer, and HIV-affected hate violence in 2016*. New York, NY: Emily Waters.

National LGBT Health Education Center. (2016). *Affirmative care for transgender and gender non-conforming people: Best practices for front-line health care staff*. https://www.lgbthealtheducation.org/wp-content/uploads/2016/12/Affirmative-Care-for-Transgender-and-Gender-Non-conforming-People-Best-Practices-for-Front-line-Health-Care-Staff.pdf

Omoto, A. M., & Kurtzman, H. S. (2006). *Sexual orientation and mental health: Examining identity and development in lesbian, gay, and bisexual people*. Washington, DC: American Psychological Association.

Parks, C. A., Hughes, T. L., & Matthews, A. K. (2004). Race/ethnicity and sexual orientation: Intersecting identities. *Cultural Diversity and Ethnic Minority Psychology, 10*(3), 241–254.

Patton, L. D., & Simmons, S. L. (2008). Exploring complexities of multiple identities of lesbians in a Black college environment. *Negro Educational Review,*
59(3–4), 197–215.

Pope, M., & Dworkin, S. H. (2014). *Casebook for counseling lesbian, gay, bisexual, and*
transgender persons and their families. Alexandria, VA: Wiley.

Riggle, E. D., Whitman, J. S., Olson, A., Rostosky, S. S., & Strong, S. (2008). The positive aspects of being a lesbian or gay man. *Professional Psychology: Research*
and Practice, 39(2), 210–217.

Ring, T. (2020). These are the trans people killed in 2019. https://www.advocate
.com/transgender/2019/5/22/these-are-trans-people-killed-2019#media
-gallery-media-9

Ritter, K., & Terndrup, A. I. (2002). *Handbook of affirmative psychotherapy with lesbi-*
ans and gay men. New York, NY: Guilford Press.

Sarno, E. L., Mohr, J. J., Jackson, S. D., & Fassinger, R. E. (2015). When identities
collide: Conflicts in allegiances among LGB people of color. *Cultural Diver-*
sity and Ethnic Minority Psychology, 21(4), 550–559.

Shelton, K., & Delgado-Romero, E. A. (2013). Sexual orientation microaggressions:
The experience of lesbian, gay, bisexual, and queer clients in psychotherapy. *Psychology of Sexual Orientation and Gender Diversity, 1*(S), 59–70.

Singh, A. A. (2013). Transgender youth of color and resilience: Negotiating oppression and finding support. *Sex Roles, 68*(11–12), 690–702.

Singh, A. A., Hays, D. G., & Watson, L. S. (2011). Strength in the face of adversity:
Resilience strategies of transgender individuals. *Journal of Counseling and*
Development, 89(1), 20–27.

Sue, D. W. (Ed.). (2010). *Microaggressions and marginality: Manifestation, dynamics,*
and impact. Hoboken, NJ: John Wiley & Sons.

Szymanski, D. M., & Gupta, A. (2009). Examining the relationship between multiple internalized oppressions and African American lesbian, gay, bisexual,
and questioning persons' self-esteem and psychological distress. *Journal of*
Counseling Psychology, 56(1), 110–118.

Tozer, E. E., & McClanahan, M. K. (1999). Treating the purple menace: Ethical considerations of conversion therapy and affirmative alternatives. *Counseling*
Psychologist, 27(5), 722–742.

Walker, J. N. J., & Longmire-Avital, B. (2013). The impact of religious faith and
internalized homonegativity on resiliency for Black lesbian, gay, and bisexual emerging adults. *Developmental Psychology, 49*(9), 1723–1731.

World Professional Association for Transgender Health. (2012). *Standards of*
Care for the Health of Transsexual, Transgender, and Gender Nonconforming
People [7th Version]. https://www.wpath.org/publications/soc

APPENDIX A. EXAMPLE OF LETTER OF SUPPORT
FOR GENITAL RECONSTRUCTION SURGERY

On Letterhead

Date

Re: Patient [Use the name Client identifies by. Discuss Client's feeling regarding a need to include deadname.]

DOB:

To whom it may concern,

I am writing this letter in support of [Client's first and last name] decision to obtain gender confirmation surgery.

Client has been in my clinical care since [start of treatment] specifically to discuss their desire to obtain surgery. Client's experience of themselves fits a diagnosis of gender dysphoria, they identify as genderqueer, and go by they/them pronouns. [Provide any detailed history of social and medical transition.] Client has expressed a persistent desire for genital reconstruction surgery. Their goals of surgery are to align their primary sex characteristics with their identity.

Client reports significant anxiety and distress due to their experience of dysphoria. By my independent evaluation of Client, I diagnosed them with gender dysphoria (ICD-10 F64.1). My impression is that Client is a well-grounded person who is of sound mind and able to make decisions fully regarding their medical care. I have no concerns that Client is currently suicidal, homicidal, or would harm himself or anyone else in any way and they have no history of such feelings. They have no issues with illicit drug use or abuse. They are stably housed and have prepared for their post-op recovery.

In my professional experience working with other transgender individuals with gender dysphoria, Client meets the WPATH criteria for genital reconstruction surgery. They are knowledgeable of the risks, benefits, and alternatives of this surgery and understands them. It is Client's expectation as well as my own that they be able to undergo surgery to fully transition as they see fit.

If you have any questions or concerns, please do not hesitate to contact me.

Sincerely,

Provider's name, license number, and contact information

CHAPTER 13

African American Women with Disabilities

Anthea A. Gray
Ngozi Ndukwe
Angela M. Kuemmel

INTRODUCTION

According to the Americans with Disabilities Act (ADA) of 1990, a person with a disability is defined as someone with a physical or mental impairment that substantially limits one or more of the major life activities of the individual. Of the six categories of disability (viz., mobility, cognition, independent living, vision, hearing, and self-care), the prevalence rates for women exceed that of males, outside of hearing and self-care disabilities (Okoro et al., 2018). According to the U.S. Census Bureau (2016), 21 million American women and girls reported having a disability, which constitutes 12.9 percent of all noninstitutionalized women. Rates of disability among African Americans (AA) range around 18.1 percent (Courtney-Long et al., 2017; Okoro et al., 2018). But what is unique about the experience of being an African American woman with a disability (AA WWD)? In this chapter, we explore factors that are remarkable to the experiences of AA WWD disabilities including biases and stereotypes, implications of multiple-minority statuses, and aspects of both AA (e.g., family, religion, and hair) and disability (e.g., Americans with Disabilities Act) culture gleaned through our clinical work as rehabilitation psychologists.

The Identity of an African American Woman
with a Disability

Identity is defined as (a) a social category that awards membership to an individual based on an implicit or explicit set of rules, as well as common shared characteristics (Fearon, 1999), such as gender, race, ethnicity, sexual orientation, and disability status (Ratts et al., 2016); and (b) a conception of self that is structured upon personal values, beliefs, and goals (Erikson, 1968). Though very few studies discuss disability, race, ethnicity, and gender through the lens of an AA WWD, available literature has suggested that the multidirectional oppressions experienced by individuals with multiple identities could contribute to a fragmented view of self, depending on the context of one's interactions and perspective of their multiple identities (Petersen, 2006). It has also been found that racial and ethnic minorities with disabilities may experience discrimination, as well as isolation from their respective racial and ethnic groups (McDonald, Keys, & Balcazar, 2007), which can further impact how the individual perceives themselves. For racial and ethnic minorities with disabilities they can also experience discrimination based on one, some, or all of their minority statuses (McDonald et al., 2007). It is believed by Stuart (1992) and Vernon (1999) that a person's dual identification as a person of color and a person with a disability impedes total membership to and by either identity group. This is likely because each group has stereotypes of the other. As a result, getting adequate social support (McDonald et al., 2007) and confronting oppression may be more challenging for these individuals (Block, Balcazar, & Keys, 2001). The impact of an additional identity (sex) infers significant difficulties for AA WWD. Of note, McDonald and colleagues (2007) note that individuals with invisible disabilities may not experience social rejection or exclusion, due to their ability to "choose" disclosure.

Two frequently referenced racial and ethnic identity models are the Black Racial (Nigrescence) Identity model (Cross, 1971, 1978, & 1991) and the Minority Identity Development model (Atkinson, Morten, & Sue, 1993). The Black Racial Identity model is comprised of five stages: preencounter, encounter, immersion-emersion, internalization, and internalization-commitment. Atkinson and colleagues' (1993) Minority Identity Development Model was later elaborated on by Sue and Sue (2012) and referred to as the Racial/Cultural Identity Development model (R/CID). The R/CID model is comprised of five stages: conformity, dissonance, resistance, introspection, and awareness. Despite the models referenced, it is clear that there are transitional phases experienced as a person gains insight into their own racial identity. Each model demonstrates a progression in racial identity development.

With respect to disability identity development, theories are often structured through an Erikson-esque (1968) informed stage model. Marcia's Identity Status model (1966, 1980) posits (a) an absence of Erikson's (1968) fifth stage—identity versus role confusion; (b) the potential for a nonlinear progression, particularly if the adolescent experiences a traumatic or life-altering event that causes them to reevaluate their identity; (c) the potential for partial completion of the stages; and (d) the possibility for varying identity statuses that are situation specific (i.e., someone could be at one stage in one environment and at another stage in another environment). Gill's model of disability identity identifies four distinct phases: "(1) 'coming to feel we belong' (integrating into society); (2) 'coming home' (integrating with the disability community); (3) 'coming together' (internally integrating our sameness and differentness); and (4) 'coming out' (integrating how we feel with how we present ourselves" (Gill, 1997, 39). Gibson's disability identity model is spaced across a lifetime, recognizes the potential for non-progression after Stage 1, and features three stages: passive awareness, realization, and acceptance (2006). Key features of Stage 1 include no role model with a disability, denial of social aspects of disability, avoidance of attention and connection with disability community. Key features of Stage 2 include a gradual awareness of one's disability, anger toward the fact that one has a disability, self-hatred, concern about appearance, and a "Superwoman/man" complex. Key features of Stage 3 include self-acceptance, having personal value, connects with others in disability community, becomes an advocate for disability rights, and integrates into the dominant majority (i.e., non-disabled) culture.

Additional factors pertaining to disability identity development include the nature of acquisition (i.e., congenital or acquired). In comparison to someone with a congenital disability, a woman that has acquired a disability is confronted with a foreign identity (viz. disability) and challenged to integrate it into her self-perception (Banks, 2018). It is also important to recognize that disability identity development can coincide with racial identity development; these processes can occur in tandem without detriment or interrupt either identity development (Mpofu & Harley, 2006). Further related, individuals with visible disabilities may be more apt to identify as a person with a disability (Bogart et al., 2017). Also, the impact of stigma—perceived or experienced—can either discourage disability identification or drive a collective sense of disability pride that fosters disability identification (Bogart et al., 2017; Bogart et al., 2018; Darling & Heckert, 2010; Nario-Redmond & Oleson, 2016).

It is essential that mental health providers understand the various theories, stages of development, and complexities of their client's identity to establish rapport and credibility with their AA WWD clients, conceptualize treatment, and offer culturally competent and beneficial care.

Intersectionality—What It Is and Psychotherapy's Role

Upon its theoretical conception, intersectionality challenged traditional feminist theory and anti-racist politics by demonstrating the diversity within cultural groups—more specifically, race and sex (Crenshaw, 1989)—and the importance of structural-level changes to promote equal rights. Several authors contend that psychotherapy with AA WWD can also take on a form of social activism—a belief also supported by some psychoanalysts and psychiatrists (Eder, 2015; Jacoby, 1983). At face value, psychotherapy is an operational tool that facilitates mental well-being, yet is a place where AA WWD can work through the *personal* effects of oppression, politics, and social issues and experience social change collectively. Psychotherapy offers AA WWD clients a forum to (a) communicate their unique experiences of oppression, (b) receive education on the psychological impact of oppression on their self-concept and everyday functioning, (c) learn how to or develop comfort in labeling their experiences in a healthy manner, and (d) get validation and empowerment from their mental health provider. Though many mental health providers do not see themselves as social activists, there is certainly cause to understand the ways in which an AA WWD experiences oppression to work more effectively with this group. Furthermore, the consequences of unaddressed and mismanaged oppression for an individual is internalization, which may manifest in poor mental (Banks, Kohn-Wood, & Spencer, 2006; Williams & Mohammed, 2009) and physical health (Diaz, Ayala, & Bein, 2004).

The Unique Experiences of Women with Disabilities

Work

In comparison to men, many women are confronted with challenges in the workplace, which include but are not limited to gaps in pay (Graf, Brown, & Patten, 2018), pregnancy discrimination (Eaton, 2019), and biases surrounding capacity for leadership (Heilman & Eagly, 2008). Though gender equality in the workplace has yet to be achieved, the current cultural climate of exposure (i.e., #METOO & #TIMESUP) and growing intolerance has called the behaviors (e.g., sexual harassment and unequal pay) of yesteryear to task. The double biases of race and gender experienced by AA women may pose risk for social exclusion (e.g., from discussions and work events–related gatherings), lack of or minimal opportunities for mentorship, disproportionately high demands and expectations, and assumptions of incompetence and lower intelligence (Hall, Everett, & Hamilton-Mason, 2012; Kwate, 2001). AA women might also feel as though they need to code-switch, work longer hours, take on additional assignments, and take less absences from work to "prove" themselves and challenge race and gender biases (Hall, Everett, & Hamilton-Mason, 2012; Scott, 2013). Richie (1992) suggests that perceptions of organizational and interpersonal discrimination might also affect AA women before they even apply for employment and as a result, limit their career aspirations and options.

Women with disabilities might also face double discrimination based on their gender and disability. Common biases include beliefs that women with disabilities aren't able to attain and maintain gainful employment, are best suited for low-level jobs, and can't compete with non-disabled individuals (Alston & McCowan, 1994). As a result, women with disabilities might also feel as though they need to work double time to counterbalance preconceived notions about their abilities. Carrying the weight of three minority statuses (gender, race, and disability) could be a heavy load to bear in the workplace and result in added stress and job-related pressure. Further, if an AA WWD also identifies with another identity group (e.g., LGBTQ+, veteran, non-dominant religious group), the individual might experience additional feelings of exclusion or feel as though they need to conceal this part of themselves.

Treatment considerations and recommendations:

- Workplace discrimination can present overtly or covertly (i.e., micro-aggression), leaving the AA WWD employee confused about their experience and or resulting in an internalization of their experiences. It is often useful to validate their discrimination, offer education on the matter, and facilitate problem-solving.
- As demonstrated in some of the aforementioned identity development models, connection with people of a similar background is often an integral component of an individual's sense of self. If an AA WWD finds herself to be a minority in her workplace, mentorship can be extremely beneficial. Discuss ways in which your client can find a mentor.
- Working with AA WWD involves good working knowledge of disability rights and policies. According to Cornish et al. (2008), ethical practitioners need to know about the Americans with Disabilities Act. The ADA was enacted in 1990 and is the most significant disability legislation in the world. Covering five domains, the ADA brought equal opportunity to qualified individuals whose disabilities interfere with designated major life activities in the areas of employment, public services, public accommodations, telecommunications, and miscellaneous. The ADA impacts psychologists in various ways from training and education of students with disabilities to hiring practices. When clinicians provide education on disability rights, it can be empowering; especially to individuals facing oppression. Research on women with disabilities indicates that when WWD learned about disability rights in a support group specifically for WWD, they felt like they had a place in the world where they frequently receive messages that they don't belong (Mejias, Gill, &

Shpigelman, 2014). In one of our social support groups, disability rights is a popular topic because of all the environmental barriers WWD face in the community; triggering stigma and oppression. The group members share educational resources, knowledge, and advocacy strategies that help them feel more empowered to handle these challenges.

Sexuality and Relationships

Conceptions of women's sexuality and femininity have evolved over time and are significantly influenced by popular culture and media. Cultural narratives of women are often based on a perception of women being weak and dependent (McDonald et al., 2007). Stereotypes pertaining to AA women have historically been portrayed in one of four ways: (1) Jezebel—sexually promiscuous, (2) Mammy —overweight, unattractive, and motherly, (3) Sapphire—dominant and angry, and (4) welfare queens—low income and has children to reap the benefits of the public welfare system (West, 2008; Woodard & Mastin, 2005). For people with disabilities, there is a perception of the person being asexual, heroic, weak, and passive based on stereotypes (Kuemmel, Campbell, & Gray, 2019). Specific to women with disabilities, they are often perceived to be vulnerable, more dependent, socially excluded, poor, less feminine, nurturing, and unfit parents (Nario-Redmond, 2010). Efforts have been made to challenge society's conceptions of sexuality through more inclusive representation by media and fashion, though it remains an exception and is far from the norm. As media and fashion inform social perception, its relative exclusion of women with disabilities runs parallel to society's conceptions about the sexuality of women with disabilities. In a society that values and emphasizes physical attractiveness and appearance in evaluating the worth of women (Roberts & Zurbriggen, 2013), the implications of exclusion for WWD and AA WWD have a profound impact on cultural standards of beauty.

For women that have greater functional limitations, sexual activity might present frustrating challenges (e.g., decreased lubrication, spasticity, difficulty with positioning, bowel and bladder issues). However, there is also opportunity for pleasure with adaptations and perhaps even a reconceptualization of and education on intimacy. DeLoach and Greer (1981) note that oral sex, masturbation, and sexual aids (e.g., anal beads, vibrators) might facilitate engagement for all parties. However, some studies suggest that AA women are less likely to engage in masturbation in comparison to other cultural groups (Laumann & Mahay, 2012; Shulman & Horne, 2003), which is attributed by Das (2007) to conflicts with moral standards. Whether for reasons related to personal preference or religious beliefs, this could leave an AA woman with a high degree of functional limitations with less options for sexual intimacy and satisfaction.

In relation to finding a partner, Rintala et al. (1997) found that women with disabilities cited less satisfaction with dating and identified more barriers to dating than non-disabled women. More specifically, the study found that those with hearing and speech impairments, certain types of disabilities (e.g., stroke, cerebral palsy, and TBI), greater functional limitations, and having a disability before their first date were related to poorer experiences with dating (Rintala et al., 1997). There is also literature to suggest that women with disabilities are less likely to marry and if they do marry, do so later in life and have a greater rate of divorce (Fine & Asch, 1988). This is likely due to stigma and stereotypes including asexuality and devaluation. Also, many typical roles of women such as caregiver, homemaker, and hostess of events have a physical component that disability may impede. If WWD are unable to fulfill these traditional roles, they may experience a loss of feminine identity, disability stigma, and a sense of rolelessness, which is the experience of a lack of definitive social roles (Fine & Asch, 1981; Merton, 1967).

Asch and Fine (1988) also found that heterosexual marriages were more likely to result in divorce if the woman acquired her disability after the wedding. By comparison, men with disability were less affected by this variable (Fine & Asch, 1988). In some ways similar to WWD compared to other women, AA women marry later than White women (median = 30 versus White women, 26 years old) (Elliot et al., 2012), have higher rates of divorce in comparison to White women, and lower marriage rates compared to all other racial groups (Raley, Sweeney, & Wondra, 2015). In a review of historical trends, Raley and colleagues (2015) found that AA marriages began to decrease around the 1960s; potential reasons might include a decrease in unemployment for AA men in the 1970s and '80s (Bound & Holzer, 1993; Wilson & Neckerman, 1986) and higher death and incarceration rates for AA men (Raley et al., 2015).

Though AA women are least likely to date outside of their race (Passel, Wang, & Taylor, 2010), casting a wider net by dating outside one's racial group might increase one's chances of finding a partner. However, in a study looking at heterosexual, interracial dating preferences, AA women were the least likely to be chosen by men of all racial groups (Bany, Robnett, & Feliciano, 2014). Findings suggest this is due to an overall preference for lighter complexions, straighter hair (versus curly), and thin body types; exclusionary factors also related to stereotypical conceptions of the AA woman (e.g., talk louder, more argumentative, and aggressive in comparison to other women) (Thomas et al., 2019; Weitz & Gordon, 1993). These factors create a challenging scenario for an AA woman with a disability and might create feelings of anxiety, low self-worth, and intimidation.

A look at abusive relationships reveals that women with disabilities experience abuse at the same rate as women without disabilities, but the abuse tends to last for longer periods of time (Nosek et al., 2001). In comparison by sex, men and women with disabilities experience similar rates of physical abuse, but men experience sexual abuse at half the rate (Powers et al., 2004). Disability-related risk factors for abuse include need for personal care assistance, increased exposure to institutions and medical facilities, environmental barriers, social isolation, financial stress, limited economic opportunities, increased disability-related stress to families, devaluation by society, and childhood exposure to abuse (Andrews & Verona, 1993; Hassouneh-Phillips, 2005; Nosek et al., 2001).

Treatment considerations and recommendations:

- As the understanding of mental health's responsibilities in addressing sexuality with patients improves, it is up to the mental health professional to educate themselves on sexuality with a disability, which includes adaptive techniques and devices, consumer and professional education resources, particular issues that AA WWD might experience, and ethical issues (Hess & Hough, 2012). Additionally, sex is still conceived by society at large as taboo (Gill & Hough, 2007). Learning to address personal apprehension and discomfort surrounding topics pertaining to sexuality will be of utmost importance before speaking with your clients.
- Resources for providers:
  - « *Sexuality and Disability: A Guide for Everyday Practice* (Cooper & Guillebaud, 1999)
  - « *Sexuality: Your Sons and Daughters with Intellectual Disabilities* (Hingsburger & Melberg-Schwier, 2000)
- Resources for clients and providers:
  - « The Center for Sexual Pleasure and Health (https://thecsph.org)
  - « RespectAbility (https://www.respectability.org/resources/sexual-education-resources/)
  - « *Regain That Feeling: Secrets to Sexual Self-Discovery* (Tepper, 2015)
  - « Brainline (https://www.brainline.org)
  - « *The Sessions* (Lewin, 2012)
- Use the PLSSIT model (i.e., ask permission, provide limited information, make specific suggestions, and refer to intensive therapy) (Annon, 1976) to initiate discussions surrounding sexuality.
- If your client is interested in dating, offer a space to discuss concerns (e.g., how to manage inappropriate questions surrounding disability on a date, whether or not to disclose disability when online dating).
- For married clients/those in a relationship, invite partners into session when appropriate to support the couple's adjustment to disability. For intensive therapy, refer them to a rehabilitation couples' therapist.
- WWD face multiple risks and barriers to reporting abuse, and thus, it is very important for care providers to routinely provide adequate screening. Examples of how and what to ask can

be found in materials such as *Personal Assistance, Disability, and Intimate Partner Violence: A Guide for Healthcare Providers* (Salwen, Gray, & Mona, 2016).

Motherhood

Though regarded as outside the realm of possibility by some, motherhood is well within reach for many women with disabilities. Stereotypes and discriminatory practices surrounding mothers with disabilities relate not only to their ability to physically conceive a child, but also to their ability to care for a child (Smeltzer, 2007). These stereotypes affect relationships, sexuality, health care, safety, and social roles. Unfortunately, WWD rarely receive information to counter these stereotypes and consequently internalize them (Nario-Redmond, 2010; Nosek et al., 2001). This phenomenon was illustrated during an ongoing, bimonthly support group for WWD (Women's Alliance for Veteran Empowerment; WAVE) (Kuemmel, Campbell, & Gray, 2019) when a young female with multiple sclerosis felt that motherhood was not possible for her, because none of her medical providers had initiated a discussion on this topic with her. The group discussed society's narrow implications of motherhood excluding mothers with disabilities. The group also shared the various ways in which they continue to maintain their roles as mothers, including receiving help from family members with the physical tasks of caregiving.

An AA family whose matriarch has a disability might also wear the archetypal badge of the Strong Black Woman, imposing the expectation she can just "jump right back in where she left off" before her injury or illness and/or "beat" her disability (Alston & McCowan, 1994). Similarly, she might also find herself subject to the "supercrip stereotype," who is portrayed as someone that "fought" their disability and "won" (Martin, 2017). The theatrics surrounding this stereotype and desire to be a nondisabled person is particularly insulting to individuals that promote an acceptance model of disability (Harnett, 2000). Though a strong will and determination can be strong values among AA WWD, approaching disability and challenges with an attitude of invincibility is dehumanizing. Additionally, it is neither realistic nor helpful and in fact might contribute to feelings of ineptitude (Alston & McCowan, 1994).

Treatment considerations and recommendations:

- Finding local mentorship or online (e.g., social media apps, blogs, podcasts) is an excellent way to find hope, validation, encouragement, and education for clients that want to become pregnant or those that are already mothers.
- Create a packet of informational resources that you might share with clients that are interested in conceiving. Empower them to ask questions on their next trip to the doctor.

- Invite family members into therapy sessions to offer education on disability and support the family's overall adjustment to disability. Refer to a family therapist that specializes in rehabilitation needs.

Body Image

In our society, physical attractiveness and appearance are not only cultural measures of beauty, but also evaluative instruments for a woman's worth (Roberts & Zurbriggen, 2013). The impact of these social standards is far-reaching. Women with disabilities experience rates of body dissatisfaction at higher rates than non-disabled women (Moin, Duvdevany, & Mazor, 2009), due to social comparison, though acceptance may develop over time (Moin et al., 2009). Literature over time has fairly consistently presented AA women's body image as somewhat paradoxical: in comparison to white women, AA women tend to be body positive regardless of weight (Miller et al., 2000; Nishina et al., 2006), yet simultaneously report feelings of self-consciousness and engagement in weight loss efforts (Befort et al., 2008; Reel et al., 2008).

For many AA women, hair is a representation and internalization of identity (Garrin & Marcketti, 2018; Thomas, Hacker, & Hoxha, 2011; Turner, 2015) whose significance is tied closely to its historical underpinnings. Dating back to slavery, women with hair more similar to Europeans (longer, straighter) reaped favor and benefits (Patton, 2006), while those with more traditional African hair (coarse, short) were subject to more physically demanding work and often covered their hair. The end of slavery led to efforts to distance themselves from slave culture by wearing a wider range of styles including straight hair (Byrd & Tharps, 2014). In the 1960s, the civil rights movement embraced being "Black and Proud," and women wore styles that showcased their natural texture. The choice in textured hairstyles was an expression of empowerment, although the trend shifted in the 1980s and 1990s (Dawson, Karl, & Peluchette, 2019) and resurfaced in the mid-2000s. AA women's utilization of natural styles is growing in prevalence, but they still may be perceived as unkempt and unprofessional in some settings (Dawson et al., 2019).

Though the concept of "good" and "bad" hair is not particularly relevant to this chapter, the notion of having a well-put-together style for its cultural importance and relevance is. For example, AA women that have had a brain injury might have scars that make it difficult to style in a natural style after rehab and injury. For those with limited upper-extremity functioning, doing up-dos and styles may prove challenging, as well. How this affects a woman in terms of her acceptance with other AA individuals is also important, as it is both a spoken and unspoken expression of communication. For those individuals with limited communication skills, it might even be a way to express themselves in a manner that their injury or disability has prohibited them from doing.

Treatment considerations and recommendations:

- Though social media can foster negative body image and negative social comparison, it might also facilitate positive associations with disability, create "roles," and normalize experiences with disability. Come up with a list of positive social media influencers that you might recommend to your clients that might benefit.
- The cultural importance of hair does not disappear in rehabilitation or skilled nursing facilities. For clients disinterested in natural styles, engage in open dialogue about how they might like to wear their hair (e.g., flat ironed, weave, wig), and research ways to execute the client's styling preferences.
- For those clients that are interested in natural hairstyles, encourage learning via YouTube and other social media (e.g., Instagram) tutorials. This is also a useful learning tool for those assisting individuals with disabilities.
- Some AA women avoid exercise to preserve the style of their hair. Natural hairstyles offer a good remedy for that concern and present an opportunity to decrease risk factors associated with AA WWD (e.g., obesity, cardiovascular issues).
- Depending on level of functioning and gym regulations, access to a public gym might be limited for WWD. Encourage clients to speak with a physical therapist and their physician about a home-health fitness plan that will support their fitness goals safely.
- Further related to lifestyle factors and potentially decreasing health risk factors, help your client come up with a recipe book of healthy meals after working with a dietitian that might help them meet their fitness goals

Religion and Spirituality

Religion and spirituality can be valuable coping tools for individuals with disability (Koenig, McCullough, & Larson, 2001; Wilson et al., 2017). Among individuals with chronic health conditions and disability, studies have found improved treatment and medical outcomes (e.g., greater cardiovascular health, more treatment engagement and follow-through with medical recommendations, and quicker alleviation of depressive symptoms) (Koenig, 2007: Mueller, Plevak, & Rummans, 2001). Studies have found that the benefits of religion and spirituality are equally beneficial to AA women (Mattis, 2000, 2002; van Olphen et al., 2003). Active devotion, which includes acts like prayer, reading the Bible, and physically going to church (Koenig, 2007), is particularly useful to AA people as they are a way to manage daily stressors, oppression, and adversity (Mattis, 2002; Neighbors, Musick, & Williams, 1998). Religion and spirituality are more than a coping skill for AA people, they are a way of life and deeply imbedded in AA culture and identity—both historically and contemporarily. As touched upon previously, daily practice can certainly be done at home, but for many within the AA community, going to service is a chance not only to worship and offer praise, but also to connect with one's social support network, which for many is considered to be part of their extended family (Krause & Bastida, 2011; Taylor et al., 2004). Though an important part of worship to many, some AA women with disabilities might find barriers to attendance such as a lack of accessible parking, trouble finding accessible and stylish church apparel, fast and loud speech/singing that individuals with low processing speed or sensitivities to loud noises might find difficult to tolerate, and sitting for long periods of time and potentially in uncomfortable pews.

Treatment considerations and recommendations:

- Encourage your client to speak with church administrators about accommodations.
- Given the significance of church attendance for many AA women with disabilities, treatment team members, particularly occupational therapists and physical therapists, might consider visiting their client's church to assess and offer solutions for accessibility—with the client's permission.

If your client is financially able, encourage them to look for accessible clothing that will improve comfort, decrease risk for adverse health issues from ill-fitting clothing (e.g., pressure ulcer from harsh fabric that might rub on the skin), and allow for easy removal of clothing in case one needs to use the restroom. If finances are limited, suggest that the individual alter or enlist a community/family member to tailor their preexisting clothing. Offer your clients guidelines for accessible fashions (e.g., seamless pants for wheelchair users, easy closures), as well.

CONCLUSION

African American women have long been regarded as "invisible" both socially (Sesko & Biernat, 2009) and politically (Fryberg & Townsend, 2008; hooks, 1981). Though they have a different history and set of challenges, women with disabilities experience many of the same consequences of invisibility. The profound impact of intersectionality of these two identities creates unique challenges for African American women with disabilities. A cloak of prevailing stereotypes and oppression keeps African American women with disabilities invisible. It is the hope of these authors that this chapter will increase awareness, offer support and resources, and make the experiences of African American women with disabilities more visible.

CASE STUDY

Brittany is a 40-year-old Black woman with a recent C5 AIS B spinal cord injury from a motor vehicle accident. She is a single mother of two young children. Brittany is also a cisgender, bisexual woman. Prior to her injury she worked as a nursing instructor. She now needs help with most of her activities of daily living and utilizes a power wheelchair to ambulate. Her mother has moved in with her and her kids to help take care of them. Prior to her spinal cord injury, she was always very well put together, wearing stylish clothes, trendy hairstyles, and makeup; but now it takes her so long to get ready, and her mom tells her she is not "[client's] personal hair stylist or make-up artist." She is referred for psychotherapy to address adjustment to disability.

Prior to her arrival, you arrange your office in a way that will allow Brittany to enter and sit comfortably in the room. When she arrives, you let her know where the accessible restrooms are located. Because this client identifies as a person *with* a disability, careful consideration will be made to use person first language when speaking to her and when documenting notes. You also notice that she describes herself as "Black," so you use that language—instead of African American, as well.

In her initial session, you introduce yourself and share a little about your competence to work with people with disabilities. She shares that she feels like a burden on her family and that she has lost her role as a mother to her children because her mother is taking care of them. She shares that she always identified as a Strong Black Woman who could overcome any adversity without depending on anyone and is experiencing a sense of feeling like a failure. She hates wearing sweatpants, which are easy to get on, and doesn't feel like herself without her hair and makeup. She is on a leave of absence from work, and returning to work as a nurse would put her at risk of losing her disability social security benefits. In addition, she hates going out in the community because "I don't want people to see me like this." Brittany said that she "barely thought about dating or sex." You reinforce that that discussion could be had when she is ready and suggest she watch the documentary *Take a Look at This Heart* if she becomes curious about the subject.

The 12 follow-up sessions focus on increasing her receptiveness to accepting help and viewing the people she depends on for personal care assistance as tools to maximize her independence through cognitive interventions focused on reframing her thoughts and perceptions. Another focus of cognitive intervention is the mind reading she does of people she interacts with in the community, as she assumes they think negatively of her when they see her in a wheelchair. You talk about behavioral interventions and problem-solving strategies that she can use to increase her involvement in her children's care by participating in their bedtime routines, reading bedtime stories, and finding more inclusive ways to play with them such as table activities; which help her feel more like a mother. Her perception of overcoming her injury is shifted from cure focused to living a full life with her disability. Her mother joins her for a session to talk about the importance of fashion, hair, and makeup to her identity of feeling like a woman. Resources for adaptive fashion and adaptive ways to apply makeup were found online and shared. Finally, the benefits and disadvantages of returning to work with disability accommodations are explored. One long-term goal is readiness to explore dating and sexuality. As she starts to redefine her identity to integrate her disability and feels she has regained confidence through dressing fashionably, doing her hair and makeup, and going out socially in the community, she expresses interest in learning how she can positively present herself to prospective partners she may meet online. Another long-term goal is to find meaning in her life post-acquired disability. She initially finds meaning in her children and being a mother, but eventually further explores vocational and volunteer activities.

Brittany's case illustrates many common experiences after acquired disability that negatively impact adjustment to disability, such as difficulty accepting help, social disability issues that impact community reintegration, identity loss, and dating and sexuality. She benefits from cognitive behavioral interventions that help facilitate the adjustment and reidentification process.

REFERENCES

Alston, R. J., & McCowan, C. J. (1994). African American women with disabilities: Rehabilitation issues and concerns. *Journal of Rehabilitation, 60*(1), 36–40.

Americans with Disabilities Act. (1990). http://www.ada.gov

Andrews, A. B., & Verona, L. J. (1993). Sexual assault and people with disabilities. *Journal of Social Work and Human Sexuality, 8*(2), 137–159.

Annon, J. S. (1976). The PLISSIT model: A proposed conceptual scheme for the behavioral treatment of sexual problems. *Journal of Sex Education and Therapy, 2*(1), 1–15.

Atkinson, D. R., Morten, G., & Sue, D. W. (1993). Counseling American minorities: A cross-cultural perspective. Dubuque, IA: Brown/Benchmark.

Banks, K. H., Kohn-Wood, L. P., & Spencer, M. (2006). An examination of the African American experience of everyday discrimination and symptoms of psychological distress. *Community Mental Health Journal, 42*(6), 555–570.

Banks, M. E. (2018). Women and disability: The role of feminist psychology. In C. B. Travis, J. W. White, A. E. Rutherford, W. S., Williams, S. L. Cook, & K. F. E. Wyche. *APA handbook of the psychology of women: Perspectives on women's private and public lives, Vol. 2* (pp. 313–330). Washington, DC: American Psychological Association.

Bany, J. A., Robnett, B., & Feliciano, C. (2014). Gendered Black exclusion: The persistence of racial stereotypes among daters. *Race and Social Problems*, *6*(3), 201–213.

Befort, C. A., Thomas, J. L., Daley, C. M., Rhode, P. C., & Ahluwalia, J. S. (2008). Perceptions and beliefs about body size, weight, and weight loss among obese African American women: A qualitative inquiry. *Health Education & Behavior*, *35*(3), 410–426.

Block, P., Balcazar, F., & Keys, C. (2001). From pathology to power: Rethinking race, poverty, and disability. *Journal of Disability Policy Studies*, *12*(1), 18–39.

Bogart, K. R., Lund, E. M., & Rottenstein, A. (2018). Disability pride protects self-esteem through the rejection-identification model. *Rehabilitation Psychology*, *63*, 155–159. http://dx.doi.org/10.1037/rep0000166

Bogart, K. R., Rottenstein, A., Lund, E. M., & Bouchard, L. (2017). Who self-identifies as disabled? An examination of impairment and contextual predictors. *Rehabilitation Psychology*, *62*, 553–562. http://dx.doi.org/10.1037/rep0000132

Bound, J., & Holzer, H. J. (1991). *Industrial shifts, skills levels, and the labor market for White and Black males* (No. w3715). Cambridge, MA: National Bureau of Economic Research.

Byrd, A., & Tharps, L. (2014). *Hair story: Untangling the roots of Black hair in America.* New York, NY: Macmillan.

Cooper, E., & Guillebaud, J. (1999). *Sexuality and disability.* London, England: CRC Press.

Cornish, J. A. E., Gorgens, K. A., Monson, S. P., Olkin, R., Palombi, B. J., & Abels, A. V. (2008). Perspectives on ethical practice with people who have disabilities. *Professional Psychology: Research and Practice*, *39*(5), 488–497.

Courtney-Long, E. A., Romano, S. D., Carroll, D. D., & Fox, M. H. (2017). Socioeconomic factors at the intersection of race and ethnicity influencing health risks for people with disabilities. *Journal of Racial and Ethnic Health Disparities*, *4*(2), 213–222.

Crenshaw, K. (1989). Demarginalizing the intersection of race and sex: A Black feminist critique of antidiscrimination doctrine, feminist theory and antiracist politics. *University of Chicago Legal Forum*, *140*, 139–167.

Cross, W. E., Jr. (1971). The Negro-to-Black conversion experience. *Black World*, *20*(9), 13–27.

Cross, W. E., Jr. (1978). The Thomas and Cross models of psychological nigrescence: A review. *Journal of Black Psychology*, *5*(1), 13–31.

Cross, W. E., Jr. (1991). *Shades of Black: Diversity in African-American identity.* Philadelphia, PA: Temple University Press.

Darling, R. B., & Heckert, D. A. (2010). Orientation toward disability: Differences over the lifecourse. *International Journal of Disability Development and Education*, *57*, 131–143. http://dx.doi.org/10.1080/ 10349121003750489

Das, A. (2007). Masturbation in the United States, *Journal of Sex & Marital Therapy*, *33*(4), 301–317.

Dawson, G. A., Karl, K. A., & Peluchette, J. V. (2019). Hair matters: Toward understanding natural Black hair bias in the workplace. *Journal of Leadership & Organizational Studies*, *26*(3), 389–401.

DeLoach, C. P., & Greer, B. G. (1981). *Adjustment to severe disability: A metamorphosis.* New York, NY: McGraw-Hill.

Diaz, R. M., Ayala, G., & Bein, E. (2004). Sexual risk as an outcome of social oppression: Data from a probability sample of Latino gay men in three U.S. cities. *Cultural Diversity and Ethnic Minority Psychology, 10*(3), 255–267.

Dunn, D. S., & Burcaw, S. (2013). Disability identity: Exploring narrative accounts of disability. *Rehabilitation Psychology, 58*(2), 148–157.

Eaton, B. L. (2019). Pregnancy discrimination: Pregnant women need more protection in the workplace. *South Dakota Law Review, 64*, 244–297.

Eder, S. L. (2015). Off the couch and into the streets: Psychotherapy and political activism. *Smith College Studies in Social Work, 85*(4), 373–386.

Elliott, D. B., Krivickas, K., Brault, M. W., & Kreider, R. M. (2012, May). Historical marriage trends from 1890–2010: A focus on race differences. SEHSD Working Paper no. 2012–12 presented at the annual meeting of the Population Association of America; San Francisco, CA, May 2012.

Erikson, E. H. (1968). *Identity: Youth and crisis.* New York, NY: Norton.

Fearon, J. D. (1999). *What is identity (as we now use the word).* Unpublished manuscript, Stanford University, Stanford, California.

Fine, M., & Asch, A. (1981). Disabled women: Sexism without the pedestal. *Journal of Sociology and Social Welfare, 8*(2), 233–248.

Fine, M., & Asch, A. (1988). Disability beyond stigma: Social interaction, discrimination, and activism. *Journal of Social Issues, 44*(1), 3–21.

Fryberg, S. A., & Townsend, S. S. M. (2008). The psychology of invisibility. In G. Adams, M. Biernat, N. Branscombe, C. S. Crandall, & L. W. Wrightsman (Eds.), *Commemorating Brown: The social psychology of racism and discrimination* (pp. 173–193). Washington, DC: American Psychological Association.

Garrin, A. R., & Marcketti, S. B. (2018). The impact of hair on African American women's collective identity formation. *Clothing and Textiles Research Journal, 36*(2), 104–118.

Gibson, J. (2006). Disability and clinical competency: An introduction. *California Psychologist, 39*(6), 6–10.

Gill, C. J. (1997). Four types of integration in disability identity development. *Journal of Vocational Rehabilitation, 9*(1), 39–46.

Gill, K. M., & Hough, S. (2007). Sexuality training, education and therapy in the healthcare environment: Taboo, avoidance, discomfort or ignorance? *Sexuality and Disability, 25*(2), 73–76.

Graf, N., Brown, A., & Patten, E. (2018, April 9). The narrowing, but persistent, gender gap in pay. Pew Research Center. http://leametz.pbworks.com/f/Gender%20pay%20gap%20has%20narrowed%2C%20but%20changed%20little%20in%20past%20decade.pdf

Hall, J. C., Everett, J. E., & Hamilton-Mason, J. (2012). Black women talk about workplace stress and how they cope. *Journal of Black Studies, 43*(2), 207–226.

Harnett, A. (2000). Escaping the "evil avenger" and the "supercrip": Images of disability in popular television. *Irish Communications Review, 8*(1), 21–29.

Hassouneh-Phillips, D. (2005). Understanding abuse of women with physical disabilities: An overview of the abuse pathways model. *Advances in Nursing Science, 28*(1), 70–80.

Heilman, M. E., & Eagly, A. H. (2008). Gender stereotypes are alive, well, and busy producing workplace discrimination. *Industrial and Organizational Psychology, 1*(4), 393–398.

Hess, M. J., & Hough, S. (2012). Impact of spinal cord injury on sexuality: Broad-based clinical practice intervention and practical application. *Journal of Spinal Cord Medicine, 35*(4), 211–218.

Hingsburger, D., & Melberg-Schwier, K. (2000). *Sexuality: Your sons and daughters with intellectual disabilities.* Baltimore, MD: Paul Brookes Publishing.

hooks, b. (1981) Ain't I a woman: Black Women and feminism. Boston, MA: South End Press.

Jacoby, R. (1983). *The repression of psychoanalysis: Otto Fenichel and the political Freudians.* New York, NY: Basic Books.

Koenig, H. G. (2007). Religion and remission of depression in medical inpatients with heart failure/pulmonary disease. *Journal of Nervous and Mental Disease, 195*(5), 389–395.

Koenig, H. G., McCullough, M. E., & Larson, D. B. (2001). *Handbook of religion and health* (pp. 276–291). New York, NY: Oxford University Press.

Krause, N., & Bastida, E. (2011). Social relationships in the church during late life: Assessing differences between African Americans, Whites, and Mexican Americans. *Review of Religious Research, 53*(1), 41–63.

Kuemmel, A., Campbell, C. P., & Gray, A. A. (2019). Women and disabilities: Maintaining womanhood in amid social challenges. In D. Dunn (Ed.), *Understanding the experience of disability.* New York, NY: Oxford University Press.

Kwate, N. O. A. (2001). Intelligence or misorientation? Eurocentrism in the WISC-III. *Journal of Black Psychology, 27*(2), 221–238.

Laumann, E., & Mahay, J. (2002). The social organization of women's sexuality. In G. M. Wingood & R. J. DiClemente (Eds.), *Handbook of women's sexual and reproductive health* (pp. 43–70). New York, NY: Kluwer Academic/Plenum Publishers.

Lewin, B., Beltrami, M., Levine, J., & Nemeth, S. (2012). *The sessions.* Twentieth Century Fox Home Entertainment.

Marcia, J. E. (1966). Development and validation of ego-identity status. *Journal of Personality and Social Psychology, 3*(5), 551–558.

Marcia, J. E. (1980). Identity in adolescence. *Handbook of Adolescent Psychology, 9*(11), 159–187.

Martin, J. J. (2017). *Handbook of disability sport and exercise psychology.* New York, NY: Oxford University Press.

Mattis, J. (2000). African American women's definitions of spirituality and religiosity. *Journal of Black Psychology, 26*(1), 101–122.

Mattis, J. S. (2002). Religion and spirituality in the meaning-making and coping experiences of African American women: A qualitative analysis. *Psychology of Women Quarterly, 26*(4), 309–321.

McDonald, K. E., Keys, C. B., & Balcazar, F. E. (2007). Disability, race/ethnicity and gender: Themes of cultural oppression, acts of individual resistance. *American Journal of Community Psychology, 39*(1–2), 145–161.

Mejias, N. J., Gill, C. J., & Shpigelman, C-N. (2014). Influence of a support group for young women with disabilities on sense of belonging. *Journal of Counseling Psychology, 61*(2), 208–220.

Merton, R. (1967). *On theoretical sociology.* New York, NY: Free Press.

Miles, A. L. (2019). "Strong Black Women": African American women with disabilities, intersecting identities, and inequality. *Gender & Society, 33*(1), 41–63.

Miller, K. J., Gleaves, D. H., Hirsch, T. G., Green, B. A., Snow, A. C., & Corbett, C. C. (2000). Comparisons of body image dimensions by race/ethnicity and gender in a university population. *International Journal of Eating Disorders*, 27(3), 310–316.

Moin, V., Duvdevany, I., & Mazor, D. (2009). Sexual identity, body image and life satisfaction among women with and without physical disability. *Sexuality and Disability*, 27(2), 83–95.

Mpofu, E., & Harley, D. A. (2006). Racial and disability identity: Implications for the career counseling of African Americans with disabilities. *Rehabilitation Counseling Bulletin*, 50(1), 14–23.

Mueller, P. S., Plevak, D. J., & Rummans, T. A. (2001, December). Religious involvement, spirituality, and medicine: implications for clinical practice. In *Mayo Clinic Proceedings*, 76(12), 1225–1235. Elsevier.

Nario-Redmond, M. R. (2010). Cultural stereotypes of disabled and non-disabled men and women: Consensus for global category representations and diagnostic domains. *British Journal of Social Psychology*, 49(3), 471–488.

Nario-Redmond, M. R., & Oleson, K. C. (2016). Disability group identification and disability rights advocacy contingencies among emerging and other adults. *Emerging Adulthood*, 4, 207–218. https://doi.org/10.1177/2167696815579830

Neighbors, H. W., Musick, M. A., & Williams, D. R. (1998). The African American minister as a source of help for serious personal crises: Bridge or barrier to mental health care? *Health Education & Behavior*, 25(6), 759–777.

Nishina, A., Ammon, N. Y., Bellmore, A. D., & Graham, S. (2006). Body dissatisfaction and physical development among ethnic minority adolescents. *Journal of Youth and Adolescence*, 35(2), 179–191.

Nosek, M. A., Howland, C. A., Rintala, D. H., Young, M. E., & Chanpong, G. F. (2001). National study of women with disabilities: Final report. *Sexuality and Disability*, 19(1), 5–39.

Okoro, C. A., Hollis, N. D., Cyrus, A. C., & Griffin-Blake, S. (2018). Prevalence of disabilities and health care access by disability status and type among adults—United States, 2016. *Morbidity and Mortality Weekly Report*, 67(32), 882–887.

Passel, J. S., Wang, W., & Taylor, P. (2015). One-in-seven new U.S. marriages is interracial or interethnic. Pew Research Center's Social & Demographic Trends Project. http://www.pewsocialtrends.org/2010/06/04/marrying-out/

Patton, T. O. (2006). Hey girl, am I more than my hair? African American women and their struggles with beauty, body image, and hair. *NWSA Journal*, 18(2), 24–51.

Petersen, A. (2006). An African American woman with disabilities: The intersection of gender, race and disability. *Disability & Society*, 21(7), 721–734.

Powers, L. E., McNeff, E., Curry, M., Saxton, M., & Elliott, D. (2004) Preliminary findings on the abuse experiences of men with disabilities. Portland, OR: Oregon Health & Science University Center on Self-Determination.

Raley, R. K., Sweeney, M. M., & Wondra, D. (2015). The growing racial and ethnic divide in U.S. marriage patterns. *The Future of Children/Center for the Future of Children, the David and Lucile Packard Foundation*, 25(2), 89–109.

Ratts, M. J., Singh, A. A., Nassar-McMillan, S., Butler, S. K., & McCullough, J. R. (2016). Multicultural and social justice counseling competencies: Guidelines for the counseling profession. *Journal of Multicultural Counseling and Development*, 44(1), 28–48.

Reel, J. J., SooHoo, S., Summerhays, J. F., & Gill, D. L. (2008). Age before beauty: An exploration of body image in African-American and Caucasian adult women. *Journal of Gender Studies, 17*(4), 321–330.

Richie, B. (1992). Coping with work: Interventions with African-American women. *Women & Therapy, 12*(1–2), 97–111.

Rintala, D. H., Howland, C. A., Nosek, M. A., Bennett, J. L., Young, M. E., Foley, C. C., Rossi, C. D., & Chanpong, G. (1997). Dating issues for women with physical disabilities. *Sexuality and Disability, 15*(4), 219–242.

Roberts, T. A., & Zurbriggen, E. (2013). The problem of sexualization: What is it and how does it happen? In T.-A. Roberts and E. Zurbriggen (Ed.), *The sexualization of girls and girlhood: Causes, consequences, and resistance* (pp. 3–21). New York, NY: Oxford University Press.

Salwen, J. K., Gray, A., & Mona, L. R. (2016). Personal assistance, disability, and intimate partner violence: A guide for healthcare providers. *Rehabilitation Psychology, 61*(4), 417–429.

Scott, K. D. (2013). Communication strategies across cultural borders: Dispelling stereotypes, performing competence, and redefining black womanhood. *Women's Studies in Communication, 36*(3), 312–329.

Sesko, A. K., & Biernat, M. (2010). Prototypes of race and gender: The invisibility of Black women. *Journal of Experimental Social Psychology, 46*(2), 356–360.

Shulman, J. L., & Horne, S. G. (2003). The use of self-pleasure: Masturbation and body image among African American and European American women. *Psychology of Women Quarterly, 27*, 262–269.

Smeltzer, S. C. (2007). Pregnancy in women with physical disabilities. *Journal of Obstetric, Gynecologic & Neonatal Nursing, 36*(1), 88–96.

Stuart, O. (1992). Race and disability: Just a double oppression? *Disability, Handicap & Society, 7*(2), 177–188.

Sue, D. W., & Sue, D. (2012). Counseling the culturally diverse theory and practice (6th ed.). John Wiley & Sons.

Taylor, R., Chatters, L., & Levin, J. (2004). Religion in the lives of African Americans: Social, psychological, and health perspectives. Thousand Oaks, CA: Sage Publications.

Tepper, M. (2015). *Regain that feeling: Secrets to sexual self-discovery*. CreateSpace.

Thomas, A. J., Hacker, J. D., & Hoxha, D. (2011). Gendered racial identity of Black young women. *Sex Roles: A Journal of Research, 64*(7–8), 530–542.

Thomas, H. N., Hamm, M., Borrero, S., Hess, R., & Thurston, R. C. (2019). Body image, attractiveness, and sexual satisfaction among midlife women: A qualitative study. *Journal of Women's Health, 28*(1), 100–106.

Turner, F. (2015). I am not my hair: A Black woman's struggle with identity through hair. *Oakland Journal, 25*, 58–82.

van Olphen, J., Schulz, A., Israel, B., Chatters, L., Klem, L., Parker, E., & Williams, D. (2003). Religious involvement, social support, and health among African-American women on the east side of Detroit. *Journal of General Internal Medicine, 18*(7), 549–557.

Vernon, A. (1999). The dialects of multiple identities and the disabled people's movement. *Disability & Society, 14*(3), 385–398.

Weitz, R., & Gordon, L. (1993). Images of Black women among Anglo college students. *Sex Roles, 28*(1–2), 19–34.

West, C. (2008). Mammy, Jezebel, Sapphire, and their homegirls: Developing an "oppositional gaze" toward the images of Black women. In J. Christer, C. Golden, & P. Rozee (Eds.), *Lectures on the psychology of women* (4th ed., pp. 286–99). New York, NY: McGraw-Hill.

Williams, D. R., & Mohammed, S. A. (2009). Discrimination and racial disparities in health: Evidence and needed research. *Journal of Behavioral Medicine, 32*(1), 20–47.

Wilson, C. S., Forchheimer, M., Heinemann, A. W., Warren, A. M., & McCullum-smith, C. (2017). Assessment of the relationship of spiritual well-being to depression and quality of life for persons with spinal cord injury. *Disability and Rehabilitation, 39*(5), 491–496.

Wilson, W. J., & Neckerman, K. M. (1986). Poverty and family structure: The widening gap between evidence and public policy issues. In S. Danziger & D. Weinberg (Eds.), Fighting poverty: What works and what doesn't (pp. 232–259). Cambridge, MA: Harvard University Press.

Woodard, J. B., & Mastin, T. (2005). Black womanhood: *Essence* and its treatment of stereotypical images of Black women. *Journal of Black Studies, 36*(2), 264–281.

CHAPTER 14

The Mental Health Needs of African American Women Enrolled in Higher Education

Mahlet Endale
Terrence Harper II

HISTORY AND BACKGROUND

For many students, the college years provide opportunities for significant identity development, personal growth, and the expanding of one's wage-earning potential. For women of African descent, these opportunities are often inextricably associated with systemic barriers designed within oppressive systems to limit their capacities to survive and thrive based on the identities they hold. In this chapter, we endeavor to elucidate the multifaceted experiences of Black women in higher education, while offering implications for treatment and support of this population during a phase of their lives in which change is often the primary constant. For this chapter, higher education is defined as postsecondary training for the purpose of earning certifications and/or an associate's, bachelor's, master's, or doctoral degree.

The U.S. Department of Education's National Center for Education Statistics' (NCES) 2019 numbers on degrees conferred give a good snapshot of who is earning what degrees in the United States. See Table 14.1 for the most recent numbers for Black women as compared to all students and females:

Table 14.1
The U.S. Department of Education's National Center for Education Statistics'
(NCES) 2019

2016–2017 Conferred Degrees	All Students	Black Students	Female Students	Black Female Students
Certificates	944, 940	158, 960	540, 227	98,938
Associate's	1,005,649	129,874	611,490	86,701
Bachelor's	1,956,032	196,300	1,119,987	125,746
Master's	804,604	89,577	477,792	62,601
Doctoral	181,352	14,067	96,706	9,267

Recent attention has been given to an oft-cited statistic that Black women are the most educated demographic by race and gender in the United States (US Department of Education, 2019b). Many point to this statistic as indicative of significant progress toward racial and gender equity. However, while the resilience of this population can certainly be understood as a factor implicated in this national trend, further extrapolation based on these statistics without recognizing these numbers within the appropriate context is likely to result in unbalanced conclusions. For example, whereas Black women make up a significant percentage of Black people earning postsecondary degrees, since 2004, increases in their graduation rates have not kept pace with the increases in graduation rates of Latinx, White, and Asian American women (Bartman, 2015; Guerra, 2013). Additionally, it cannot be said that these enrollment numbers ensure equitable participation in the free market, as Black women in the aggregate experience annual and lifetime earnings significantly lower than that of many of their comparably educated counterparts with respect to race and gender (Guerra, 2013). What these statistics may then speak to is a capable population, which has not seen the expected progression in educational attainment and the achievement of educational success, or the result of fair pay. At the very least, such conclusions are sobering when considering what it may be like for Black women to excel while dealing with both challenges related to the intersectional identities of Black women and the myriad of issues common to college students.

Stressors Faced in Higher Education Enrollment

There are common stressors faced by most students enrolled in higher education. Students are learning new study skills, fine-tuning their time management, developing new relationships, possibly away from support systems for the first time, and learning how to live as independent adults (Parker et al., 2004). One study exploring existing research found the following common stressors for students in higher education: academic pressure, financial burdens, and increased maladaptive technology use (Flatt, 2013).

Studies have shown an increase in mental health symptoms like depression and anxiety in students enrolled in higher education as compared to their experiences before enrollment (Bayram & Bilgel, 2008; Bewick et al., 2010; Keyes et al., 2012). In fact, Bewick et al. (2010) found students' distress rises in their first year of enrollment and never returns to their pre-enrollment levels. Students can face different types of consequences if they are not able to manage their stress and mental health concerns. Often, their relationships and levels of engagement are negatively impacted (Salzer, 2012). Further, any untreated symptoms have the potential to become a chronic concern, and undertreated stress and mental health concerns are correlated with lower graduation rates (Ghio et al., 2014). This potentially has long-term implications for lifetime career and income potential.

Bartman (2015) conducted a literature review of articles published between 2002 and 2015 and identified four main issues specifically impacting African American women enrolled in higher education:

Holding Multiple Marginalized Identities

This community faces "issues of dual oppression" as students who identify both as Black and as women. In other words, in addition to the common stressors in higher education mentioned previously, Black women also must navigate the cumulative impact of gendered racism (Howard-Hamilton, 2003). Per Howard-Hamilton (2003), African American women have been invited to enroll into institutions of higher education in larger numbers but continue to be seen and treated as outsiders without much say in the quality of their experience.

Further, the intersection of race, sexual orientation, and gender identity in combination influence the stressors faced by students. As an example, one study looked at reported campus sexual assault prevalence rates from 2000 to 2015; the results appear in Table 14.2.

Fedina et al. (2018) noted the studies they found focus primarily on White, cisgender female, heterosexual participants at predominantly four-year residential colleges. In searching for data on the experiences of

Table 14. 2
Reported Campus Sexual Assault Prevalence Rates from 2000 to 2015

Type of Assault	Prevalence Found
Unwanted Sexual Contact	1.8% to 34%
Attempted Rape	1.1% to 3.8%
Completed Rape	0.5% to 8.4%
Incapacitated Rape	1.8% to 14.2%
Total Sexual Assault	5.2% to 60.4%

Source: Fedina, Holmes, & Backes (2018).

Black women in higher education with sexual assault, the research was lacking. Despite Fedina et al. (2018) calling sexual assault on campuses an epidemic, researchers are not looking at the specific experiences of Black women. Krebs et al. (2011) is one study showing a lower rate of reported sexual assault by Black women attending historically Black colleges and universities (HBCUs) as compared to reports by women at predominantly White institutions (PWIs), but much more research is needed to more fully understand the experiences of Black women.

In looking at additional identities, one campus study found women identifying as bisexual reported experiencing sexual assault at a notably higher rate than heterosexual women within their group of participants (37.8 percent as compared to 24.7 percent) (Ford & Soco-Marquez, 2016). Further, another study using the National College Health Assessment-II examined the rates of violence reported by transgender, cisgender male, and cisgender female students (Griner et al., 2017). The authors found "transgender students experienced the highest odds in crimes involving sexual victimization" (Griner et al., 2).

All this is to say, race, gender identity, and sexual orientation come together to give students unique experiences. To better understand the needs of students, it is important to understand their experiences as informed by the intersection of their identities rather than based on single aspects of their identities.

Absence of a Critical Mass of Black Female Students

Guerra (2013) notes, "African American women held 8.58 percent of bachelor's degrees held by women in 2012 though they constituted 12.7 percent of the female population" (2). In addition to the students' sense of community, there is a need for a critical mass, so students are seen for themselves rather than representations of their race (Hughes & Howard-Hamilton, 2004). According to Hughes & Howard-Hamilton (2004), when there isn't a large enough community, individual students are more likely to experience "burnout, which negatively impacts retention and attainment rates and adds to the lack of critical mass of this particular student group."

Disproportion in Male-Female Enrollment

According to Bartman (2015), low enrollment of Black men "negatively [impacts] student interactions and social life on campus" for women who date men. Many Black women choose not to date or marry outside their race for a variety of reasons. For some, it is important to have a partner and family that reflect their culture of origin. For others, there is a fear of rejection by one's [Black] and other communities if they date outside of their race. The disproportionate numbers of male and female students combined with the stressors of what it could mean to date outside one's race can force some Black college women to choose not to date at all. The stress of navigating these nuanced factors in a dating life can put some Black college women "at risk for depression, anxiety, anger, guilt, shame, and despair" (Henry, 2008, 20). It is hard to imagine this stressor does not also impact Black sexual orientation and gender minority students as their numbers tend to be smaller than that of heterosexual and cisgender students. Some may minimize dating stress in the larger context of life stressors, but this is a meaningful component of life for young adults. When institutions of higher education miss this unintended impact of the disproportionate numbers of enrollment for Black students, they also fail to see the potential mental health impact.

Small Number of Black Faculty

In 2016, 6 percent of full-time faculty were African American, of which 3 percent were African American women. That same year, 8 percent of full-time assistant professors were African American, and 4 percent were African American women. These statistics show a drop in the number of Black faculty and Black female faculty from 2012 (U.S. Department of Education, 2018). At least one study has shown students' academic self-confidence is directly related to their relationship with an African American mentor (Rosales & Person, 2003). However, based on the statistics, there are not enough Black faculty, especially Black female faculty, to provide mentorship for the number of enrolled Black students. According to Bartman (2015), "this adds to the isolation, lack of belonging, and stress so prevalent within this subset of students."

IMPACT OF DIFFERENT TYPES OF HIGHER EDUCATION SETTINGS

When considering the variable experiences of Black women in higher education, a significant contributing factor to this variability is the differences unique to the particular institutional setting. The discussion below focuses on experiential differences in academic settings and their impact for Black women.

Undergraduate, Graduate, and Professional Settings

The beginning of one's undergraduate career is often marked by significant change. Within U.S. society, the transition out of high school and the 18th birthday often signify entry into adulthood. Recently, scholars have more explicitly defined the ages of 18–25 as being indicative of "emerging adulthood" in recognition of the unique transitional experiences marking this stage of development (Munsey, 2006). For Black women,

responsibilities and tasks of this stage of development are best conceptualized as multifaceted and demanding. In describing these demands,
Arnold (1993) writes of Black women students, "Caught in the juncture
where economics of class, gender, and race converge, they juggle full- and
part-time jobs, a multiplicity of family roles, and overall, an economically
precarious lifestyle" (200). The legacies of institutional oppression result
in multiple barriers limiting access to opportunities that serve to increase
upward mobility. Thus, individuals with multiple marginalized identities
often prioritize access when seeking institutions of higher learning. These
students may also have family, occupational, and community obligations,
which make remaining close to their homes essential.

There are additional considerations for first-generation students. Families of these students may not fully grasp the demands of being in an academic setting and the energy expended acclimating to different cultural
expectations that call into question their sense of belonging. This lack of
understanding of the academic rigor with which students must engage
can be doubly taxing for students who do not experience any difference in
the responsibilities they are expected to manage at home. Members of the
students' support network may also struggle with providing appropriate
guidance given their lack of familiarity and discomfort with university
culture (Hinderlie & Kenny, 2002).

For students who choose and can attend schools farther from home, it
can often be the first time being away from family and community. College may also be the first time students are exposed to different value sets,
which can be experienced positively and negatively. Exposure to new values may assist students with exploring aspects of their identities that may
have been less likely to have been explored previously. However, changes
in values can often put Black women at odds with members of their support networks, who have certain expectations about who they are based
on earlier phases of their identity development.

At the graduate and professional level, Black female students are often
faced with noteworthy new experiences. Often these programs have significantly lower enrollment of minority students than do their undergraduate
counterparts when situated within PWIs. The experience of being one of
a smaller population often entails that there are less options for building
community among people who may share similar racial and gender identities. These opportunities may be limited within and outside of an individual's program of study. While not universal, feelings of isolation as well as a
lack of belonging can often typify such an experience. It is also sometimes
the case that Black women experience pressure to be the "spokesperson"
for the underrepresented identities they hold in these spaces. Overall, there
usually are fewer opportunities for mentorship for Black women in higher
education if seeking guidance from people who share similar identities.
Black women comprise just 1 percent of tenured full professors and 3 percent of assistant or associate professors (Johnson, 2017).

Historically Black Colleges and Universities, Predominantly White Institutions, and Single-Sex Institutions

Most African American college students attend coeducational PWIs, while historically Black colleges and universities (HBCUs) award a higher proportion of bachelor's degrees to African Americans (Watt, 2006). HBCUs and single-sex institutions emphasize leadership development and holistic growth (e.g., academic and social) via culturally based educational efforts (Zamani, 2003). Even though more students attend PWIs by number, some research indicates HBCUs and single-sex institutions offer safer, more supportive, accessible, and affirming educational environments for Black collegians (Borum & Walker, 2012; Williams & Johnson, 2019). Percentages of sexual assault and violence perpetrated against Black women tend to be lower at HBCUs (Krebs et al., 2011). HBCU graduates tend to be more likely to pursue graduate, professional, and post-baccalaureate education (Haag, 1997; Zamani, 2003; Williams & Johnson, 2019). Conversely, PWIs tend to be larger and often are better resourced than HBCUs; these larger numbers may also mean some PWIs have greater numbers of Black students than smaller HBCUs, potentially allowing more opportunities for connection. Climate issues at HBCUs may disproportionately affect support for Black women identifying as lesbian, gay, bisexual, transgender, or queer (LGBTQ) (Williams & Johnson, 2019). Research additionally suggests Black women may face racial discrimination at predominantly White single-sex institutions and gender discrimination at HBCUs (Perkins, 1998; Zamani, 2003).

School Size

Although resources at larger institutions can be numerous, some students may experience larger schools as overwhelming, which might limit their ability to access these resources. Smaller schools may offer opportunities for closer relationships, as smaller class sizes may lend themselves more easily to developing relationships with mentors and faculty (especially in classes with Black women instructors). Diversity in student organizations may be limited at smaller schools; this issue is compounded when further developing culturally relevant programs and organizations is stymied due to administrative resistance (e.g., administrators may question the allocation of resources for smaller populations). Even the largest HBCUs have student enrollment numbers resembling mid-sized PWIs (around 10,000 students for the top five), which means Black female students seeking a large institution experience may be required to enroll at a PWI. Private institutions tend to be smaller, more expensive, and more selective, which may mean limited access for Black women who have working-class backgrounds, average grades, and financial disadvantages (Haag, 1997; Zamani, 2003).

Community Colleges, Proprietary Colleges, and Four-Year Colleges

Proprietary institutions and community colleges, often situated in urban areas and less selective, tend to account for large enrollments of Black female students (Zamani, 2003). Accordingly, community colleges may offer more opportunities for balancing demands of home and school due to their geographical convenience, affordability, and accessibility. While these schools may provide educational opportunities to a significant number of Black women, the extent to which they provide the most practical educational option for students who aspire to further pursue education beyond an associate's degree is less certain. Some research indicates students entering a two-year college with the intent of eventually pursuing a bachelor's degree are less likely to earn a bachelor's degree than those attending a traditional four-year college (Zamani, 2003). Four-year colleges also typically have better funding and more opportunities for extracurricular engagement, which can be critical to positive adjustment and community building. Students attending commuter and community colleges may have fewer opportunities to engage with their college communities due to the possibility of different and conflicting demands on their time in academic, occupational, and family domains (Melendez & Melendez, 2010).

Like community colleges, proprietary (for-profit) colleges tend to enroll large numbers of women and racial minority students. Proprietary college students may be better prepared for certain trades in programs with high levels of specificity. When programs are more general or less well-established, the efficacy of degrees earned at proprietary colleges is diminished. The cost of education tends to be higher at proprietary institutions than at public community colleges. Overall rates of degree completion, accumulated debt, and labor market competitiveness tend to compare unfavorably with public postsecondary alternatives (traditional four-year and two-year institutions) (Deming, Goldin, & Katz, 2013).

CAMPUS MENTAL HEALTH SERVICES

Most campuses depend on mental health professionals to attend to the mental health needs of their students. If a campus is resourced enough, there are licensed mental health professionals paid by the school to provide psychotherapy to students on campus. If this is not possible, campus staff members refer students to nearby providers.

Campus counseling centers generally offer individual and group counseling, campus outreach services, crisis appointments, and consultation (for students, faculty, and staff). Some campuses also offer couples and family therapy options. Often, medication management is available by psychiatrists in the counseling center and/or a student health center.

Many campuses employ multidisciplinary teams to provide mental health care for students. Others also offer trained students to provide paraprofessional mental health support and outreach programming. The demographics of counseling center staff are also more diverse than ever. In 2018, counseling centers reported to the Association for University and College Counseling Center Directors (AUCCCD) that 27.6 percent of staff identified as a person of color, 3.8 percent of staff identified as trans or nonbinary, 16 percent identified as LGBTQ, and 10.6 percent identified as differently abled (AUCCCD, 2018).

There is also increasing diversity within students accessing services. According to the AUCCCD's 2018 survey, on average, campus mental health centers serve about 11.8 percent of students on non-community college campuses, and 5 percent of students on community college campuses. The Center for Collegiate Mental Health's (CCMH) 2018 report stated approximately 2 percent of students served in this year identified as gender nonbinary. According to the 2018 CCMH report, 9.6 percent of students served identified as African American or Black, and 34.7 percent identified as a person of color. The 2018 AUCCCD and CCMH surveys found the top four concerns typically bringing students in for counseling were anxiety, depression, stress, and specific relationship problems.

TREATMENT CONSIDERATIONS AND RECOMMENDATIONS

Recommendations for Mental Health Professionals in Higher Education Systems

As has been detailed previously, African American women face unique stressors in the pursuit of higher education. The intersection of gendered racism (and potentially other marginalized identities) with stress associated with being a college student is perhaps one of the most prominent factors of which clinicians in college settings must remain mindful. The identities held by Black women and their status as students might predispose this population to stress and mental health concerns as a function of experiencing dual oppression. Gendered racism can result in microaggressive experiences unique to the individual's social group membership (Lewis et al., 2016). Longmire-Avital and Robinson (2018) point out that women, emerging adults, and racial minorities all tend to have higher rates of depression compared to other populations. Based on these findings, these authors suggest intersecting systems of oppression can contribute to depressive symptomology.

Clinicians should be especially attentive to the nuances of Black women's intersectionality. In their exploration of the multiple marginalities of an immigrant Black Muslim woman at a PWI, McGuire, Casanova, and Davis (2016) highlight the need to avoid subsuming multiple identities based on one identity that an individual may possess (e.g., the erasure of Malcolm X's embodied religious identity as it is subsumed by his Blackness). Jackson (2013) also highlights the potential for losses of identity when transitioning among different levels of postsecondary education, noting women who transferred from a community college to a four-year HBCU expressed how important it was for them to retain aspects of their identities while pursuing a scholarly identity.

Clinicians must also be aware of and acknowledge the stigma often associated with mental health help-seeking that exists for this population. Considering decades of mistreatment by said professionals, such recognition should be accompanied by validation of the justified reasons African American women have for being leery of health professionals and researchers. College counseling centers and clinicians who work with college students may be required to engage in initiatives that are effortful in reaching out to students and decreasing stigma. Such efforts would do well to humanize the person of the therapist, thereby increasing how accessible these services can feel for this population. The provision of psychoeducational outreach designed specifically to address the concerns of this population can also demonstrate multicultural and social justice values in action (e.g., providing information about the unique nature of stressors particular to this population; providing validation of experiences with gendered racial microaggressions and resources for coping; Lewis et al., 2016), thereby diminishing stigma and barriers to access.

Flexible treatment options and approaches also play a role in decreasing stigma for mental health services for African American women. The pervasiveness of institutional oppression affects the university setting, the training of psychotherapists, and the clinicians socialized to internalize racist and sexist ideologies. As such, counseling centers and clinicians who work with college students should consider nontraditional and decolonized treatment approaches (see Chapter 2) that better imagine empowering mental health solutions for Black women. Innovation can include adapting current treatment approaches (e.g., individual counseling, group counseling, workshops, crisis work, etc.) in culturally relevant ways. It also can entail a reexamination of the status quo in college mental health, potentially with more flexible service delivery, including possibilities such as sister circles (support groups for Black women), embedded models (in which counselors are housed in campus buildings outside of the counseling center), and preventative community health programming that may more relevantly address the needs of Black women.

The framing of Black women as highly successful in educational settings, while speaking to an extent to their resilience, may also undermine institutional efforts to provide support that can enable academic thriving (Winkle-Wagner et al., 2019). Such institutional efforts are paramount in light of how historically research has focused on individual factors for academic success, which can inadvertently place the onus for change on

Black women, rather than addressing the institutional and sociostruc-
tural issues so often implicated in the academic success of Black women
(Winkle-Wagner, 2015). These institutional measures can also serve the
purpose of decreasing the harmful impact and pressure Black women
often face based on stereotypes about their strength and perseverance
(Lewis et al., 2016). Such measures may also need to maintain a certain
amount of specificity, as research suggests common support systems (e.g.,
Black student unions, multicultural resource centers), while helpful, may
not be sufficient to provide the space for successful intersectional identity
exploration (Watt, 2006; Winkle-Wagner et al., 2019).

Identity exploration and development, as a hallmark of emerging adulthood, are also key considerations for Black women students. Black women
may feel pressure, both external and self-imposed, in responding to societal expectations. This pressure can result in efforts to work harder, prove
others wrong, be "twice as good" as others, and make good impressions
in the hope of overcoming the negative expectations held by peers, faculty, and staff (Hanon et al., 2016). Engagement in compensatory behavior
may have variable effects on one's identity development and well-being.
Watt (2006) notes that when Black women are exploring their identities,
they score lower on self-reported measures of self-esteem. Watt cites bell
hooks's (1981) hypothesis that Black women often feel forced to choose
commitment to racial equality over and above the struggle for women's
rights and the value of womanhood. Such conflict is difficult to navigate,
but with successful identity consolidation, Black women can expect positive outcomes. Watt (2006) notes women with positive attitudes about
being Black also appeared to feel positively about being women; they also
report higher levels of self-esteem when they reject negative images of the
Black race and of male supremacy. Thus, clinicians working with Black
women students may play a role in providing perspective that assists students with adaptively negotiating identity development.

Additional Campus Options for Supporting Student Mental Health

African Americans experience mental illness at the same rate as other
racial groups, but only a third of African Americans who need mental
health care receive it (American Psychiatric Association, 2017). Barriers to
care include stigma and self-concealment, distrust of health providers, the
lack of racially and ethnically diverse providers, lack of multiculturally
competent providers, and not having health insurance (American Psychiatric Association, 2017; Masuda, Anderson, & Edmonds, 2012).

One benefit to being in an educational setting is that there usually are
a variety of resources available to support students' social and emotional
development. Systems of higher education have an opportunity to use
student support services and resources to help foster resilience for their

Black female students before or while they interface with mental health counseling as part of fostering overall wellness.

Support Identity-Based Student Organizations

Identity-based student organizations are organizations constructed around a student's single or multiple identities. These organizations provide opportunities to connect with fellow students who share aspects of one's identity (Museus, 2008; Renn & Ozaki, 2010). This is particularly important for marginalized students, especially if they "have been negatively stereotyped by their peers or unwelcome in predominantly White organizations" (Kodama & Laylo, 2017, 73). Often, identity-based student organizations form when there is a discriminatory or unwelcoming campus climate, or to help educate members of the community about specific concerns impacting a specific student group (Harper & Quaye, 2007). At other times, these organizations are used as an opportunity for students to learn more about an aspect of their identity (Kodama & Laylo, 2017). These organizations provide peer support, a sense of belonging, and frequently a necessary safe space for marginalized students (Deo, 2013; Moreno & Sanchez Banuelos, 2013).

In applying this to the idea of supporting African-descended women on campus, higher education systems can foster social engagement and community by supporting student organizations for African-descended cis and trans women. Systems can do this in multiple ways. First, support Black or African–descended ethnicity organizations like a Caribbean Student Union (CSU), African Student Union (ASU), or Black Student Union (BSU). CSUs and ASUs generally are made up of students who are immigrant or first generation. BSUs are generally made up of a variety of African diaspora members especially including African American students. Supporting LGBTQ student organizations is also key in supporting a dimension of some Black female students' identities. These organizations help create community for specific intersections of race, sexual orientation, and/or gender identity. Historically Black sororities represent another set of organizations serving students at the intersection of race and gender identity (Greyerbielh & Mitchell, 2014).

Support Campus Resource Centers

Supporting student-run identity-based organizations is a great start; however, adding identity-focused resource centers adds another layer of support, protection, and resources. As students matriculate, attend to fluctuating academic demands, and then graduate, the consistency and effectiveness of student organizations can vary semester to semester. Further, faculty and staff have more power than students. Resource centers provide a more consistent and resourced space that can provide a variety of services for Black female students, faculty, and staff. Resource centers help institutionalize the commitment to the specific interests and needs of specific populations existing on a campus.

Foster Mentorship Programs for Black Women Students

A 2008 multidisciplinary meta-analysis comparing mentored to non-mentored individuals found "mentoring is associated with a wide range of favorable behavioral, attitudinal, health-related, relational, motivational, and career outcomes" (Eby et al., 2008, 254). The effect size was especially high for educational and career-related mentorship. According to Louis et al. (2014), African American women often are not afforded and/or are aware of support available to help them succeed academically, socially, and personally during their matriculation in higher education. The authors suggest mentorship is an effective way to help Black women students navigate both traditional college stressors and the unique stressors they experience due to their intersecting identities. However, the authors point out there is a shortage of African American female faculty to meet the mentorship need of African American female students. The authors insist there is a need for faculty who do not identify as African American to be more proactive in helping African American women students in their academic, social, and professional development. However, it is imperative that faculty doing so invest in as much training as needed to ensure their cultural competence in attending to this population of students (Louis et al., 2014). Such competencies need to span across students' identities, including race, ethnicity, gender identity, and sexual orientation.

CASE STUDY

Jemele is a 23-year-old, Black bisexual, able-bodied, agnostic, cis-woman who is a junior in communications. Jemele's mother and grandmother lived together and raised her for the first 11 years of her life, until Jemele's mother passed away from sickle cell anemia complications. She didn't know much about her father, who she heard had been financially supportive, even though he and Jemele's mother chose not to remain together. Jemele's father passed away in a car accident when she was a toddler. Jemele remembered a loving home, in which hard work and education were highly valued. Until the last years of her life, Jemele's mother regularly worked multiple jobs in order to provide for Jemele and Jemele's grandmother. Shortly after her mother's death, Jemele and her grandmother moved to live with her mother's sister and her uncle. Her once-close relationship with her grandmother became distant in recent years, which Jemele attributed to invalidation during her coming-out process. Jemele felt invalidated by her grandmother's disclosure that her sexual identity "was just a phase." Their relationship feels further complicated because Jemele is the primary caretaker for her grandmother. A significant reason why she began her collegiate career at a community college was the convenience and flexibility this afforded her to attend to responsibilities at home.

After earning her associate's degree, Jemele transferred to a four-year public PWI. It is her first time living on a residential campus, and she reported being interested in having a "real college experience." She reported being unsure about how much to focus on her interests within a minor or major (e.g., women's studies), when she's been advised by her uncle that a communications major makes better fiscal sense. Jemele also expressed concerns about belonging related to her status as a transfer and slightly "older" student. She felt as if her life experiences were different enough from those of her peers that she might feel out of place (e.g., she cited a lack of familiarity with pop and hip hop cultures as an impediment to developing social connections).

Jemele additionally noted she'd been having difficulty finding spaces in which she felt able to authentically be herself. She disclosed that her sexual identity was particularly salient for her, but that at many of the LGBTQ student organization interest meetings, she noticed she was one of one or two people of color in attendance. Worse yet, she'd experienced racial microaggressions in one of the meetings, which she found confusing due to the organization's espoused value of social justice. Jemele added her particular sexual identity often made her feel invisible in these settings, noting some people were less likely to prioritize her inclusion depending on her current dating partner. She reported that in LGBTQ spaces she feels the need to emphasize the privilege she holds regarding her bisexual identity. She wondered if she'd feel even less included if she chose to share experiences of alienation as much as she discussed her privilege.

Jemele is seeking assistance at the counseling center to address pervasive low mood, chronic fatigue, low motivation, and difficulty with concentration. She shared she's had ongoing questions about her identity associated with grief/loss in her life. She reported having briefly participated in counseling in the past at her community college, noting a slightly negative experience in which her counselor, a White woman, was often prescriptive and made sweeping generalizations about her religion and sexual identity based on her race. Jemele was hesitant to seek counseling services again but had an opportunity to interact with counseling center staff of color during her transfer orientation, which provided her with the hope of being better understood.

Working with Jemele

Jemele would likely be best supported with a collaborative, culturally responsive treatment approach. Meaningful collaboration requires that her perspective, experience, and expertise are instrumental in informing conceptualization of her concerns and the subsequent treatment approach. As discussed in treatment recommendations and considerations, adapting one's established therapeutic orientation/approach to be culturally responsive is one way this can be accomplished. For example, if a practitioner were to attempt to use a cognitive-behavioral approach with Jemele, this could entail examination of the ways in which the development of schemas and maladaptive thought patterns implicated in Jemele's experience of adjustment and depressive symptoms are influenced by oppressive societal norms—situating aspects of the presenting concern as less intrapsychic. The importance of joining with Jemele in recognizing the impact of oppressive structures and systems on her individual experience cannot be emphasized enough. Jemele's experience of symptoms like low mood and chronic fatigue can potentially be normalized as appropriate psychological responses to existing in an oppressive society. Such an approach is also likely to validate her experience while empowering her to consider the role her help-seeking plays in combating the very systems designed to oppress her. As Audre Lorde (1988) put it, "Caring for myself is not self-indulgence. It is self-preservation, and that is an act of political warfare" (131).

One might also consider engaging in consultation or supervision in decolonized and multicultural/feminist approaches in working with Jemele, as the egalitarian stance these approaches embody might lend itself to quickly establishing rapport and providing empowerment for the client. A decolonized approach has the added benefit of interrogating the tenets of psychotherapeutic practice that have been informed by White supremacy, acknowledging the structures of mental health provision itself that could likely reenact oppressive injury in treatment, so as to adequately challenge these structures with implementation of transformative intervention reconstructed upon a bedrock of ancestral knowledge, respect for human dignity, justice, and equity. Practical examples of decolonized approaches could be reinclusion of cultural healing practices, such as the sharing of food, engaging in body awareness/movement, and gift-giving in a therapeutic space (Chapman, 2019). This may also entail a blending of healing practices from multiple perspectives, such as considering how providing Jemele with recommended coping strategies to explore could be understood as a gift empowering her to learn more about her unique healing process.

Jemele's social concerns might be best addressed within group therapy. Her experience as a transfer student is not uncommon, but the unique way in which this status intersects with other aspects of her identities (e.g., racial and sexual identities) may suggest her experience of social isolation is multifaceted, and exponentially burdensome in light of her context. Sister circle interventions could be optimal in providing a supportive space to explore Jemele's identity concerns, to gain perspective regarding meaningful living, and to build community.

Special attention should be given to the conceptualization of grief/loss in Jemele's life. She's experienced significant personal loss, which likely has implications for relationship development. Additionally, a broadening of a grief/loss conceptualization could be helpful, highlighting how grief and loss can be experienced culturally and sociopolitically (perhaps examining experiences of communal grief/loss associated with marginalized identities—traumatic grief associated with the erasure of the lives of queer and trans people of color).

Many counseling centers have adopted short-term models for individual counseling, which favor increasing the number of students seen. These models have implications for the time clinicians can afford to allocate toward acclimating clients to the frame of therapy. Given Jemele's past negative experience with counseling, an egalitarian approach would demonstrate transparency with regard to session limits while also highlighting the value for honoring the client's expertise in the pacing of sessions. Frequent check-ins regarding the extent to which the client's therapeutic needs are being met can facilitate changes in course, if necessary. This approach would entail intentionality with the scope of material that can be covered in therapy. Jemele's experience of traumatic loss is extensive, meaning she may be able to complete "a piece of the work" within a short-term model, thereby laying a foundation for ongoing work in a setting that may be less restrictive with regard to the number of sessions. This frame would also be appropriate for the amelioration of Jemele's depressive symptoms in that certain symptoms (e.g., difficulty with concentration) may be more amenable to immediate, short-term interventions than other, more long-standing symptoms (e.g., pervasive low mood). For clinicians working in private practice, there may be more flexibility available with pacing that can more gradually acclimate the client to therapy. However, it would be important to consider the financial viability of such an approach for the client. Some counseling centers make provisions to allow for longer-term therapy with individuals who lack the financial means to pursue such treatment in the community. It also bears mentioning that support for a nontraditional decolonized approach within a college counseling center may be difficult to procure, in light of the fact that counseling centers being systems themselves (which again are inundated with the structures of White supremacy) would be resistant to changes that fundamentally call central pillars into question. In such cases, one can also consider how nontraditional healing practices can be sought after outside of the walls of the counseling center.

Ideally, these interventions would provide Jemele with a corrective emotional experience that would empower her to continue with her education. Termination issues would likely entail providing referrals if Jemele is interested in pursuing open-ended counseling services (potentially further addressing traumatic loss) and/or providing resources that would facilitate the maintenance of therapeutic gains (e.g., grounding, positive affirmations to combat pervasive messages of anti-Blackness).

REFERENCES

American Psychiatric Association. (2017). *Mental health disparities: African Americans.* https://www.psychiatry.org/psychiatrists/cultural-competency/education/african-american-patients

Arnold, F. W. (1993). "Time is not on our side": Cultural vs. structural explanations of Black American women students' achievement in the urban, non-elite university. *Urban Review, 25,* 199–220.

Association for University and College Counseling Center Directors (AUCCCD). (2018). *The association for university and college counseling center directors annual survey—public version 2018* (Reporting period July 1, 2017, through June 30, 2018). https://www.aucccd.org/assets/documents/Survey/2018%20AUCCCD%20Survey-Public-June%2012-FINAL.pdf

Avent Harris, J. R., & Wong, C. D. (2018). African American college students, the Black church, and counseling. *Journal of College Counseling, 21*(1), 15–28.

Bartman, C. C. (2015). African American women in higher education: Issues and support strategies. *College Student Affairs Leadership, 2*(2), Article 5. http://scholarworks.gvsu.edu/csal/vol2/iss2/5

Bayram, N., & Bilgel, N. (2008). The prevalence and socio-demographic correlations of depression, anxiety and stress among a group of university students. *Social Psychiatry and Psychiatric Epidemiology, 43,* 667–672. https://doi.org/10.1007/s00127-008-0345-x

Bewick, B., Koutsopoulou, G., Miles, J., Slaa, E., & Barkham, M. (2010). Changes in undergraduate students' psychological well-being as they progress through university. *Studies in Higher Education, 35*(6), 633–645. https://doi.org/10.1080/03075070903216643

Borum, V., & Walker, E. (2012). What makes the difference? Black women's undergraduate and graduate experiences in mathematics. *Journal of Negro Education, 81*(4), 366–378. https://doi.org/10.7709/jnegroeducation.81.4.0366

Center for Collegiate Mental Health (CCMH). (2019, January). *2018 Annual Report* (Publication No. STA 19–180). https://sites.psu.edu/ccmh/files/2019/01/2018-Annual-Report-1.30.19-ziytkb.pdf

Chapman, R. (2019, October). *Decolonizing Therapy 102: Advanced Clinical Practice with BIPOC.* Presented at the 2019 Carolina Conference on Queer Youth, Charlotte, NC.

Deming, D., Goldin, C., & Katz, L. (2013). For-profit colleges. *The Future of Children, 23*(1), 137–163.

Deo, M. E. (2013). Two sides of a coin: Safe space & segregation in race/ethnic-specific law student organizations. *Washington University Journal of Law and Policy, 42,* 83–129.

Eby, L. T., Allen, T. D., Evans, S. C., Ng, T., & DuBois, D. (2008). Does mentoring matter? A multidisciplinary meta-analysis comparing mentored and non-mentored individuals. *Journal of Vocational Behavior, 72*(2), 254–267. https://doi.org/10.1016/j.jvb.2007.04.005

Fedina, L., Holmes, J. L., & Backes, B. (2018). Campus sexual assault: A systematic review of prevalence research from 2000 to 2015. *Trauma, Violence, & Abuse, 19*(1), 76–93. https://doi.org/10.1177/1524838016631129

Flatt, A. K. (2013). A suffering generation: Six factors contributing to the mental health crisis in North American higher education. *College Quarterly, 16*(1). https://files.eric.ed.gov/fulltext/EJ1016492.pdf

Ford, J., & Soco-Marquez, J. G. (2016). Sexual assault victimization among straight, gay/lesbian, and bisexual college students. *Violence and Gender*, *3*(2), 107–115.

Ghio, L., Gotelli, S., Marcenaro, M., Amore, M., & Natta, W. (2014). Duration of untreated illness and outcomes in unipolar depression: A systematic review and meta-analysis. *Journal of Affective Disorders*, *152–154*, 45–51. https://doi.org/10.1016/j.jad.2013.10.002

Greyerbiehl, L., & Mitchell, D. (2014). An intersectional social capital analysis of the influence of historically Black sororities on African American women's college experiences at a predominantly White institution. *Journal of Diversity in Higher Education*, *7*(4), 282–294.

Griner, S. B., Vamos, C. A., Thompson, E. L., Logan, R., Vázquez-Otero, C., & Daley, E. M. (2017). The intersection of gender identity and violence: Victimization experienced by transgender college students. *Journal of Interpersonal Violence*, *35*(23–24), 5704–5725. https://doi.org/10.1177/0886260517723743

Guerra, M. (2013). Fact sheet: *The state of African American women in the United States*. https://www.americanprogress.org/issues/race/reports/2013/11/07/79165/fact-sheet-the-state-of-african-american-women-in-the-united-states/

Haag, P. (1997). Women and the path to college. *ERIC Review*, *5*(3), 10–13.

Hannon, C. R., Woodside, M., Pollard, B. L., & Roman, J. (2016). The meaning of African American college women's experiences attending a predominantly White institution: A phenomenological study. *Journal of College Student Development*, *57*(6), 652–666.

Harper, S. R., & Quaye, S. J. (2007). *Student organizations as venues for Black identity expression and development among African American male student leaders.* http://repository.upenn.edu/gse_pubs/166

Henry, W. J. (2008). Black female millennial college students: Dating dilemmas and identity development. *Multicultural Education*, *16*(2), 17–21.

Hinderlie, H. H., & Kenny, M. (2002). Attachment, social support, and college adjustment among Black students at predominantly White universities. *Journal of College Student Development*, *43*(3), 327–340.

hooks, b. (1981). *Ain't I a woman: Black women and feminism*. Boston, MA: South End Press.

Howard-Hamilton, M. F. (2003). Theoretical frameworks for African American women. *New Directions for Student Services*, *104*, 19–27.

Hughes, R. L., & Howard-Hamilton, M. F. (2004). Insights: Emphasizing issues that affect African American women. *New Directions for Student Services*, *2003*(104), 95–104.

Jackson, D. L. (2013). A balancing act: Impacting and initiating the success of African American female community college transfer students in STEM into the HBCU environment. *Journal of Negro Education*, *82*(3), 255–271. https://doi.org/10.7709/jnegroeducation.82.3.0255

Johnson, H. L. (2017). Pipelines, pathways, and institutional leadership: An update on the status of women in higher education. https://www.acenet.edu/Documents/Higher-Ed-Spotlight-Pipelines-Pathways-and-Institutional-Leadership-Status-of-Women.pdf

Keyes, C. L., Eisenberg, D., Perry, G. S., Dube, S. R., Kroenke, K., & Dhingra, S. S. (2012). The relationship of level of positive mental health with current mental disorders in predicting suicidal behavior and academic impairment in college students. *Journal of American College Health, 60*(2), 126–133. https://doi.org/10.1080/07448481.2011.608393

Kodama, C. & Laylo, R. (2017). The unique context of identity-based student organizations in developing leadership. *New Directions for Student Leadership, 2017*(155), 71–81.

Krebs, C. P., Barrick, K., Lindquist, C. H., Crosby, C. M., Boyd, C., & Bogan, Y. (2011). The sexual assault of undergraduate women at historically Black colleges and universities (HBCUs). *Journal of interpersonal violence, 26*(18), 3640–3666.

Lewis, J. A., Mendenhall, R., Harwood, S. A., & Browne Huntt, M. (2016). "Ain't I a woman?": Perceived gendered racial microaggressions experienced by Black women. *Counseling Psychologist, 44*(5), 758–780.

Lilly, F. R., Owens, J., Bailey, T. C., Ramirez, A., Brown, W., Clawson, C., & Vidal, C. (2018). The influence of racial microaggressions and social rank on risk for depression among minority graduate and professional students. *College Student Journal, 52*(1), 86–104.

Longmire-Avital, B., & Robinson, R. (2018). Young, depressed, and Black: A comparative exploration of depressive symptomatology among Black and White collegiate women. *Journal of College Student Psychotherapy, 32*(1), 53–72.

Lorde, A. (1988). *A burst of light: Essays.* Ithaca, NY: Firebrand Books.

Louis, D. A., Russell, S. S., Jackson, D. L., Blanchard, S. J., & Louis, S. L. (2014). Mentoring experiences of African American female students: Navigating the academy. *National Journal of Urban Education & Practice, 7*(3), 232–246.

Masuda, A., Anderson, P. L., & Edmonds, J. (2012). Help-seeking attitudes, mental health stigma, and self-concealment among African American college students. *Journal of Black Studies, 43*(7), 773–786. https://doi.org/10.1177/0021934712445806

McGuire, K., Casanova, S., & Davis, C. (2016). "I'm a Black female who happens to be Muslim": Multiple marginalities of an immigrant Black Muslim woman on a predominantly white campus. *Journal of Negro Education, 85*(3), 316–329. https://doi.org/10.7709/jnegroeducation.85.3.0316

Melendez, M. C., & Melendez, N. B. (2010). The influence of parental attachment on the college adjustment of White, Black, and Latina/Hispanic women: A cross-cultural investigation. *Journal of College Student Development, 51*(4), 419–435.

Moreno, D. R., & Sanchez Banuelos, S. M. (2013). The influence of Latina/o Greek sorority and fraternity involvement on Latina/o college student transition and success. *Journal of Latino/Latin American Studies, 5*(2), 113–125.

Munsey, C. (2006). Emerging adults: The in-between age. *Monitor on Psychology, 37*(7). http://www.apa.org/monitor/jun06/emerging

Museus, S. D. (2008). The role of ethnic student organizations in fostering African American and Asian American students' cultural adjustment and membership at predominantly White institutions. *Journal of College Student Development, 49*(6), 568–586. https://doi.org/10.1353/csd.0.0039

Parker, D., Summerfeldt, M., Hogan, S., & Majeski, S. (2004). Emotional intelligence and academic success: Examining the transition from high school to university. *Personality and Individual Difference, 36*, 163–172.

Perkins, L. (1998). The racial integration of the Seven Sister Colleges. *Journal of Blacks in Higher Education, 19*, 104–108. https://doi.org/10.2307/2998936

Renn, K. A., & Ozaki, C. C. (2010). Psychosocial and leadership identities among leaders of identity-based campus organizations. *Journal of Diversity in Higher Education, 3*(1), 14–26. https://doi.org/10.1037/a0018564

Rosales, A.M., & Person, D. R. (2003). Programming needs and student services for African American women. *New Directions for Student Services, 2003*(104), 53–65.

Salzer, M. S. (2012). A comparative study of campus experiences of college students with mental illnesses versus a general college sample. *Journal of American College Health, 60*(1), 1–7.

U.S. Department of Education, Institute of Education Sciences, National Center for Education Statistics. (2019a). *Status and trends in the education of racial and ethnic groups 2018* (NCES 2019–038). https://nces.ed.gov/pubs2019/2019038.pdf

U.S. Department of Education, National Center for Education Statistics. (2018). *The condition of education 2018* (NCES 2018144). https://nces.ed.gov/programs/coe/indicator_csc.asp

U.S. Department of Education, National Center for Education Statistics. (2019b). *Status and trends in the education of racial and ethnic groups 2018* (NCES 2019–038). https://nces.ed.gov/fastfacts/display.asp?id=72

Watt, S. K. (2006). Racial identity attitudes, womanist identity attitudes, and self-esteem in African American college women attending historically Black single-sex and coeducational institutions. *Journal of College Student Development, 47*(3), 319–334.

Williams, M. S., & Johnson, J. M. (2019). Predicting the quality of Black women collegians' relationships with faculty at a public historically Black university. *Journal of Diversity in Higher Education, 12*(2), 115–125. https://doi.org/10.1037/dhe0000077

Winkle-Wagner, R. (2015). Having their lives narrowed down? The state of Black women's college success. *Review of Educational Research, 85*(2), 171–204.

Winkle-Wagner, R., Kelly, B. T., Luedke, C. L., & Reavis, T. B. (2019). Authentically me: Examining expectations that are placed upon Black women in college. *American Educational Research Journal, 56*(2), 407–443.

Zamani, E. M. (2003). African American women in higher education. *New Directions for Student Services, 2003*(104), 5–18.

CHAPTER 15

Culturally Competent Counseling with Clients Identifying as Multiracial

Jasmine H. Winbush

It was less than 55 years ago that the U.S. Supreme Court officially allowed interracial marriage. A landmark case known as *Loving v. Virginia* put an end to laws that previously forbade interracial unions. Following this ruling, the number of interracial marriages surged from 150,000 (in 1960), to 1.6 million (in 1990), to 11 million (in 2015) (Jones & Bullock, 2012; Parker et al., 2015). This surge in interracial unions, in part, led to a significant increase in the number of multiracial babies, known as the "biracial baby boom." Recent estimates purport that multiracial adults make up more than 7 percent of the general population (Parker et al., 2015). The multiracial population continues to be one of the quickest-growing populations, with the U.S. Census Bureau projecting that the number of multiracial individuals will triple by 2060 (Parker et al., 2015).

Though there is increasing visibility of multiracial individuals, this is not a new population of people. In fact, there is an extensive, complicated, and painful history of multiracialism in the United States. We cannot understand multiracialism in the United States without discussing the agonizing history of Black–White relations in this country. While the years of slavery, Reconstruction era, and Jim Crow laws might seem like a distant memory to some, the residue remains in the consciousness and everyday experiences of Black and Black multiracial Americans.

It is necessary to briefly discuss terminology. In this chapter, the term *multiracial* will be used to describe individuals who identify as having roots from two or more different racial backgrounds. Due to the nature and content of this book, the word multiracial in this chapter refers to those who are Black multiracial—individuals who have African American heritage plus one or more additional racial backgrounds. There are varying views on the currently accepted way to describe individuals identifying as having one or more races, including mixed-race, multiracial, biracial, and mixed, just to name a few. The use of multiracial in this chapter is for simplicity purposes and in no way attempts to erase or simplify the complexity surrounding the multiracial community. Words that some view as derogatory and have a painful historical connotation, such as mulatto, are used in this chapter when providing historical context. Also, when describing certain studies or references, the terminology used by those authors will be replicated.

HISTORY

Having a Black multiracial identity can lead to a diverse number of racial backgrounds. Although Black and White biracial individuals only encompass one manifestation of Black multiracial individuals, it is imperative to explore the deep-rooted history of Black–White relations in this country. Dating back to the Colonial era, marriage and cohabitation between "non-Whites"[1] and Whites was made illegal through anti-miscegenation laws. These laws were intended to reinforce separation between Whites and Blacks and uphold the racial hierarchy wherein Whites maintained power and dominance. It's important to mention that while interracial sexual contact was technically illegal, interracial sex was not a rarity. Because those enslaved were considered property, it was not uncommon for White slave owners to rape those they enslaved. Though White slave owner/ Black slave rape was certainly not the only form of interracial sex during this time, it was very common (Pilgrim, 2000).

In fact, interracial sexual contact happened so frequently that a large number of biracial babies, or "mulattos" as they were termed at the time, were born. This class of Black–White biracial people needed to be categorized into racial groups because the current systems and structures that delineated freedom, power, and privilege were all race based. Traditionally, the paternal heritage defined the child's heritage and freedom status (Moran, 2004). This would mean a large number of biracial individuals (with predominantly White fathers and Black mothers) would be considered White and free. However, this worried White slaveholders because it would lead to an increasing number of free biracial people—with potential loyalties to their Black, enslaved mothers. A rise of biracial people

---

[1] Anti-miscegenation laws primarily targeted relationships between Blacks and Whites, though some Western states also banned unions between Whites/Asians and Whites/ Native Americans (Moran, 2004).

with power and freedom would also mean a reduction in the number of enslaved biracial individuals. As a result, the people in power (White men) changed the rules surrounding heritage, lineage, and freedom status. It was decided that a biracial child's heritage and freedom status would be based on the maternal lineage, resulting in an increase in the number of enslaved rather than free people (Moran, 2004). This is one of the early examples of how multiracialism was decided and defined by those in power, in direct relation to social standards and pressures of the time.

Linking a biracial child to their (typically) Black mother was one way to perpetuate the notion that any amount of Blackness eliminates all Whiteness. The "one-drop rule" formally and structurally decided that White and Black blood were fundamentally different. One drop of Black blood would, in essence, contaminate any amount of White blood, heritage, and lineage (Davis, 2005). This maintained the pseudoscientific notion of White purity and ensured that Whites maintained their position at the top of the power structure. It also meant that Whites continued having authority to define what it meant to be Black or White.

Though mulattos were officially deemed Black, they often had more privileges than Black individuals who did not have (or appear to have) any White heritage. Enslaved Blacks were bought, sold, deeded, insured, gifted, and mortgaged the same way we manage our assets today. Physique, work ability, age, fertility, and behavior were just some of the categories that were valued in the slave trade. In many slave markets, an enslaved mulatto female was sold at a high price due to her alleged sexual seductiveness, physical features, and accessibility to Blackness yet association with Whiteness. To be clear, both enslaved Black and mulatto females were objectified, sexualized, and raped. However, enslaved mulattos were seen as a status symbol and indicator of wealth for many White slave owners (Pilgrim, 2000).

The "tragic mulatto" (most often portrayed as a Black–White woman with lighter skin) became a pervasive trope. This descriptor designates Black–White biracial women as fundamentally and hopelessly confused, sad, and lost between a White and Black world. The image of a tragic mulatto aims to highlight how unnatural and harmful it is for Blacks and Whites to procreate. In other words, the challenges faced by the tragic mulatto are inherently related to the non-humane mixing of races rather than a racist, sexist, White-supremacist environment and society (Pilgrim, 2000).

Even after the institution of slavery "ended," a social and political need existed to define one's multiraciality and find one's place within the racial hierarchy. Segregation between Whites and Blacks wasn't the only line in the sand being drawn. Dissonance among people of color existed. Free people of color (Blacks and mulattos who already had their freedom) felt threatened that their status and opportunities were now in competition with newly freed Blacks and mulattos.

The Black community used physical features, primarily skin color, to separate classes of Blacks and mulattos. For example, some social clubs only allowed Blacks whose skin color was lighter than a brown paper bag, also known as "paper bag tests." The "blue vein test" asserted that if your veins were visible through your skin, then you were seen as a part of the more privileged class of people of color. Though a lighter skin color was the primary determinant of status, the "comb test" was also used. If a comb passed through your hair without too much effort, then you were allowed many more privileges (Kerr, 2005). Understanding this history about within-community bias—which almost always exists due to external systematic injustices and discrimination—gives some context to the complicated importance of skin color, and other physical characteristics, within the Black and Black multiracial community today.

A central theme to notice from this brief historical overview of Black multiracialism in the United States is the vehement need to define, classify, and even monoracialize multiracial individuals. This defining of multiracial identities has happened throughout time by way of laws, social standards, pseudoscience, linguistics, institutions, and politics. The Black multiracial history is unique: in some ways, multiracial people were just as oppressed as other Black people; in other ways, multiracial people were given preferential status and privilege; and, at times, multiracial people were doubly oppressed via objectification, sexualization, and exoticization.

MULTIRACIAL IDENTITY

Identity Development

Racial autonomy (the ability to decide one's racial identity) has been taken away from Black multiracial people, both formally (e.g., one-drop rule) and informally (e.g., tragic mulatto propaganda) over the years. Although there has been an increase in visibility of multiracial people in recent years, misconceptions and stereotypes still prevail (e.g., multiracial individuals in chronic identity distress). In order to better understand the inner world of multiracial people, it's helpful to discuss multiracial identity development. Racial identity development refers to a complex process of how an individual understands, labels, and experiences their race/ethnicity (Poston, 1990).

In the wake of the civil rights era and Black power movement, identity development models for people of color emerged (Cross, 1971). Many of these models include a progression from conformity with majority culture, dissonance and rejection of majority culture, immersion and pride in minority culture, and integration of all aspects of one's identity (Atkinson, Morten, & Sue, 1979; Helms, 1995). However, these models do not necessarily holistically capture the experience of multiracial individuals because they "do not recognize the social complexity of adopting a biracial [or multiracial] identity in a monoracially defined social world" (Miville, 2005, 303).

Poston (1990) and Root (1990, 1996) were two of the first scholars to research multiracial identity development. Poston was groundbreaking in delineating that multiracial identity development differed from minority monoracial identity development. His model asserted that the multiracial experience is not one comprised of deficits and that a biracial identity can, in fact, result in a healthy racial identity. Though Poston's model was innovative, it assumed a relatively fixed developmental progression through stages and failed to explicitly incorporate the role that a discriminatory and racist society plays in one's identity development. Root's model (1990, 1996) did take into consideration the fluid and contextual nature of multiracial identities. She also assumed there could be multiple healthy expressions of multiracial identity, which differed from most other multiracial identity development models that assumed integration of all identities was the only healthy identity outcome. In recent years, there has been a growing interest in the different factors that can impact multiracial peoples' identity development.

Factors Impacting Identity Development

A multiracial individual might identify with one, both, or all of their different racial backgrounds. Although there is no single narrative or specific formula that predicts how a multiracial individual will identify, there are known factors and variables that can affect multiracial identity development. Physical appearance, cultural knowledge, social class, gender, family of origin, community, geographic region, first name/surname, and age are just a few of these factors.

Physical appearance—including skin color, hair (e.g., texture, color, style), eye (e.g., shape, color), facial features, and body type and size—can affect multiracial identity development. One reason physical appearance is so frequently tied to racial identity is because it is one of the initial ways that society perceives one's racial group membership. In a country founded on racism, colorism, and White supremacism, one's outward appearance is often directly tied to how others classify one's racial group membership. A landmark Pew Research Center study reports that 47 percent of multiracial individuals surveyed said they did not identify as multiracial because they only "look like" one race (Parker et al., 2015). Of these same people surveyed, 21 percent mentioned that at some point in their lifetime they changed something about their physical appearance (e.g., their hair or how they dressed) in order to influence how others perceived their racial identity. These findings speak to the significant role appearance plays in racial group identification.

Social environment (family, peers, neighborhood, school systems, and online social networks) is another huge factor that impacts multiracial identity development. Some research has shown that family influence is the most significant contributor to multiracial identity development (Quintana, 2007). Specifically, parental racial socialization—how parents approach issues surrounding race, racial identity, racial knowledge, and racial pride—can significantly impact how a multiracial child perceives their own racial group membership (Peters, 1985). Peters (1985) emphasizes that racial socialization with children of color is more than simply just discussing race; rather, it is "a set of overt and covert behaviors parents use, over and above those responsibilities shared by all parents, to psychologically prepare children for success in a racially stratified American society" (562). Many multiracial people realize at some point in childhood that they look different than one or both of their parents or other family members. How parents and family respond to this realization can affect a child's racial identity development process.

The diversity of one's neighborhood and school also influence racial identity development. Racially diverse communities tend to lead to fewer negative experiences (e.g., discrimination, questioning of one's race, alienation, etc.) for multiracial people (LaBarrie, 2007). Because social networks are much more expansive than they were at one time (through social media, for example), it's possible for multiracial people to find social networks either similar or dissimilar to their actual physical environments/communities, which can aid in their identity development.

One's *cultural knowledge and exposure* can also affect multiracial identity development. Cultural knowledge and exposure refers to awareness of and experience with the history, values, language, music, current events, and the struggle of their unique heritage groups. The assumption is that increased cultural knowledge and exposure to a particular racial/heritage group will increase one's identification and connection with that group (Peters, 1985).

Age is another factor that plays a role in multiracial identity development. Root (2004) suggests that the sociopolitical time in which a multiracial woman is raised significantly impacts her identity development process. She outlines three generations of multiracial women: the Exotic Generation (born before the late '60s), the Vanguard Generation ('60s and late '70s), and the Baby Boomer Generation (born after the late '80s/post-civil rights).

The Exotic Generation did not have a visible cohort of other multiracial people and were born during segregated times, prior to many racial pride movements. Root (2004) explains that some dealt with their invisibility by using their "mixed appearance [as a] part of their specialness" (24). This exoticness was a double-edged sword; although it gave multiracial women a form of identity, it also perpetuated their otherness and chances of objectification. Root (2004) notes that this generation might currently struggle with the heightened visibility of the Baby Boomer Generation. Root (2004) explained a woman from the Exotic Generation "may feel replaced not only due to age, but also due to the greater acceptance that the younger cohort experiences. The public media deals with the young cohort of mixed race people as though they are new" (Root, 2004, 24).

The Vanguard Generation were coming of age after the *Loving v. Virginia* ruling and attended desegregated schools. Root (2004) describes this generation as less "traumatized" than the previous generation due to increased visibility, acceptance, and racial discourse (e.g., through ethnic minority pride movements, race-based campus organizations, etc.). She explains this generation felt less tied to monoracial identities and began to explore multiracial identities and question the concept of race.

The Baby Boomer Generation is characterized by their significant visibility (in their friend groups, family, classmates, media, etc.) compared to previous generations. As a result, Root (2004) describes this generation as more comfortable with bending racial boundaries in the way in which they identify, discuss, and challenge racial notions. However, Root (2004) notes this generation can face challenges when they move to new communities (e.g., go to college) that differ from their home environments as they might have to face their multiracial identity for the first time. Though this cohort still does experience racism and otherness based on their multiracial identities, the multiracial baby boomers might find it harder to interpret these experiences of oppression and racism as they are more covert.

Root (2004) only outlines three generations of multiracial women, due to the time of her publication. There is another generation of multiracial women coming of age in the alleged "post-racial" society in which we currently live. A potential and fitting name for this generation of multiracial women is the Visible Generation. The increase in visibility of multiracial people in media, politics, sports, the arts, and so on affords the younger generations of multiracial people opportunities to see other people who are like them. Though this increased visibility is largely positive, there are a few drawbacks that are worth discussing.

Increasing visibility can, at times, lead to a larger stage for objectification, exoticization, and stereotyping. For example, in 2019, a show called *Mixed-ish* premiered. It was the first of its kind to chronicle a multiracial (Black mother, White father, three multiracial children) family's experience living in the '80s. Many people who identify as multiracial, or are close to the multiracial experience (e.g., a monoracial parent of a multiracial child), find comfort, humor, and representation in the show. However, some suggest that shows like this might make "outsiders" (none multiracial people) feel like they have an understanding of the multiracial experience simply through watching the show. They may not understand that some of the stereotypes or jokes used might be appropriate for in-group members, but should not infiltrate out-group members' understandings, colloquialisms, or assumptions about multiracial individuals.

One drawback of the Visibility Generation is the increased risk for exploitation. In recent years, industries such as the fashion industry, advertising, and film have attempted to diversify in terms of race, ethnicity, gender, body size and type, and so on. Many racially ambiguous women are sought out in casting, esteemed in music videos, and seen as physical status symbols. Though an immense privilege comes with this visibility, it can also replicate the objectification of multiracial women as it implies their worth is due to their physical appearance. Some posit that in advertising, racially ambiguous multiracial women are used as ways to sell products to a mass audience, as they have physical features that can reach multiple racial groups. There is also an undercurrent that multiracial people are used in advertising and the media to promote the (dangerous) myth of a utopian, color-blind society.

The Visibility Generation is also tasked with curing racism. The narrative that it is multiracial people's job or calling to end racism is not only wrong, but potentially harmful. Though the United States is becoming more diverse, the simple presence of more multiracial people or the increase in multiracial children will not end White supremacy. Those who benefit from White supremacy hold the primary responsibility of, first, acknowledging White supremacy and, then, working toward deconstructing systematically racist power structures. Unfortunately, in recent years, the increase of multiracial people and immigrants has been used as political propaganda to instill fear about the increase in Black and Brown people and the diminishing White race—inciting fear, hatred, and violence. Our pseudo "post-racial" society, allegedly initiated by having our first Black multiracial president, has created a false folklore that denies the current presence of structural racism. The post-racial society fantasy has the potential of liberating people of privilege from their guilt. A passive blending of racial lines is now expected to end racism, as opposed to an active dismantling of White supremacy.

There are many examples of multiracial people who are provided a visible platform and a seat at the table, when their monoracial Black brothers and sisters are not. While this certainly can cause tension, discord, and resentment among communities of color, many multiracial people feel being a part of the fight for Black equality utilizes their unique position of being both the oppressor and the oppressed (e.g., in the case of Black–White biracial individuals).

While multiracial people can certainly play an important role in this fight, implying that they are solely responsible for fixing the long, painful racial history in this country is overly simplistic and a disservice to everyone involved. Those at the top of the power structure and benefiting the most from White privilege must play an active role.

Fluidity of Identity

Because factors influencing multiracial identity development can change (e.g., cultural knowledge and exposure, geographic location, one's peer group, etc.), so can one's racial identification. One of the unique and, arguably, most salient aspects of the development and expression of multiracial identity is how fluid it can be. Fluidity refers to one's ability to shift their racial identification across time, space, and situations. While some multiracial people have racial identities that are unchanging with all social contexts and consistent across time, it is also common for multiracial people to have fluid identities that change over time and/or change as a function of their immediate environment. The Pew Institute reports, "About three-in-ten adults with a multiracial background say that they have changed the way they describe their race over the years—with some saying they once thought of themselves as only one race and now think of themselves as more than one race, and others saying just the opposite" (Parker et al., 2015, 8). Though some might wonder if this fluidity is associated with confusion and distress, plenty of multiracial people (particularly those born in later generations) see their racial fluidity as a strength. So, one might ask, "What *is* a healthy multiracial identity?" One of the most important factors in healthy multiracial identity development is that individuals' racial identity "fit" both their internal world (e.g., self-perceptions) and external world (e.g., social environment). A sense of "fit" leads to higher self-esteem, a higher sense of efficacy, and lower stereotype vulnerability (Bracey, Bámaca, & Umaña-Taylor, 2004; Shih & Sanchez, 2009). A significant part of a multiracial person's feeling of "fit" is how others validate or invalidate their identity.

Validation and Invalidation

Root (1990) explains "self–concept is in part internalized by the reflection of self in others' reactions" (579). Rockquemore and Brunsma reiterate that "identities are interactionally validated self-understandings" (2004, 93). It is often through social interactions that multiracial identities are tested, ascribed, and validated/invalidated. When our social environment validates our self-defined racial identity, there is a level of congruence that leads to feelings of acceptance, belongingness, and psychological well-being (Rockquemore & Brunsma, 2004). When our social environment invalidates our self-defined racial identity, there is a level of incongruence that can lead to feelings of rejection, a constant need to defend one's authenticity to desired racial group, and "cultural homelessness" (i.e., being a perpetual out-group member) (Gillem & Thompson, 2004, 10).

Family relationships play a large role in validation/invalidation of one's self-defined identity. As noted earlier in the chapter, family and parental socialization is one of the largest contributing factors to multiracial identity development. It can be particularly painful when one's family is the invalidating source. It is common for multiracial people to experience explicit invalidation and microaggressive rejection within their families. Sometimes this is related to extended family members who may or may not have any direct experience with the multiracial person's "other side" of the family (Nadal et al., 2013). One Black–White biracial client expressed shock and confusion as she recalled the first time she heard the "White side" of her family make racist remarks about Black people.

Looking "different" from other members in one's nuclear and/or extended family can lead to validation/invalidation. Experiences of favoritism within families are noted by many multiracial people. For example, if a multiracial girl has lighter or darker skin than the rest of their family members, they might get either overvalued or undervalued, either of which can cause feelings of otherness, distress, and disdain from other family members.

While invalidation from family members is certainly painful, having your identity invalidated by others in your social environment (strangers, coworkers, bosses, romantic interests, friends, etc.) can also cause distress. Many multiracial people have heard that they are "too this" or "too that." For example, "You're not Black, you talk too proper"; "You're not a real Dominican, you don't even have an accent"; "You date White guys, so that makes you White"; "Are you sure you're mixed? You don't have mixed hair!"

Authenticity Testing

Many multiracial people face pressure to pass authenticity tests. Authenticity testing is an injunction for one to prove that they are an insider within a particular racial group. These authenticity tests can be in the form of peer pressure, joking, teasing, or hazing the multiracial person to demonstrate knowledge of and attachment to the culture, history, and political interests of the racial group in question. Conforming to certain cultural norms related to language, accent, clothing, music, food, romantic partners, hobbies, and so on are all fair game to prove/disprove authenticity. Root (1998) explains "the standards for passing such a test are fluid and determined by the one giving the test; thus, whether one passes or fails the authenticity test is largely determined not by one's insider knowledge, but often by the tester's assumptions about the individual or about mixed-race people in general" (243).

Though not exclusive to one particular racial group, authenticity tests frequently occur within the Black community and are rooted in the ways Blacks have been historically excluded and oppressed by Whites (Root, 1998). Racially ambiguous people, lighter-skinned Black multiracial people, and/or Black multiracial people who don't appear to have Black cultural experiences are often the target of authenticity tests (Root, 1998). This makes sense if we think back to how mulattos and lighter-skinned Blacks were provided more privilege and opportunities than other Black individuals (i.e., preferential treatment, increased value in slave trade, admittance to social clubs, etc.). The history of competition among minority group members due to scarcity of opportunity and resources plays a role in why many Black multiracial people now need to prove their Blackness.

Passing

The painful history of mistrust and skin color–based privilege also provides context for the modern dilemma and controversy surrounding "passing" within the Black and Black multiracial community. Many times, passing isn't a choice at all—others just assume your race and treat you accordingly. For example, if you are multiracial with physical characteristics that others immediately "validate" as Black/African American, then you are likely living a Black experience, which in America is an experience wrought with discrimination, oppression, and a constant threat of violence. However, if you are multiracial with lighter skin or racially ambiguous, the notion of passing might be considered a privilege that one has. Along with this privilege comes an inherent conflict. For example, if you can pass as White (say, at job interviews, when getting pulled over by the cops, when living everyday life), does that mean you *should* pass (i.e., by denying your Black heritage)? Having the ability to make this choice is an innate privilege (and, likely, will require authenticity testing from those without this privilege).

Triple Jeopardy

Multiracial women face a "triple jeopardy": sexism, racism, and the pressures of monoracialism (Rockquemore & Brunsma, 2004). Multiracial women, like all women, have to navigate a sexist society, which can impact them in many different ways. One manifestation of this is that the Black multiracial woman's physical appearance becomes even more complicated as physical traits and beauty are often associated with a woman's value and worth. Some multiracial women's racial ambiguity (not looking like any identifiable racial group) or racial ubiquity (simultaneously looking like multiple racial groups) leads to the label of looking "exotic" (Hall, 2004). To some, the label of exotic can increase feelings of uniqueness, beauty, and pride. To others, the exotic label can perpetuate feelings of objectification and otherness. Being exoticized can distance the multiracial woman from the racial group with which she seeks acceptance. For example, "some believe the subdued features afford multiracial women better treatment by Whites . . . this pits mixed-race women against monorace women" (Hall, 2004, 241). This can be an even more painful experience if being exoticized leads to tension among friends and family members, resulting in perpetual invalidation, othering, and/or authenticity testing.

Multiracial women have to navigate a racist society like other people of color (though skin color absolutely plays a role in the level of racism/

colorism experienced). There can be an additional layer of stress living in a traditionally monoracial society as there are frequent experiences of inval- idation and a search for belongingness (Rockquemore & Brunsma, 2004). Many racial identity development models for people of color discuss that immersion in one's own racial minority group can provide a refuge from a racist society; however, a multiracial person may never find complete acceptance and similarity in one of their racial background groups.

It is also essential to mention that there is a quadruple jeopardy for multiracial women who do not identify as heterosexual or cisgender. Lesbian, bisexual, pansexual, queer, and transgender multiracial women are exposed to sexism, racism, monoracialism, and heterosexism/ transphobia. Bisexual and lesbian women of color are more likely to experience violence (as compared to bisexual and lesbian White women) (Bing, 2004). Some multiracial women have noted the exhaustion of hav- ing to repeatedly "come out" and explain their racial identity across vari- ous spaces and places while also having to "come out" in regard to their sexual identity (Bing, 2004). Others have noted that their racial and ethnic "bi-ness" impacted their ability to see sexuality and gender on a spectrum, facilitating their process of later identifying as lesbian or bisexual (Israel, 2004). Though not within the scope of this chapter, it is critical to note that there is a dire need for more attention, research, and care in regard to the multiracial gender nonconforming and trans communities as they experi- ence increased levels of violence, oppression, and attempted suicide rates (Herman, Brown, & Haas, 2019).

Strengths

Though identity challenges are common among multiracial women, it is important to note that these challenges are contextual. In other words, being multiracial is often a problem with the environment, not an intrinsic flaw with multiracialism itself. A client of mine once confidently and wryly said, "I don't have identity problems. They have problems identifying me." Ironically, having to undergo frequent social pressure, authenticity testing, and searching for belongingness can lead to a strong sense of self. Though trying at times, this can lead a multiracial woman to feel strong, rooted, resilient. Another client once likened her identity development process to test-driving cars, explaining, "If you've been forced to test drive every car on the lot, three times over, you're going to have an upper hand on every- one else who hasn't had to do that." She was alluding to the notion that she feels an unwavering sense of confidence and sense of self due to having to examine her own identity frequently and from an early age.

Research demonstrates that multiracial individuals often navigate diverse environments with more ease than monoracial individuals. Hav- ing a flexible worldview informed by various racial backgrounds can facil- itate the multiracial woman's ability to adapt to different environments.

Research suggests that many multiracial individuals have increased cognitive flexibility and creative problem-solving skills (Latson, 2019).

Many multiracial people have astute social skills due to their experiences in reading others' reactions, assumptions, and perceptions. Sometimes feeling "othered," or like an outsider looking in, can increase multiracial people's ability to quickly and accurately read others' verbal and nonverbal behavior. This can lead to a diverse and flexible set of social skills that can positively impact one's ability to navigate various challenges (Garbarini-Philippe, 2010).

MULTIRACIAL WOMEN IN THERAPY: TREATMENT CONSIDERATIONS AND RECOMMENDATIONS

Rapport and Intake

At the first point of contact, it is crucial that the provider and therapeutic atmosphere convey safety, openness, cultural awareness, and sensitivity. This is particularly important when working with Black multiracial women as they can be incredibly perceptive of environmental indicators of cultural openness and intuitively sense how others are perceiving them (Remedios & Chasteen, 2013). The vigilance it can take to be perpetually keyed into others' reactions and nonverbal behaviors can be an exhausting experience for the multiracial woman. To have a therapeutic relationship that does not perpetuate this exhausting dynamic can be powerful. Thus, building rapport is essential and should be the therapist's primary focus early on. Allowing the client to feel truly heard and seen, without having to defend, explain, or authenticate, requires intentionality and multicultural savviness of the therapist.

The therapist must remember that they themselves might represent a particular group of people from which the client might be seeking/ expecting racial identity validation/invalidation. Within a matter of seconds, the multiracial client might be asking themselves questions such as: "Can my Black therapist understand my experience?" "Will my multiracial therapist resent me for 'passing'?" "Will my White multiracial therapist judge me for wanting to be monoracial?" "Will my Latinx therapist speak English or Spanish to me first?" If a strong rapport exists, the therapist and client can discuss the multiracial client's expectations, experiences, desires, and fears related to the therapist's validation/invalidation of the client, if relevant.

Just because the therapist might be confused or caught off guard by the multiracial woman's presentation in therapy, this does not necessarily mean the client herself is confused. Root (2004) notes that in therapy, multiracial women might consciously or unconsciously adjust their behavior (e.g., code switching, changing the way they're wearing their hair, etc.) to assess the person with whom they're interacting. Root explains that this behavior "is often a survival skill used to assess the social environment and search for cues of danger. The woman who uses this a lot does not feel safe; this needs to be processed" (2004, 26). Additionally, some multiracial women might present as skeptical about the world or intentions of others. This could be related to being frequently judged or misperceived by others, experiencing cultural homelessness, or being privy to racist remarks from those who do not recognize their racial affiliation. The therapist's patience, transparency, genuineness, and authenticity are helpful in healthily disarming the client's skepticism.

Use intake forms with options where clients can write in their own responses rather than having to choose races/ethnicities, sexual identities, genders, religions, and so on. Simply encouraging racial autonomy and allowing the client to describe herself, without any forced choices, can be a corrective experience and indicate that the therapist makes no assumptions. Demonstrate flexibility, openness, and fluidity with a more unstructured intake interview that encourages the multiracial woman to tell her own story about herself and her mental health.

Conceptualization

There are two important points to prioritize when conceptualizing your client. Your conceptualization should be 1) contextual and 2) strengths based. Because multiracial women's lived experiences are so often affected by their environments, contextual and sociocultural factors must be included in the clinical conceptualization to avoid over pathologizing the client's struggles. Taking a strengths-based approach involves identifying how a client's strengths, internal resources, and protective factors contribute to her overall history and presentation. Although multiracial identity is contextualized within treatment, it should not be assumed that Black multiracial women's presenting concern is related to their racial identity. Clinical conceptualizations must move away from the one-dimensional perspective of multiracial women as "other," "confused," and marginalized and move toward viewing her as dimensional, adaptable, resilient, and whole (Edwards & Pedrotti, 2004). Utilizing a multicultural feminist lens can be a helpful framework for conceptualizing your multiracial client in an informed, empowered way.

Therapy Models

In terms of treatment modalities, therapeutic approaches, and interventions, I recommend using *relational* and *narrative* approaches. Relational theories posit that relationships and connection are the motivating force for humans (DeYoung, 2015). Thus, relationships play a significant role in both our suffering and our healing. Principles of relational approaches involve the therapist intentionally using empathy, attentiveness, collaboration, and authenticity to identify sources of relational disconnection related to suffering and discern how this relates to the client's understanding of themselves and others. Multiracial women do not exist within a cultural vacuum, and their relationships with themselves and others are almost always intricately related to their presenting concern.

Relational approaches assert that the therapeutic relationship can be a powerful tool for healing (DeYoung, 2015). The therapeutic relationship might be the first relationship where the client can openly explore their thoughts and feelings about self-perceptions and others' perceptions. Validation, here-and-now processing, interpretation, and thoughtful challenging can increase insight and provide a source for reparative experiences. This requires the therapist to do their own work to ensure they are culturally informed, culturally literate, and aware of their biases and assumptions.

Narrative approaches are also incredibly useful with multiracial clients. Narrative therapy asserts that "each individual creates her own reality and understands it from her own unique perspective. This reality is in constant flux, changing as the individual gains new experiences and information" (Edwards & Pedrotti, 2004, 39). Narrative approaches maintain that the client is not the problem; the problem is the problem. This assumption that psychopathology is socioculturally rooted allows for a holistic understanding of the multiracial client and a flexible, individualized treatment approach. Externalization of issues can be a powerful experience for the multiracial woman who has internalized feelings of objectification, lack of belonging, cultural homelessness, oppression, and so on. Additionally, narrative approaches see the client as the expert of their experience and utilize their strengths and internal resources to help them be the author of their own story, through collaborative work with the therapist. This can be empowering for the multiracial woman who has experienced a lack of racial autonomy, cultural homelessness, or frequent misunderstanding and misperceptions by others. When a therapist helps a multiracial client look back toward past experiences and examine their current experiences, new meaning can be made.

CASE STUDY

Let's consider the case of Lucita, a 24-year-old self-identified biracial, bisexual, cisgender female with a Mexican American father and African American mother. She was raised by her African American mother in a predominantly Black neighborhood in a suburban East Coast city. Growing up, her friend group was predominantly African American. Lucita's parents never married, and her father passed away when she was two years old. She explained her only connection with her Mexican American side of her family was with her paternal grandmother, with whom she spent every summer throughout her childhood. Lucita describes herself as having "medium brown" skin, brown eyes, and black, thick, straight hair.

Lucita indicated that growing up, she always identified as Black as she looked similar to many of her African American peers, and few realized she had Mexican heritage as her father was not around. However, she explained there were "small things" (like using different hair products than her mother, her Spanish-sounding name, enjoying being in the sun to "get darker") that often made her "feel different" from her mother and friends. During summers with her paternal grandmother, she described being filled with excitement about exploring her Mexican heritage but often felt like a "fraud" because she talked, dressed, and acted slightly differently than she did when she was back home. She explained that her paternal cousins often commented on how "American" she was. Although Lucita was confident in her appearance, generally happy, well-adjusted, and had a strong support system, she couldn't help always feeling like "something was missing" or like she was "playing the role of Lucita, not actually being Lucita."

When Lucita went away to a predominantly White college, she found herself inundated with her new peers' questions regarding her racial and ethnic identity. Her new Black peers were thrown off by her "Spanish-sounding" name, her Latino peers were thrown off by her Black physical appearance, and her White peers seemed fascinated by the "wonderful contradictions" in her physical appearance (as one of her White peers stated). She found herself surprised that, given this new opportunity, she was uncertain how to label herself. After a few positive experiences with the Latinx student organization on campus, she immersed herself in friend groups, student activities, and experiences that were centered around other Latinos. She eventually decided to major in Spanish and Latin American Studies. She began identifying as Afro-Latina as she felt this encompassed her attachment to both her African and Mexican ancestry.

At the time she presented for treatment, she had recently graduated from college and was experiencing grief over the recent death of her mother. Without her mother and father alive, she described feeling like she was "floating alone" in the world. She was experiencing sadness, insomnia, bouts of crying, overeating, weight gain, difficulties concentrating, feelings of hopelessness, and irritability. During the first session, she indicated she felt like most of her current suffering was related to regret that she "spent so long searching for [her]self and wanting to connect with [her] father, in whatever way possible, that [she] missed time with [her] mom that [she'll] never get back."

Initial therapy sessions focused on allowing Lucita a safe space to grieve. She needed a space to unload all of her regret, anger, and doubt freely. Rapport was built through the therapist aligning with Lucita in validating her feelings, without changing, challenging, or interpreting any of Lucita's thoughts, feelings, or experiences. This alignment and validation set the stage for later narrative work in that it allowed Lucita to be an expert of her current experience without having to defend, explain, or justify. The therapist focused first on providing stability, support, and nurturance through Lucita's grieving. During this early stage, the therapist made it known that all her identities were important but encouraged Lucita to talk about this in session when it felt relevant to her. This intentional decision was made in an effort to let Lucita know that the therapist was aware that her grief might also be tied to her race/ethnicity but allowed Lucita to determine when this felt important to discuss. When these identity topics were discussed, the therapist reflected nonjudgmentally, facilitated conversation about common themes related to her racial/ethnic/sexual identities, assessed Lucita's level of congruence with her identities, and self-disclosed thoughtfully and intentionally. The therapist was intentionally authentic and appropriately transparent as a way to allow Lucita to focus on grieving and reduce her worry about the therapist's perceptions. The therapist's thoughtful self-disclosure, patience, and stability encouraged Lucita to start to see herself as a knowledgeable, essential, and collaborative contributor to the therapeutic experience.

As therapy progressed, the therapist used narrative interventions to better understand Lucita's story about her childhood, her racial/ethnic identity, and her current sense of self. First, the therapist focused on understanding Lucita's narrative and how it has served her and/or caused her suffering. Then the therapist worked alongside Lucita to empower her to reauthor her story in a way that reduced turmoil, dissonance, and disconnection with herself and others.

Through validation, understanding of Lucita's reality, challenging, processing of difficult emotions, externalization, and deconstruction of problems, the therapist helped Lucita make meaning of her new reality through a narrative that better captured her truth. She was not a woman floating. She was actually quite grounded and secure in her identity, even though it became more complex and complicated with the loss of both of her parents. The therapist normalized and validated that she was terribly sad, of course, to be without her mother and father—overwhelmed, of course, with a wish to have more time with both of her parents. But the therapist worked alongside her to include in her narrative that she was still complete, whole, and capable of dealing with the struggles associated with her current reality. Her current feelings of confusion, loss, and anger were processed and understood within the context of her history, racial/ethnic/sexual identities, and grief.

Lucita was introspective, psychologically minded, confident, open, resilient, and compassionate. The therapist not only emphasized these strengths with Lucita (with the hopes of her incorporating them into her self-narrative) but used these strengths in the therapeutic work. Lucita's ability to be compassionate and understand multiple perspectives helped her practice more self-compassion. Her resiliency and confidence helped her take an active role in reconstructing narratives that made sense to her.

For this client, what seemed to be most useful was 1) allowing her time at the beginning of therapy to grieve without a rush to pathologize, interpret, or challenge in any way; 2) the therapeutic relationship—the creation of trust, understanding, safety, and alignment that allowed the therapist to join in as an active collaborator in Lucita's healing process; and 3) narrative techniques that helped Lucita make meaning of her experiences, using her unique strengths.

Toward the end of treatment, Lucita became pregnant. She was, like most women, full of conflicting emotions of excitement, fear, anxiety, love, and hope. But, most importantly, she was thrilled for this next part of her life narrative and couldn't wait to tell her future baby how lucky she was to have all of this beautifully wonderful Black, Mexican, Afro-Latina heritage.

REFERENCES

Atkinson, D., Morten, G., & Sue, D. W. (1979). *Counseling American minorities: A cross-cultural perspective.* Dubuque, IA: W. C. Brown Company.

Bing, V. M. (2004). Out of the closet but still in hiding: Conflicts and identity issues for a Black–White biracial lesbian. In A. R. Gillem & C. Thompson (Eds.), *Biracial women in therapy: Between the rock of gender and the hard place of race* (pp. 185–202). New York, NY: Haworth Press.

Bracey, J. R., Bámaca, M. Y., & Umaña-Taylor, A. J. (2004). Examining ethnic identity and self-esteem among biracial and monoracial adolescents. *Journal of Youth and Adolescence, 33*(2), 123–132. https://doi.org/10.1023/b:joyo.0000013424.93635.68

Cross, W. E., Jr. (1971). Toward a psychology of Black liberation: The Negro-to-Black conversion experience. *Black World, 20*(9), 13–27.

Davis, F. J. (2005). *Who is Black? One nation's definition.* University Park, PA: Pennsylvania University.

DeYoung, P. A. (2015). *Relational psychotherapy: A primer.* New York, NY: Routledge.

Edwards, L. M., & Pedrotti, J. T. (2004). Utilizing the strengths of our cultures: Therapy with biracial women and girls. In A. R. Gillem & C. Thompson (Eds.), *Biracial women in therapy: Between the rock of gender and the hard place of race* (pp. 33–43). New York, NY: Haworth Press.

Garbarini-Philippe, R. (2010). Perceptions, representation, and identity development of multiracial students in American higher education. *Journal of Student Affairs at New York University, 6*, 1–6.

Gillem, A. R., & Thompson, C. A. (2004). *Biracial women in therapy: Between the rock of gender and the hard place of race.* New York, NY: Haworth Press.

Hall, C. C. I. (2004). Mixed-race women: One more mountain to climb. In A. R. Gillem & C. Thompson (Eds.), *Biracial women in therapy: Between the rock of gender and the hard place of race* (pp. 237–246). New York, NY: Haworth Press.

Helms, J. E. (1995). An update of Helm's White and people of color racial identity development models. In J. G. Ponterotto, J. M. Casas, L. A. Suzuki, & C. M. Alexander (Eds.), *Handbook of multicultural counseling.* Thousand Oaks, CA: Sage.

Herman, J. L., Brown, T. N., & Haas, A. P. (2019). Suicide thoughts and attempts among transgender adults: Findings from the 2015 US Transgender Survey. Los Angeles, CA.

Israel, T. (2004). Conversations, not categories: The intersection of biracial and bisexual identities. In A. R. Gillem & C. Thompson (Eds.), *Biracial women in therapy: Between the rock of gender and the hard place of race* (pp. 173–184). New York, NY: Haworth Press.

Jones, N. A., & Bullock, J. (2012). *The two or more races population: 2010*. Washington, DC: U.S. Dept. of Commerce, Economics and Statistics Administration, U.S. Census Bureau.

Kerr, A. E. (2005). The paper bag principle: Of the myth and the motion of colorism. *Journal of American Folklore, 118*(469), 271–289.

LaBarrie, T. L. (2007). *Explorations of variables influencing the racial self-identification of multiracial individuals*. Symposium conducted at the annual meeting of the American Psychological Association, San Francisco, CA.

Latson, J. (2019, May). The biracial advantage. *Psychology Today*. https://www .psychologytoday.com/us/articles/201905/the-biracial-advantage

Miville, M. L. (2005). Psychological functioning and identity development of biracial people: A review of current theory and research. In R. T. Carter (Ed.), *Handbook of racial–cultural psychology and counseling* (pp. 295–319). Hoboken, NJ: Wiley.

Moran, R. F. (2004). Love with a proper stranger: What anti-miscegenation laws can tell us about the meaning of race, sex, and marriage. *Hofstra Law Review, 32*(4), 22.

Nadal, K. L., Sriken, J., Davidoff, K. C., Wong, Y., & McLean, K. (2013). Microaggressions within families: Experiences of multiracial people. *Family Relations, 62*(1), 190–201.

Parker, K., Morin, R., Menasce Horowitz, J., & Lopez, M. H. (2015). Multiracial in America: Proud, diverse and growing in numbers. Washington, DC: Pew Research Center.

Peters, M. F. (1985). Racial socialization of young Black children. In H. P. McAdoo & J. L. McAdoo (Eds.), *Black children: Social, educational and parental environments* (pp. 159–173). Beverly Hills, CA: Sage.

Pilgrim, D. (2000, November). *The tragic mulatto myth*. https://www.ferris.edu /jimcrow/mulatto/

Poston, W. C. (1990). The biracial identity development model: A needed addition. *Journal of Counseling & Development, 69*(2), 152–155.

Quintana, S. M. (2007). Racial and ethnic identity: Developmental perspectives and research. *Journal of Counseling Psychology, 54*(3), 259–270.

Remedios, J. D., & Chasteen, A. L. (2013). Finally, someone who "gets" me! Multiracial people value others' accuracy about their race. *Cultural Diversity and Ethnic Minority Psychology, 19*(4), 453–460.

Rockquemore, K., & Brunsma, D. L. (2004). Negotiating racial identity: Biracial women. In A. R. Gillem & C. Thompson (Eds.), *Biracial women in therapy: Between the rock of gender and the hard place of race* (pp. 85–102). New York, NY: Haworth Press.

Root, M. P. (1998). Experiences and processes affecting racial identity development: Preliminary results from the Biracial Sibling Project. *Cultural Diversity and Mental Health, 4*(3), 237–247.

Root, M. P. (2004). From exotic to a dime a dozen. In A. R. Gillem & C. Thompson (Eds.), *Biracial women in therapy: Between the rock of gender and the hard place of race* (pp. 19–32). New York, NY: Haworth Press.

Root, M. P. P. (1990). Resolving "other" status: Identity development of biracial individuals. *Women and Therapy, 9*(1–2), 185–205.

Root, M. P. P. (Ed.). (1996). The multicultural experience: Racial borders as a significant frontier in race relations. In *The multiracial experience: Racial borders as the new frontier* (pp. 129–146). Thousand Oaks, CA: Sage.

Shih, M., & Sanchez, D. T. (2009). When race becomes even more complex: Toward understanding the landscape of multiracial identity and experiences. *Journal of Social Issues, 65*(1), 1–11.

About the Editors and Contributors

EDITORS

KIMBER SHELTON, PhD, is a licensed psychologist and owner of KLS Counseling & Consulting Services. She provides psychotherapy, professional consultation, workshops and trainings, and mentoring. Dr. Shelton specializes in the areas of cultural competence, ethnic minority and LGBTQ issues, trauma, and relationship concerns. Additionally, she serves as an adjunct instructor in Yorkville University's Masters in Counseling Psychology program. Dr. Shelton previously served as the cochair of the Texas Psychological Association Diversity Division and as a committee member on the American Psychological Association Committee on Sexual Orientation and Gender Diversity. She earned her PhD in counseling psychology from the University of Georgia and MS in mental health counseling from Niagara University.

MICHELLE KING LYN, PhD, is a licensed psychologist with work experience in a variety of clinical settings including private practice, collegiate mental health, and veterans' affairs. Dr. Lyn earned her doctorate in counseling psychology from the University of Georgia and obtained her master's degree from the University of Missouri–Columbia in educational psychology. Currently she provides consultation services and operates a private practice in the Atlanta area specializing in cultural diversity, identity development, women's issues, relationship issues, and grief and loss. In the past, she served on the Council on the Psychology of Women and Girls as part of the Georgia Psychological Association. Her other professional activities include scholarly writing and presenting at local and national conferences.

MAHLET ENDALE, PhD, is a counseling psychologist and board-certified telemental health provider. She serves clients in Georgia, Florida, and some countries abroad. Over the course of her career she has served as instructor, clinical supervisor, consultant, and psychotherapist. She opened a private practice in 2017 and primarily serves adult clients holding intersecting marginalized identities. The biggest portion of her clients identify as Black women of African descent. Prior to opening her practice, Dr. Endale worked in university mental health for 10 years in settings ranging from private liberal arts colleges to large research-one institutions.

CONTRIBUTORS

AYANNA ABRAMS, PsyD, is an Atlanta-based licensed clinical psychologist. She received her master's and doctorate degrees from the Chicago School of Professional Psychology (Chicago Campus) and completed her APA-accredited internship and postdoctoral fellowship at Emory University's Counseling and Psychological Services. Dr. Abrams is the CEO and founder of Ascension Behavioral Health, a solo mental health and consultation practice in Atlanta, specializing in the treatment of individuals and couples. Her specialty populations include culturally appropriate work with persons across the African diaspora, undergraduate and graduate students, entrepreneurs, and perinatal health in persons of color.

ROSIE PHILLIPS DAVIS, PhD, ABPP, is a professor of counseling psychology at the University of Memphis, where she has worked for more than 30 years. Previous roles include serving as the vice president for student affairs, assistant vice president for student affairs/student development, and director of the Center for Student Development. She was the 2019 president of APA, and previously served on APA's Finance Committee and Board of Directors, the American Psychological Foundation Board, the Council of Representatives, and the Society of Counseling Psychology (Division 17). She is a cofounder of the National Multicultural Conference and Summit. Davis has served on the editorial boards of multiple journals, including the *Journal of Career Assessment*, and has authored numerous articles, book chapters, and coauthored two books. Her research and advocacy projects address the power of inclusion, multicultural vocational psychology, psychological ethics, and living well in a diverse society. One of her 2019 APA Presidential Initiatives was Bringing Psychologists to the Fight Against Deep Poverty. Davis has received numerous awards including the Janet E. Helms Award for Mentoring and

Scholarship, the Arthur S. Holman Lifetime Achievement Award, the Distinguished Professional Contributions to Institutional Practice for APA Award, an APA Presidential Citation, and was named an Elder by the National Multicultural Conference and Summit.

MARIA ESPINOLA, PsyD, is assistant professor in the Department of Psychiatry at the University of Cincinnati College of Medicine. She is a licensed psychologist with expertise in diversity, women's issues, and trauma. She completed her doctorate in clinical psychology at Nova Southeastern University, her predoctoral fellowship in multicultural psychology at Boston University Medical Center, and her postdoctoral fellowship in trauma psychology at McLean Hospital and Harvard Medical School. She has received over 25 awards.

GEMARI EVANS, MA, is a family-oriented, movie-loving, psychologist-in-training. She is enrolled in the Clinical Psychology PsyD program at the Chicago School of Professional Psychology. Gemari has externed at Malcolm X College, Chicago Recovery Alliance, and Touch of Wholeness Psychological Services. Her passion involves working with Black clients and within the Black community, with the hope of making mental health services more accessible to this population.

ANTHEA A. GRAY, PsyD, is an assistant professor in the Department of Physical Medicine and Rehabilitation at the Ohio State University where she works as a rehabilitation psychologist. Her clinical work includes individuals across the spectrum of disability, but primarily brain injuries and burns. Her research interests largely pertain to the intersection of culture and disability. Dr. Gray holds an MA from Columbia University's Teachers College and a PsyD in clinical psychology from Pepperdine University. She also serves as a clinical consultant to OSU's Chronic Brain Injury Program's Neuro Night's series and chairperson to the American Psychological Association's Division 22's (Rehabilitation Psychology) Diversity Committee. In her free time, she enjoys watching her one-year-old Aussiedoodle, Lilac, chase (and never catch) squirrels in the park and visiting the latest exhibits at the Columbus Museum of Art.

CANDICE NICOLE HARGONS, PhD, is an award-winning assistant professor of counseling psychology at the University of Kentucky, where she studies sex, social justice, and leadership—all with a love ethic. She is also the founding director of the Center for Healing Racial Trauma.

LAUREN SIMONE HARPER, PhD, is a psychologist and behavioral health provider in primary care behavioral health with Providence Medical Group near Portland, Oregon. She completed her APA-Accredited doctoral internship and residency with the George Fox Integrated Care Consortium also near Portland. Dr. Harper earned her PhD in counseling psychology and a certificate in interdisciplinary qualitative studies from the University of Georgia. Her research and clinical areas of interest are in doctoral education and training of Black women, interventions for mental health treatment of Black people, love and sexual pleasure of Black LGBTQ+ persons, and clinical training in integrated health care.

TERRENCE HARPER II, PhD, serves as a staff psychologist at the Price Center for Counseling & Psychological Services at the University of North Carolina at Charlotte (UNCC). Dr. Harper has a PhD in clinical psychology from Eastern Michigan University. He has worked in college counseling since 2013 in a variety of settings including public and private, liberal arts and research, and Midwestern and Southern institutions. As a student affairs professional, Dr. Harper has had the opportunity to facilitate multiple groups, workshops, and outreach presentations with the focus of addressing the mental health and well-being of marginalized communities, including people of color, women, and LGBTQ folx. He currently serves as a cochair of UNCC's Black Student Mental Health Task Force.

NATALIE D. HASLEM, DNP, RN, CNE, PMHNP-BC, works as a staff psychiatric nurse practitioner at Ridgeview Institute and Fulton County Jail in Atlanta, Georgia. She also is a part-time nursing professor at Georgia State University in Atlanta. Dr. Haslem obtained a BS in psychology from Spelman College, a BS in nursing from Kennesaw State University, and MS and DNP in nursing from the University of South Alabama. Her areas of interest include working with chronic mental illness and social skills training.

MELISSA G. JOHNSON, PsyD, is a California-licensed clinical psychologist with over 15 years of experience in the field, specializing in forensic, correctional, and military psychology. Dr. Johnson has worked extensively with the severely mentally ill, incarcerated, and inpatient populations. Dr. Johnson has specialized training in the area of psychodiagnostic, neuropsychological, and forensic evaluations, to include suicide and violence risk assessments. Her responsibilities also include providing individual and group psychotherapy as well as research.

ANGELA M. KUEMMEL, PhD, ABPP (Rp), is a rehabilitation psychologist in spinal cord injuries and disorders and the chair of the Psychology Service Diversity Committee at the Louis Stokes Cleveland VAMC. In her nine years at the Cleveland VAMC, Dr. Kuemmel has pioneered a variety of interdisciplinary programs for veterans with SCI/D, including telehealth chronic pain management and sexuality programs, a community education project on wheelchair accessibility, and an annual birthday party celebrating the Americans with Disabilities Act.

NATALIE MALONE, MS, is a third-year counseling psychology doctoral student at the University of Kentucky. Broadly, her research interests include social justice topics and love, sex, and spirituality among Black folx.

TICILY MEDLEY, PhD, LMFT-S, LPC, has over 19 years of experience in higher education teaching and administration, as well as mental health. Her passion is providing engaging public speaking and learning opportunities. Her analytical approach, empathic engagement, and light humor help her to simplify topics that may seem complex, such as conflict resolution, and topics that can be emotionally uncomfortable, such as racial and gender oppression and personal identity awareness. Dr. Medley holds degrees from Texas Woman's University, Southern Methodist University, and the University of Texas at Austin.

CHESMORE MONTIQUE, MA (he/him/his), is a third-year doctoral candidate in counseling psychology at the University of Kentucky. Originally from New Jersey, by way of Trinidad and Tobago and Aruba, Chesmore moved to Atlanta for his BA in psychology at Morehouse College and then Washington, DC, for his MA in psychology at American University. Chesmore's research interests includes Black love and the impact of cultural and ethnic identities on romantic and other interpersonal relationships. Chesmore hopes to be a practicing psychologist with aims of helping Black couples, families, individuals, and other minorities achieve optimal well-being.

SHAVONNE J. MOORE-LOBBAN, PhD, is a licensed psychologist, training director, and assistant professor in Washington, DC. She earned her doctorate in counseling psychology from Purdue University, completed her predoctoral internship at Boston University School of Medicine/Center for Multicultural Training in Psychology, and completed her posdoctoral fellowship at the Boston Veteran Affairs Healthcare System and Harvard Medical School. Dr. Moore-Lobban specializes in trauma, severe mental illness, and providing services to marginalized communities.

NGOZI NDUKWE, PsyD, completed a bachelor of science in psychology from the University of Georgia, a master's in rehabilitation counseling from the Illinois Institute of Technology, and doctorate in clinical psychology from the Georgia School of Professional Psychology. For over 20 years, Dr. Ndukwe has worked with individuals with disabilities, with her more recent work being with individuals with spinal cord injuries, traumatic brain injuries, and neurocognitive impairments.

KAREN POWDRILL, MA, earned her bachelor of arts degree in psychology at Hampton University, master of arts degree in counseling psychology at Towson University, and a master of arts in clinical psychology at the Chicago School of Professional Psychology. Currently, she is a third-year doctoral clinical psychology student at the Chicago School of Professional Psychology. She has worked for four years in Maryland as a licensed clinical professional counselor (LCPC) and is a board-approved supervisor.

DANIELLE SIMMONS, PhD, is a licensed psychologist and owner of Simmons Counseling & Consulting Services in Chicago, Illinois. As a clinician, educator, and facilitator, she works primarily with Black and Brown folks, queer- and trans-identified individuals, couples and families to empower the making of sustainable growth, change, and healing. She has an extensive background in supporting queer folks of color growing through generational and historical trauma often exacerbated by enduring systemic oppression. She is particularly interested in assisting other practitioners through processes of honest self-reflection and awareness to increase unconditional self-compassion and acceptance of strengths and limitations to ultimately provide quality service with marginalized populations.

TAMARA D'ANJOU TURNER, PhD, is a licensed psychologist in private practice and clinical assistant professor at Georgia State University. She received her BA in psychology from Columbia University and PhD in clinical psychology from the University of Miami. She completed her predoctoral internship at UNC-Charlotte and postdoctoral fellowship at the University of Georgia. Professionally, Dr. Turner has served as the director of the Counseling Center at Georgia Gwinnett College and was awarded a SAMHSA grant for suicide prevention.

JUDI-LEE WEBB, PhD, is a licensed psychologist and certified eating disorders specialist and supervisor, providing therapy to adolescents, adults, couples and families. Dr. Webb earned her degrees from University of Georgia, Howard University, and the University of Florida. She completed her internship/residency training from Medical College of Georgia & Augusta Veterans Affairs Medical Consortium and her postdoctoral fellowship training at the Atlanta Center for Eating Disorders (now known as Walden Behavioral Care).

COURTNEY WILLIAMS, PhD, is a staff psychologist at the Vanderbilt University Counseling Center (VUCC). She earned her doctorate in counseling psychology from the University of Georgia. Dr. Williams earned her master's degree from North Carolina Central University and her bachelor's degree from the University of North Carolina at Greensboro, both in psychology. She has worked in university counseling centers, residential treatment facilities, and community mental health. Resultant of personal experiences and clinical training, she places multiculturalism, social justice, and advocacy at the forefront of her work, which is highlighted by her passion of working with Black women and girls in school and university settings.

STEPHANIE N. WILLIAMS, PhD, obtained her master's in forensic psychology from the Chicago School of Professional Psychology and her PhD from Palo Alto University. She has worked in the field of forensic psychology for over 15 years. She specializes in suicide risk, forensic evaluations, and the personality assessment of ethnic minorities. She has several peer-reviewed publications and book chapters that focus on improving mental health treatment for people of color and women. She has a private practice in the San Francisco Bay Area that provides therapeutic interventions for BIPOC (Black Indigenous persons of color) and public safety professionals.

JASMINE H. WINBUSH, PsyD, is a licensed clinical psychologist and owner of Amethyst Psychological Services, a group practice in Atlanta, Georgia, that provides psychotherapy to women. Dr. Winbush specializes in multicultural psychology and trauma. In her practice, she works with women presenting with identity concerns, depression, anxiety, trauma, relationship issues, and life transitions. She completed her master's of clinical psychology from Loyola University Maryland, her doctorate of psychology from Roosevelt University (Chicago), and completed her predoctoral fellowship at Emory University.

Index